About the Author

Angela Stafford has had a passion for cooking, painting and drawing ever since she can remember. After the release of her first book, Wild Vegan (AKA Wild Morsels), she studied Kinesiology. A large part of that study involved gaining an even deeper knowledge of nutrition and wholistic health. With this knowledge and a passion for children's health she embarked on the creation of this book. Her panel of recipe testers include her own children, Ethan and Ryan, her nieces and nephews and the children of friends. Her husband Mitchell also taste tested every recipe, however he will literally eat anything....

Angela lives with her family in South-East Queensland. They share their little piece of paradise with a group of happy chooks and spend most of their time either in the kitchen or the garden.

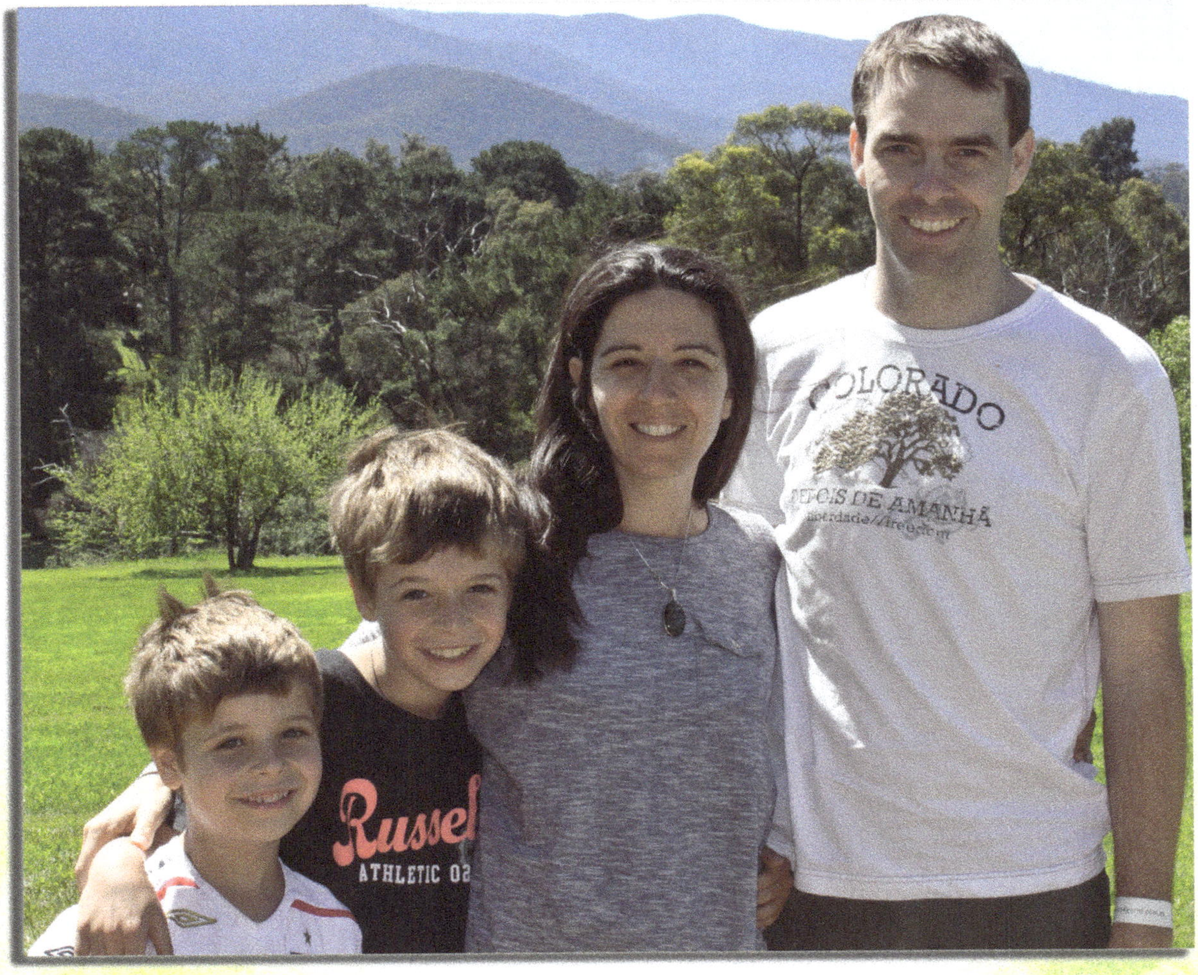

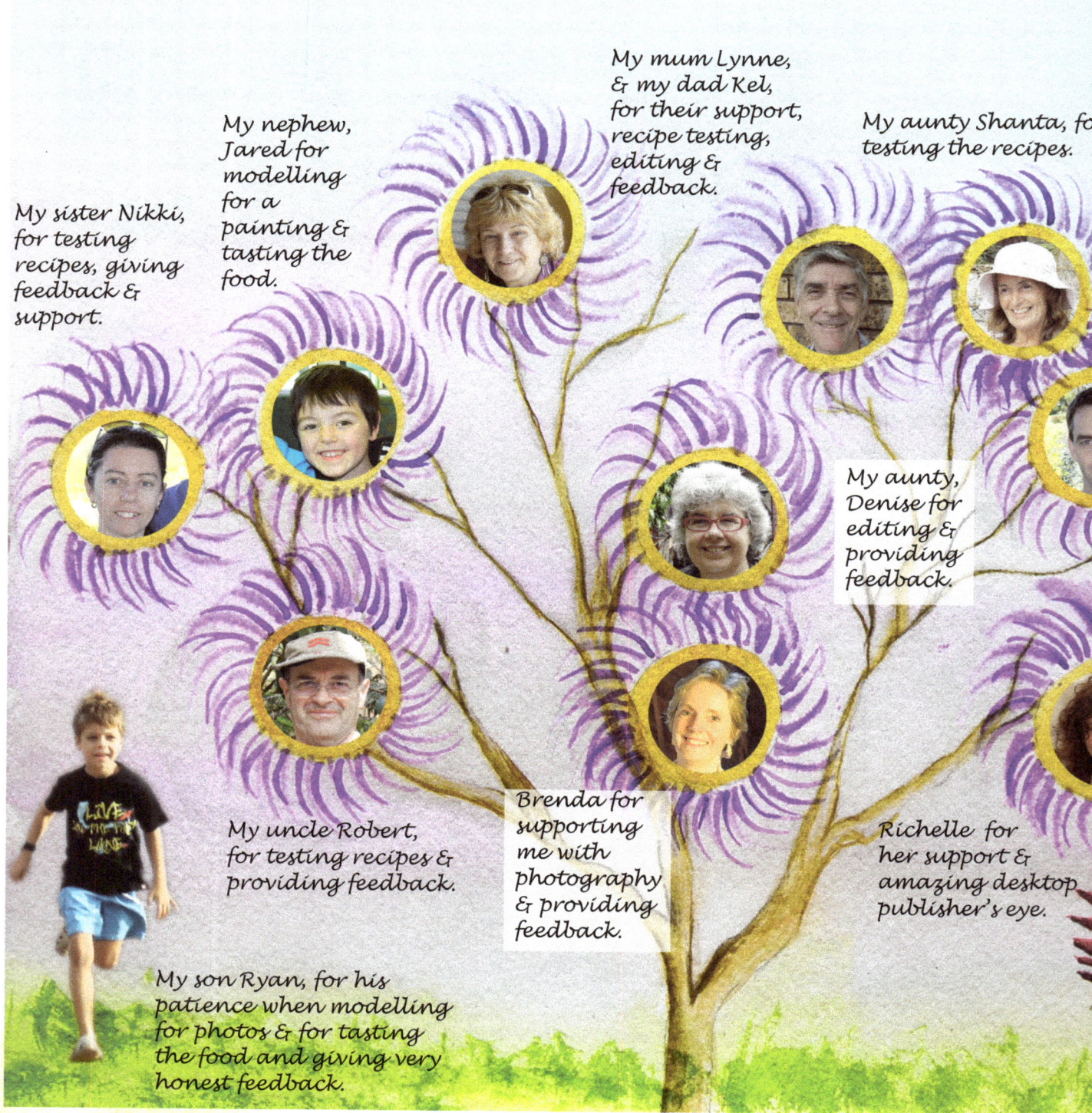

Wouldn't it be great if instead of asking for chocolate or a hot dog, your child asked for an apple or stir fry vegetables? Does this sound impossible?

I want to show you how to inspire your children to love healthy food.

This is the greatest gift you can give them. A healthy start in life gives them the best chance of a healthy adult life. As you will see, education starts in the garden, progresses to the kitchen and ends with that good feeling in the tummy after a meal that is cooked with nutritious foods and loving hands....

Many parents say that fast food once a week won't kill their child, or that eating lollies is just what kids do! The thing is, as children we develop our tastes. Those foods we are exposed to when we are young, determine to a larger extent, the foods we choose to eat as adults. We as parents are responsible for what goes into our child's mouth. We are their caretakers until they become old enough to make choices for themselves. So let's do the best job possible. Lets give them the greatest chance at a full and healthy life.

Help your children to develop a passion for foods their bodies will love!

Following are a collection of vegetarian recipes that suit a variety of palates. Why vegetarian? Because that is the kind of food that I make. This book is not specifically about vegetarianism though. My focus is on whole, healthy foods. Most of us are either omnivores or vegetarians anyway so just because you like to eat meat, doesn't mean that you cannot include the recipes in this book as part of your repertoire.

These recipes are also designed to vary palates that are used to plain food. Some are for adults to prepare with a little help from children where safe, while others are designed to allow the child to do most or all of the work. They will be marked with special symbols according to difficulty. See the section on **"How To Use This Book"** on page 8. You will also find tips on a variety of topics from dealing with fussy eaters to family ritual ideas based around food.

It is my hope that this book will not only help you and your child to cook but also to create a way of life that combines healthy food, family togetherness and a deeper knowledge of how what we eat affects our minds, our bodies and our spiritual well-being...

First published in 2013
by Angela Stafford.
Ligare, Sydney NSW
Printed in China by Red Planet.

Published in paperback 2018
by Guiding Change Press

Copyright © 2018 in text: Angela Stafford
Copyright © 2018 in images: Angela Stafford

http://www.angelaswildkitchen.com
info@angelaswildkitchen.com
ISBN: 978-0-9875035-1-0

All rights reserved. No part of this publication may be reproduced, stored in a retrieval system, or transmitted in any form or by any means, electronic, mechanical, photocopying, recording or otherwise without the prior permission in writing of the author.

Cataloguing-in-publication Entry is available from The National Library of Australia.
http://catalogue.nla.gov.au

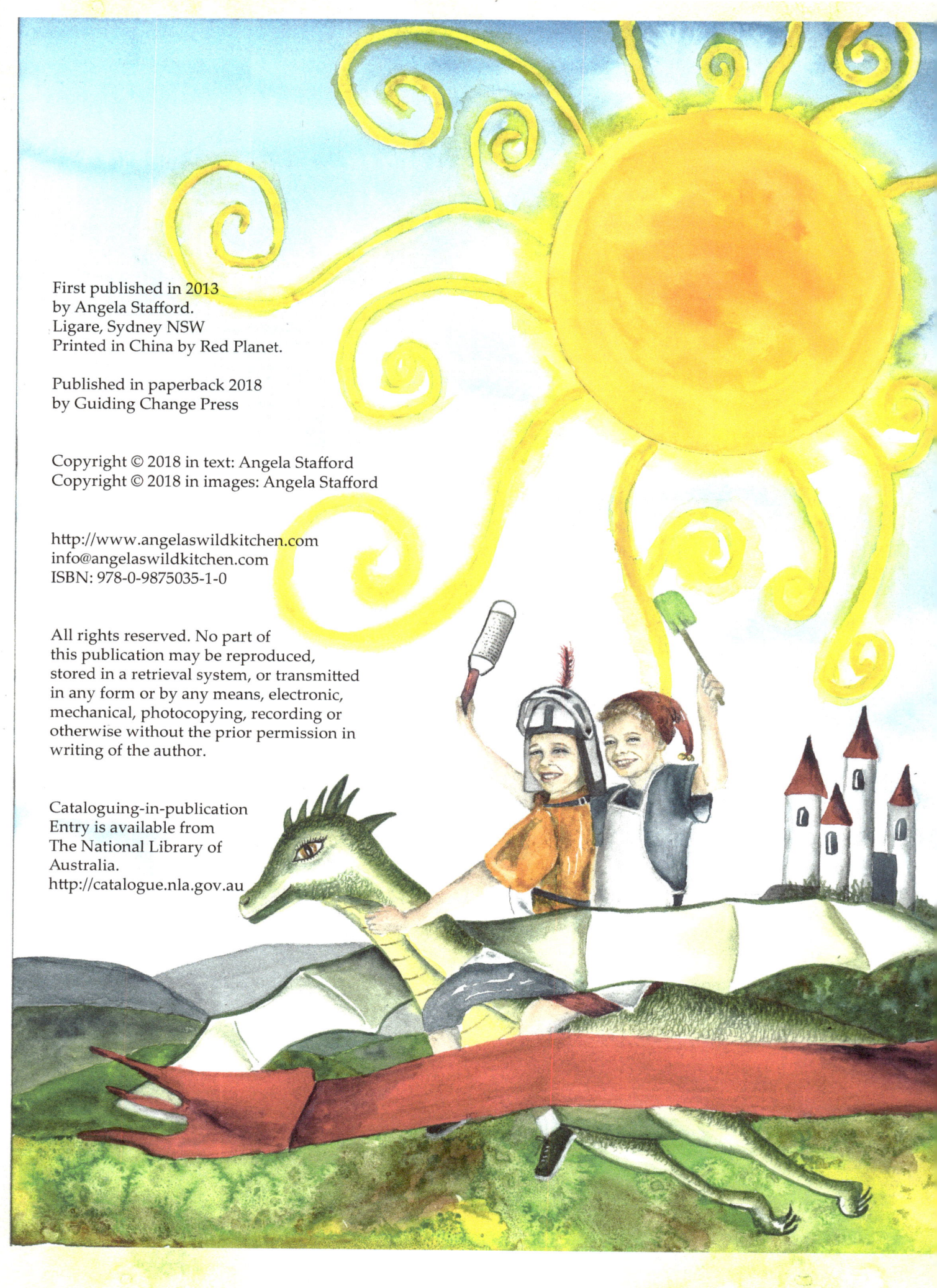

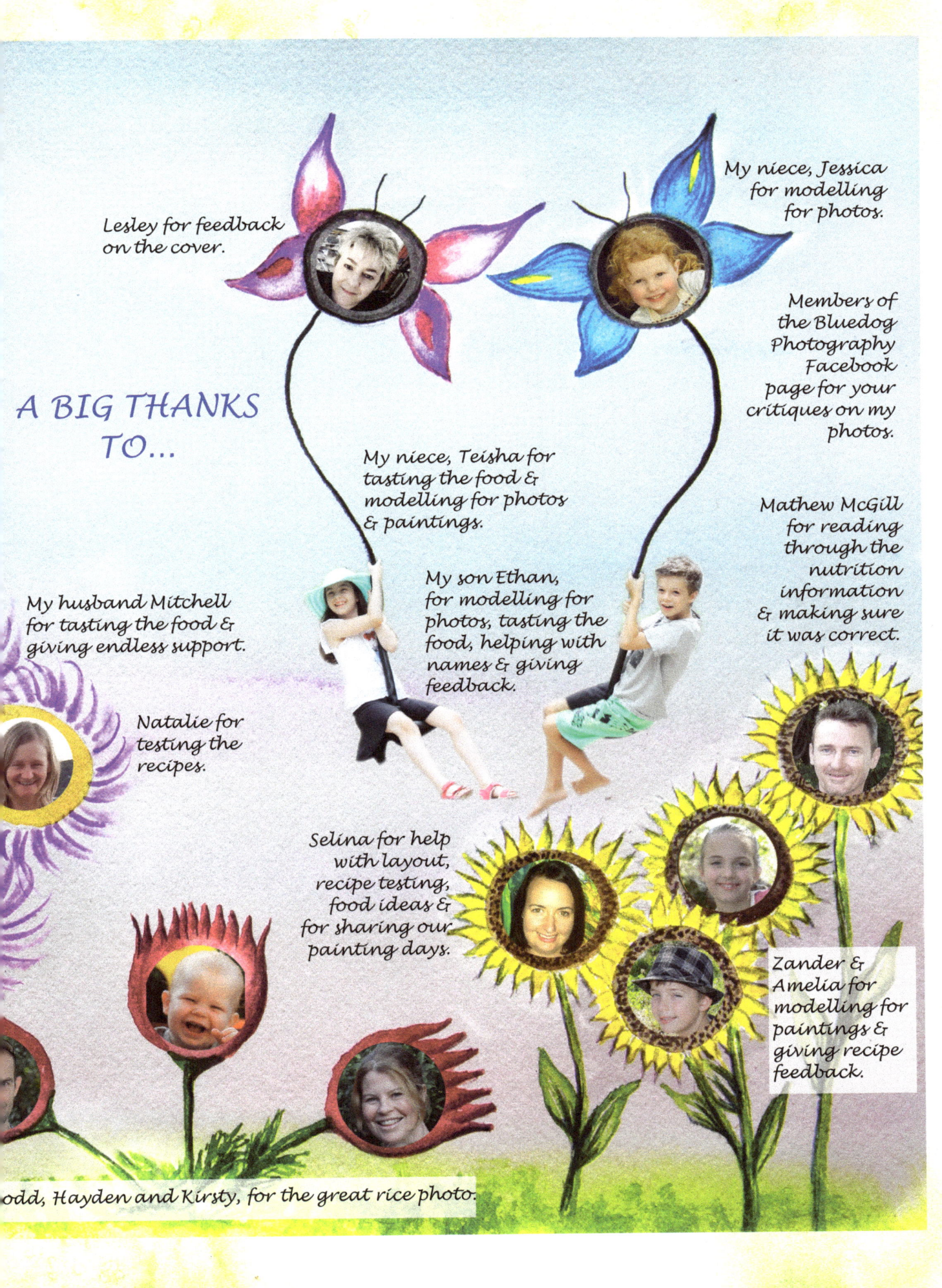

The Treasures You Will Find

How To Use This Book..8

Join the Food Safari..11

What Do Our Bodies Need?..12

- Our Own Personal Armies..15
- Superfoods..16
- Good Fats and Bad Fats..20
- What Is Wrong With Eating Too Much Junk Food?.......23
- RAW-Some Food..24
- How Do Your Taste Buds Work?..26
- Where Does Your Food Come From?..28
- Eating For a Happier Earth..33
- Your Own Fresh Eggs..34

Lets Get Started!..36

- Cooking Equipment..38
- Creating a Safe Kitchen..40
- Ambience in the Kitchen..42
- Cooking Terms..44
- Alternative Ingredients..46
- All About Flour..50
- Which Milk?..53
- Which Oil?..53
- What Do Hormones Have To Do With Canned Food?...54
- Cooking With Herbs..56
- Regional Flavours..58
- Cooking and Sprouting Techniques..64
- Varieties of Rice..66
- Cooking Great Rice..68
- Getting Creative and Expanding Your Knowledge..........71
- A Word Before You Begin..71

Beautiful Beginnings...73

- Marvelous Toasted Muesli..............................74
- Swiss Muesli..76
- Gluten Free Toasted Muesli............................77
- Berry Apple Porridge....................................78
- Omelettes...80
- Fruit Salad with Coconut Snow Cream.............81
- Waffles..82
- Perfect Pikelets...84
- LSA..86
- Powerful Banana Smoothie............................87
- Green Smoothie..88
- Tropical Bliss Smoothie................................88

Little Morsels...91

Dips..92

- Sunset Dip..92
- Smoky Baba Ghanoush.................................94
- Enchanted Forest Dip..................................94
- Stain-Your-Clothes Dip.................................96
- Guacamole..98
- Sassy Salsa...98
- Hummus..100
- Baby Bear Hummus....................................100
- Herby Tomato Hummus...............................101
- Almondy Hummus.....................................101
- Cinderella Hummus....................................102
- And Still More Hummus Ideas......................102
- Making Your Own Crackers.........................104
- Potato and Rosemary Crackers....................106
- Popeye Crackers......................................108
- Cheesy Crackers......................................109
- Heart's Desire Crackers.............................110
- Platters and Other Savoury Snacks..............111

Introduction   3

Entrees, Lunches and Appetisers.

Rice Paper Spring Rolls...112
Never-Lasting Nori Rolls..114
Not-Sausage Rolls with a Twist..................................116
Better 'n' Bought Tomato Sauce...............................117
Golden Corn Cakes...118
Greek Beanies..120
Tzatziki...120
Nutty Chick-a-pea Burgers...122
Garden Burgers...124
Mini Quiches..126

Kids Eating Green!...128
Side Dishes

Slow Roasted Tomatoes..130
Garlicky Beans...130
Maple Glazed Treasures..132
Honeyed Carrots...134
Rose-Married Potatoes..135
Beautiful Brassicas..136
Lemony Peppered Greens..138
Shanta's Sesame Rice...138
Crazy Coconut Rice..139
Queen Bee Wedges..140

Gifts from the Garden..143

Couscous Medley..144
Lime, Pumpkin & Quinoa Salad................................146
Aladdin's Salad..148
Rainbow Salad...150
Tomato Salad...152
Posh Cucumber Salad..152
Tabbouleh With a Spin..154

Sesame Rice Salad...156
Wild Salad...158
Asian Noodle Salad...160
Rainbow Spaghetti Salad................................162

Beastly Brews...165

Vegetable Stock Concentrate..........................166
The Forest King's Soup...................................168
Fire Engine Soup...170
The Soup of Endless Possibilities....................172
Hearty Lentil Soup..173
Mushroom Soup..174
Tomato and Beetroot Soup.............................176
Pumpkin Soup...178
Turkish Red Lentil Soup..................................180

Magical Mains..183

Pizzas..184
Nachos..188
Shepherd's Pie..190
Beautiful Bolognaise.......................................192
Tomato Sunrise Slice......................................194
Better Baked Beans..196
Golden Chickpea Curry...................................198
Dreamy Dahl...200
Coconut Dahl..202
Turkish Casserole...203
Awesome Adzuki Curry...................................204
Mexican Pie..206
Gado Gado..208
Pumpkin and Sweet Pea Risotto.....................210

The Land of Sweet 213
    Wholemeal vs. White Flour 214
    A Great Baking Tip 214
    Oven Settings 214
    Cake Tin Sizes 214
    Bliss Balls 216
        The Original Bliss Ball 218
        Chocolate Goji Balls 220
        Almond and Cashew Balls 221
        Chocolate Mint Balls 222
        Almond and Apricot Balls 223
        Chocolate, Honey Almond Balls 224
        Cranberry and Apple Balls 224

Baking
    Gingerbread Biscuits 226
    Chocolate Chip Pecan Biscuits 228
    Jam Drops 230
    Muesli Bars 232
    Basic Scone 234
    Lime and Coconut Scones 236
    Pumpkin Scones 238
    Cranberry and Vanilla Cake Bars 239
    Honey and Apple Cake 240
    Carrot Cake 242
    Chocolate Cupcakes 244
    Once Upon a Time Muffins 246
    Lemon Syrup Muffins 248
    Blueberry and Apple Muffins 250
    Happily Ever After Muffins 252

Raw Treats
    Crispy Cashew Rice Treats 253
    Divine Raw Brownies 254
    Raw Coconut Rough 256

From the Freezer
- Frozen Fruit...258
- Home-Made Ice blocks...258
- Multicoloured Ice blocks...258
- Tropical Bliss...259
- Banana and Berry fluff...260
- Chocolate Banana Cream..260

Desserts
- Saucy Banana Pudding..262
- Cinderella Custard..262
- Peach Pie..265
- Chocolate Chia Pudding..266
- Apple Crumble..268

The Roots of Health: Information for Parents...........271
- The Roots of Healthy Eating....................................272
- Being Healthy Is Not Just About What We Eat..........272
- Inspiring Children's Choices....................................273
- Diversifying Your Child's Palate...............................274
- Where Does Food Come From?..............................277
- Healthy Children are Happy Children......................278
- Dealing with Fussy Eaters.......................................279
- Always Something Good to Eat...............................280
- Kids in the Kitchen; Dinner Nights...........................282

Glossary..284
Bibliography...290
Suggested Reading List..291
Index..292

How To Use This Book

The recipes contained in this book are suitable for children and adults to work together. Depending on a child's age, some may even be prepared without adult help.

In the beginning for a cook starting out, it is essential to stick to the instructions in the recipes. In this way, the process of cooking is learned and the basics become a foundation for later exploration. However you will notice that below most recipes is a "Play Time" box.
This contains ideas on how to change the recipes and is just a starting point to allow the imagination to flow. The idea is, as any cook gains confidence, young or old, skills increase and creativity becomes a part of the whole process.

Child Involvement/Adult Teamwork

Each of the recipes have an indicator to you let you and your child know what level of adult help is needed. In the table of contents, the recipe name is coloured and on the recipe page, you will see a small indicator circle at the bottom of the page. Of course this is a rough guide and the age and maturity of your child will play a large role in their ability in the kitchen. Ultimately this system is to be used at your discretion.

Little or no use of sharp instruments or heat	🟢
Around Half the preparation involves sharp instruments and/or heat	🟠
High use of sharp instruments and/or heat	🔴

Dietary Requirements

Each recipe has a dietary indicator at the bottom of the page. This lets you know at a glance, suitability for allergies or food choices. Some of the recipes are free from certain ingredients outright and others can be adapted using the "Play Time" box. The indicator does take into account the "Play Time" suggestions. I have not specified the use of egg replacers or gluten free flours. If you do use either of these ingredients, then more of the recipes will be suitable for both vegans and those following a gluten free diet.

Vegan - also covers egg and dairy allergies	
Gluten Free	
Nut Free - doesn't include pine nuts or coconut	

The first chapter, *Join the Food Safari*, is directed at children and covers nutritional information as well as general cooking guidelines. Also included is information about ingredients and where they come from. If you would like to know more about a particular ingredient and have not found it listed in this first chapter, be sure to read the glossary beginning on page 284, where there are details of many ingredients.

The last chapter, *The Roots of Health*, is information for parents. This includes tips and tricks for dealing with fussy eaters and ideas for moving over to a healthier lifestyle.

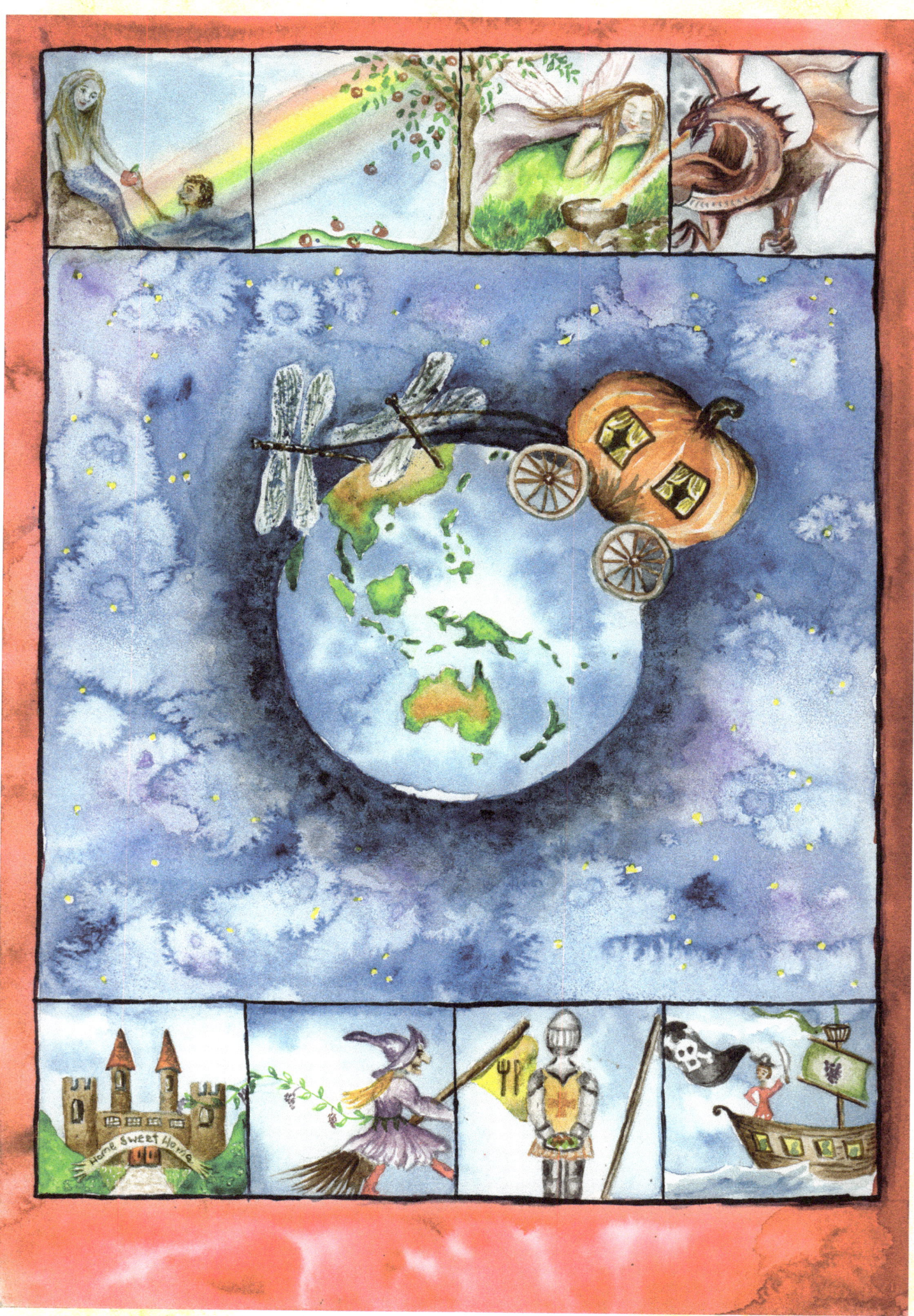

Join the Food Safari

Join the Food Safari

The Food Safari begins right now and if you choose, can continue for the rest of your life. It is called a safari because along the way you will learn, see, taste, smell and create a variety of meals, snacks and sweet treats.

You will learn how to cook in a fun and creative way, turning it into an artistic experience. However we don't use paints and paper, we use ingredients, cooking tools and lots of love and joy. Not only that, you will discover where foods come from and how different eating habits affect our bodies. Finally, you will find out how to eat in a way that is supportive to our beautiful planet.

You will see, taste and smell a variety of different ingredients. Your senses can transport you to the food markets of different countries, they can remind you of special people in your life and they can create future memories which all revolve around that very important aspect of our lives: FOOD!

You will learn to create your own combinations. Once you have followed a recipe successfully a few times, be brave and try altering the recipe with the creative tips at the bottom of each page. As you gain confidence, you may come up with your own changes. Just be sure when baking, to maintain the same ratio of wet to dry ingredients. What this means is that if you want to change the milk in a recipe for apple juice, as long as you add the same amount, the recipe will still work, however if you change the milk for more flour, the recipe will no longer work because flour is not a liquid. These are things you will learn along the way.

Most importantly, when travelling on your food safari, **BE PATIENT** with yourself. Making mistakes is an important part of your journey and is the only way to learn. Every time you make a mistake, you have given yourself an opportunity to learn what not to do next time!

What Do Our Bodies Need?

Before we decide what to cook or how, lets first find out what our bodies need to stay healthy and strong. Healthy foods contain building blocks as shown below. Your body needs these because it is growing fast. Even when you stop growing, your body is constantly repairing itself and regrowing what is already there. Building blocks make your body strong and efficient. They are made up of vitamins, minerals, amino acids, omega oils, proteins and carbohydrates (carbs for short). Every time you take in food that lacks these essential building blocks your body fails to get what it really needs in order to function well.

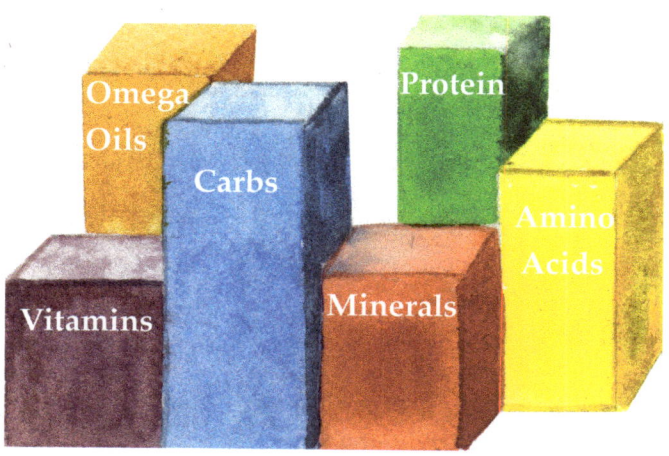

We can divide foods into 2 groups: whole foods and processed foods.

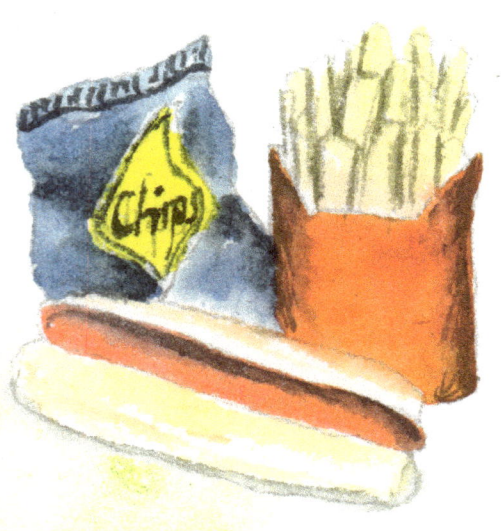

Processed foods: are foods that have been altered from their raw, natural state into some other form for convenience, longer shelf life or taste. Examples are white bleached flour, lollies, chocolates, mass-produced cakes, pastries, packaged snacks and packaged meals. The goodness of the original ingredients has been stripped away and many of these foods have added table salt, sugar, fat and chemicals.

Unfortunately the more you eat these foods, the more you want them, even when you don't feel healthy. That is because these foods are addictive, meaning your body gets so used to them that it asks for more and more and MORE! As these foods lack the building blocks that your body needs, you still feel hungry even though your tummy is physically full. This is because your cells are literally starving!

Whole foods are those that have not been changed much or at all from their natural state. A potato is a whole food, but a potato chip out of a packet is not, even though it is still part of the potato. Examples of whole foods are fruits, vegetables, whole grains and whole grain flour, beans, lentils, organically raised meat, free-range eggs, some milk and cheese. These foods still contain a powerhouse of nutrients and flavour!

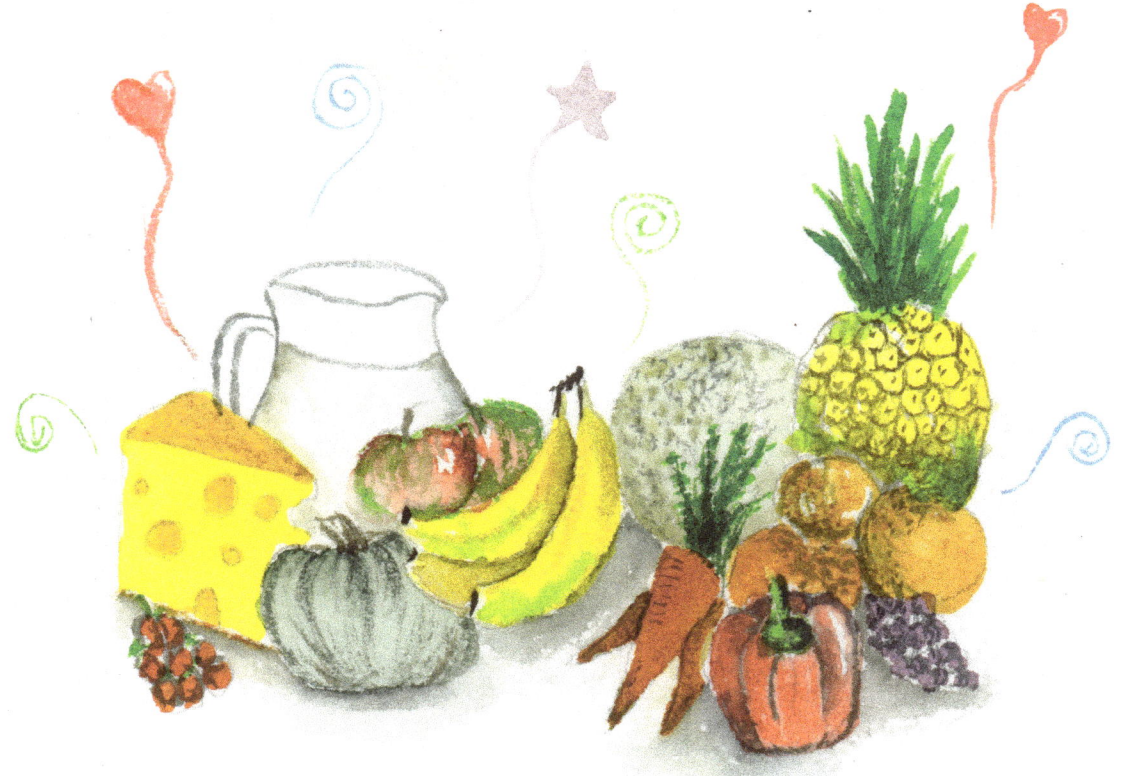

Interesting fact: Did you know that the colours of fruits and vegetables can often tell you what nutrients are in that food? Orange vegetables contain a nutrient called beta-carotene which is essential for healthy skin and eyes. Green vegetables contain chlorophyll which cleans your blood.

The Fairytale Food Safari is about making meals and snacks out of whole foods. You wouldn't catch a knight eating a chocolate bar, or a fairy eating a hot dog would you? How would the knight have the energy to fight in battles? How would the fairy feel light and healthy enough to fly? Whole food recipes can also become addictive, but in a good way. Your body will crave more nutrients, which will just make you stronger, healthier and smarter!

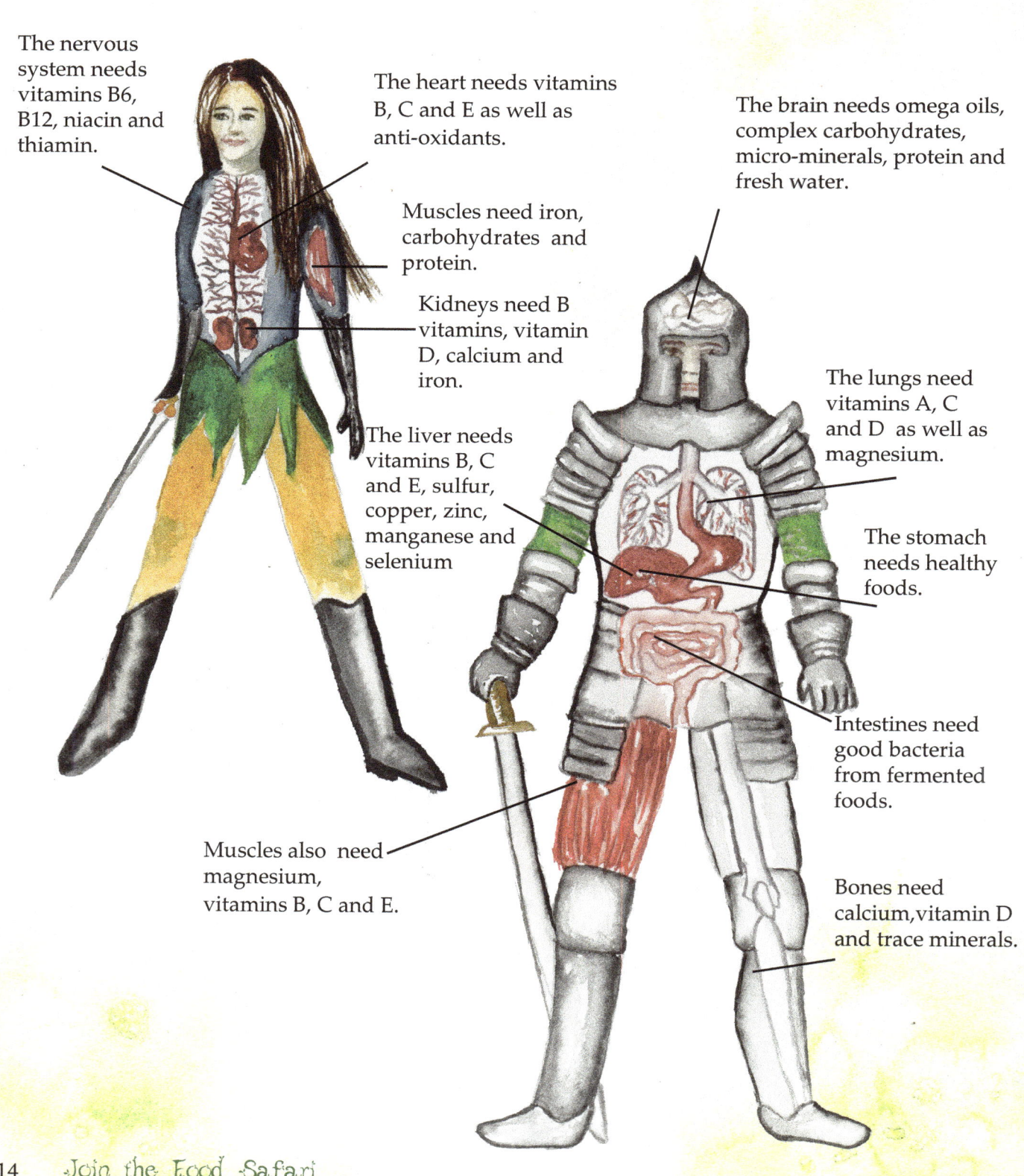

The nervous system needs vitamins B6, B12, niacin and thiamin.

The heart needs vitamins B, C and E as well as anti-oxidants.

The brain needs omega oils, complex carbohydrates, micro-minerals, protein and fresh water.

Muscles need iron, carbohydrates and protein.

Kidneys need B vitamins, vitamin D, calcium and iron.

The lungs need vitamins A, C and D as well as magnesium.

The liver needs vitamins B, C and E, sulfur, copper, zinc, manganese and selenium

The stomach needs healthy foods.

Intestines need good bacteria from fermented foods.

Muscles also need magnesium, vitamins B, C and E.

Bones need calcium, vitamin D and trace minerals.

Our Own Personal Armies

Inside each of us, we have our own personal army. This army is called the immune system. Whenever a bug or virus tries to attack our body and make it sick, our army does its best to fight it off. Sometimes it is successful and we don't even know that the sickness was trying to attack us. Sometimes the army is a little bit successful and we only get a little bit sick before the bugs are dead. Other times, the army loses and we get very sick and feel bad.

If you want your army to be strong, it will need good food. You cannot expect your army to fight for you if you are only feeding it junk foods which contain no nutrients. Give your army plenty of fresh, whole foods and it will be full of all those building blocks which allow the little soldiers to fight hard to keep those nasties away and keep you feeling good! Other kids around you may get sick, but if your army is strong there is no need for you to join them.

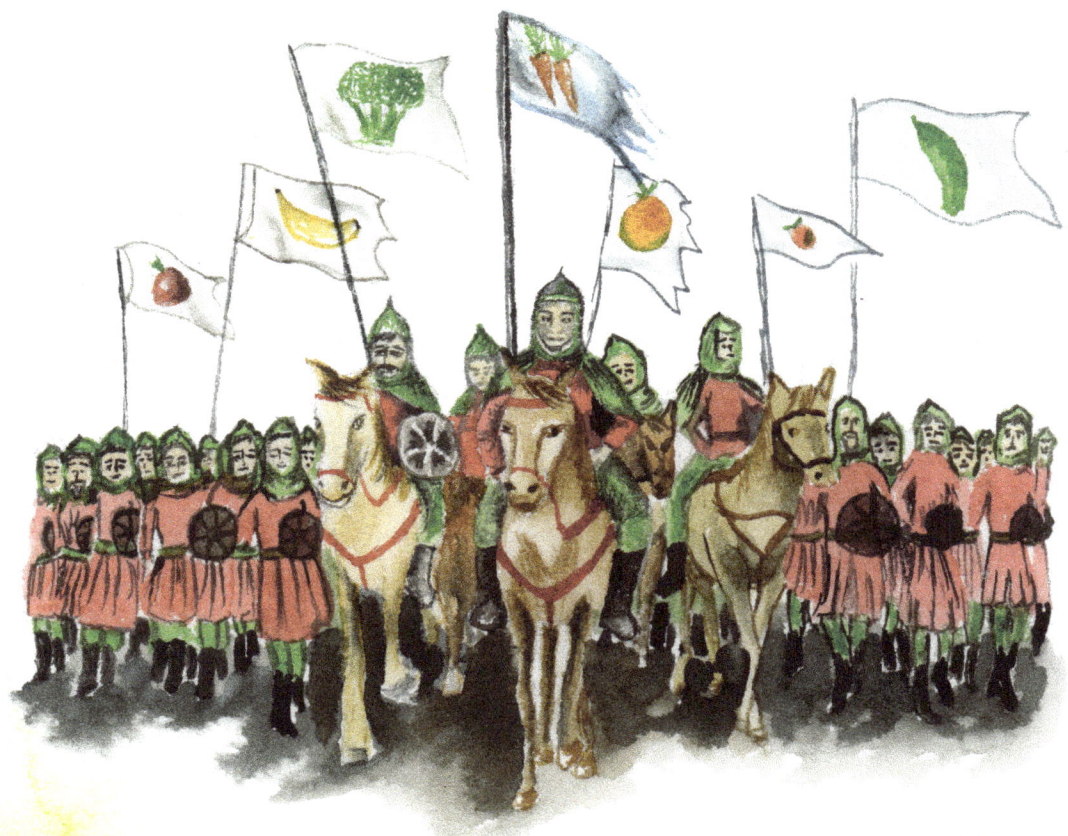

Interesting fact: Sugar makes your army weak. Researchers have found that your body will remember the sugar for two weeks after you have eaten it!

Superfoods

There are some foods that are like super heros. They have so many nutrients in them that they stand out from other whole foods. Eating lots of superfoods is like running your car on the cleanest, best fuel available. Your car will last longer and run better. So too will your body if it is full of superfoods. Here are some of the great ones. There are many more though. Why not do some of your own research to expand your superfood knowledge?

Broccoli- contains vitamins C, K, A, B6, B2 and folic acid. Minerals such as manganese, potassium, phosphorus and calcium as well as plenty of fibre to help your digestive system. It also contains chlorophyll which cleans your body from the inside. Be aware though, the more you cook your broccoli, the more of these nutrients you lose, especially the chlorophyll which will turn the cooking water green. Just lightly steam or stir-fry your broccoli for maximum nutrition!

Blueberries- are very high in vitamins C and K and contain an abundance of the mineral, manganese, which is important for bone development and for converting food into energy that your body can use. They provide fibre to maintain a healthy digestive system and are near the top when it comes to antioxidants. Antioxidants are like an army that comes into your body through your food. They kill the bad guys, called free-radicals. Free radicals are linked to the development of disease and are a result of consuming too much junk food or alcohol or suffering from too much stress. Blueberries are only rich in nutrients when eaten raw.

Goji Berries- it has been found that these sweet little berries are one of the most nutritionally dense foods on earth. They contain more vitamin C than oranges, more beta-carotene than carrots and more iron than steak.
They also contain an abundance of B vitamins, anti-oxidants and amino acids. Goji Berries have been used in China to improve blood circulation, protect the liver, improve eyesight and boost the immune system.

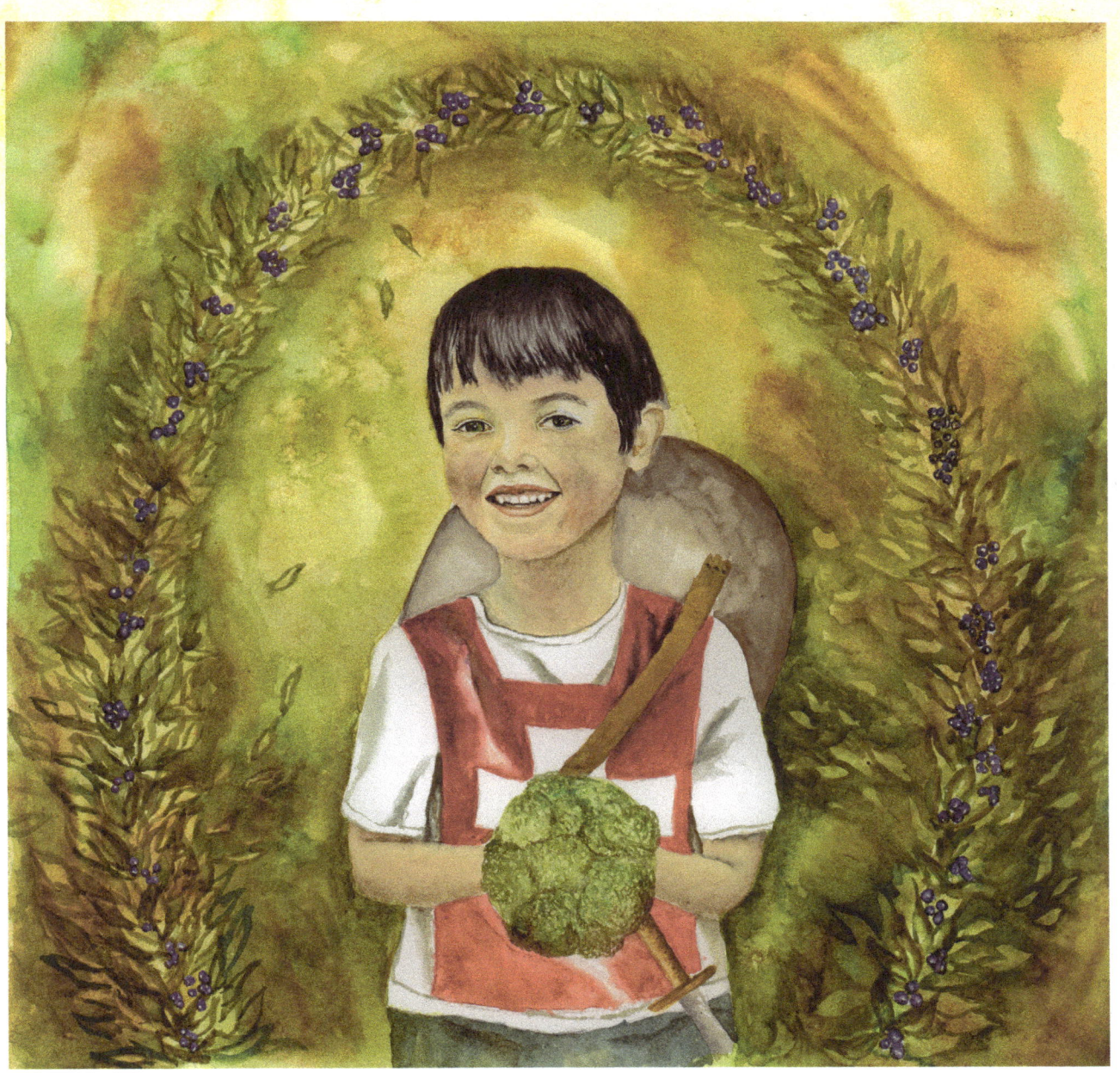

Kale- is a dark green leafy vegetable that is high in vitamin C, iron, folate and beta-carotene. As with other vegetables it also contains a good dose of fibre. The particularly special thing about this vegetable is the presence of iron and vitamin C together. Your body needs vitamin C to absorb iron, and here it is all in one package.

Garlic- is like a medicine, direct from nature. It is anti-bacterial and anti-fungal. This is why it is great for killing colds and treating sore throats. It is rich in antioxidants, manganese, vitamin B6, and vitamin C as well as thiamin, phosphorus, selenium, calcium, potassium, iron and copper. As with blueberries, these qualities are lost with cooking, so garlic is best eaten raw. Try it in a salad dressing or dip where the flavour will not be too strong.

Chia Seeds - are high in omega 3 and 6 fatty acids. Fatty acids are very important for so many bodily functions, including brain development, healthy blood, a healthy immune system, a healthy nervous system and healthy skin. Chia seeds are also high in fibre, antioxidants, minerals including iron, potassium, calcium, phosphorus, zinc, manganese, magnesium, niacin and folic acid. To top it off, the protein content of chia seeds exceeds all other grains!

Olives - are one of the most mineral rich fruits on earth. They contain vitamins A and E as well as loads of calcium, magnesium, antioxidants and omega oils. Olives help to regulate blood sugar, control blood cholesterol, and contain substances that help to ward off cancer. When using olive oil, it is best to buy extra virgin. Use it in cooking or in salad dressings.

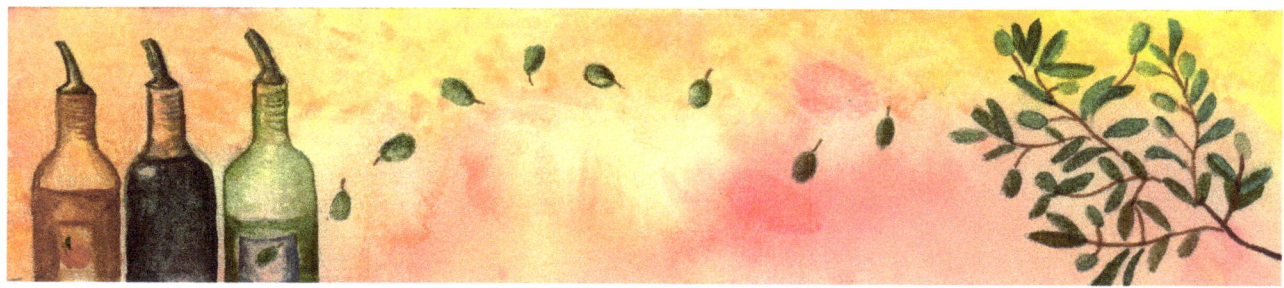

Raw Cacao - is one of the most exciting superfoods. This means chocolate is good for you! Well some of it anyway. The chocolate from the shops which is made from processed cocoa, milk and sugar is definitely no superhero, however if you use raw cacao in your food preparation at home, you can make healthy chocolate. There are recipes in this book that use it. Raw cacao is very high in antioxidants, vitamin C, iron and magnesium. Magnesium is important for the nervous system, repair of cells in the body, a healthy heart and blood vessels, and it helps to keep bones and teeth strong.

> **Interesting fact:** Monkeys were the first to discover the delicious taste of the cacao bean, not man. Lucky for us, people followed their example!

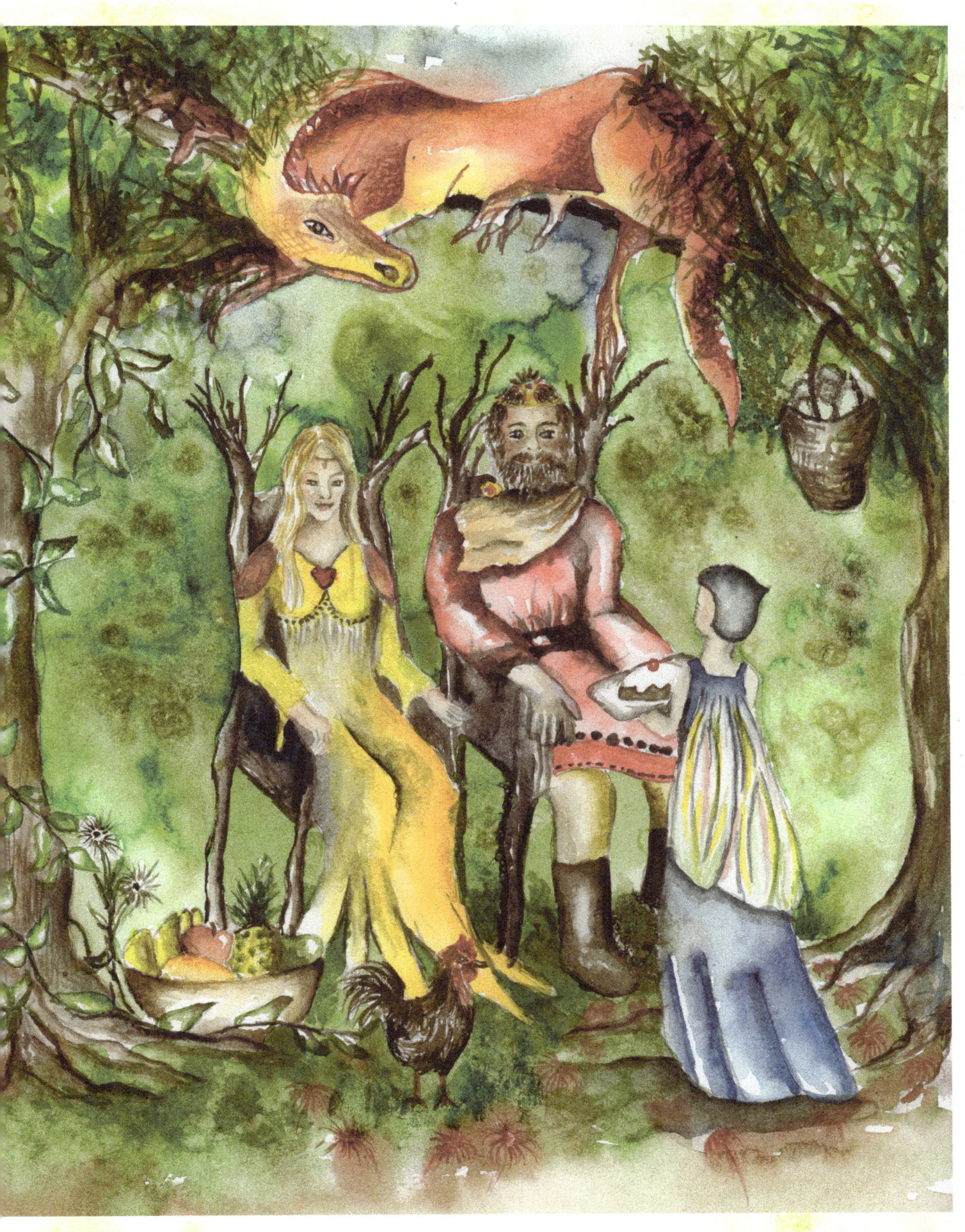

Food fit for the Royals of the Enchanted Forest

Good Fats and Bad Fats

Fat is a word that people often use in a negative way but did you know that not all fat is bad for you? There are fats that are good for your body and help it to work better and to grow stronger. There are also fats that are good in small amounts but can be very bad in larger amounts and then there are the fats you shouldn't eat at all.

Omega Oils or **Unsaturated Fats** - First lets look at the good guys. Omega oils are very important for helping your body remove excess saturated fat. They are also great for your blood, heart and immune system as well as your nervous system and brain. You know what that means? They make you smarter!

Foods that contain omega oils - include fish, avocados, walnuts, sunflower seeds, sesame seeds, pumpkin seeds (pepitas), chia seeds, and hemp seeds as well as linseeds and olives. Remember if you cook nuts and seeds, you lose a lot of the goodness in them, so the best way to eat them is raw.
When oils made from unsaturated fats are heated to high temperatures as in deep frying, the oil is often changed into a form that will do you harm. This is why it is good to limit the amount of fried food that you eat.

Saturated Fats - Provide the body with vitamins and minerals but are dangerous to eat in large quantities over a long period. Saturated fats can clog up your arteries and make it hard for your heart to pump blood around your body. When you eat foods containing saturated fat it is important to balance them with fresh fruit and vegetables and omega oils, which will help your body to clean itself of excess saturated fat. An example of a balanced meal including this group of fats would be homemade lasagne and a salad with raw vegetables, seeds and a light dressing including cold pressed oil. An unbalanced meal of saturated fat would be steak, eggs, bacon and cheese without any vegetables or salad. The first meal would be no problem for the average person to digest. The second would leave too much of the unwanted fat in the arteries.

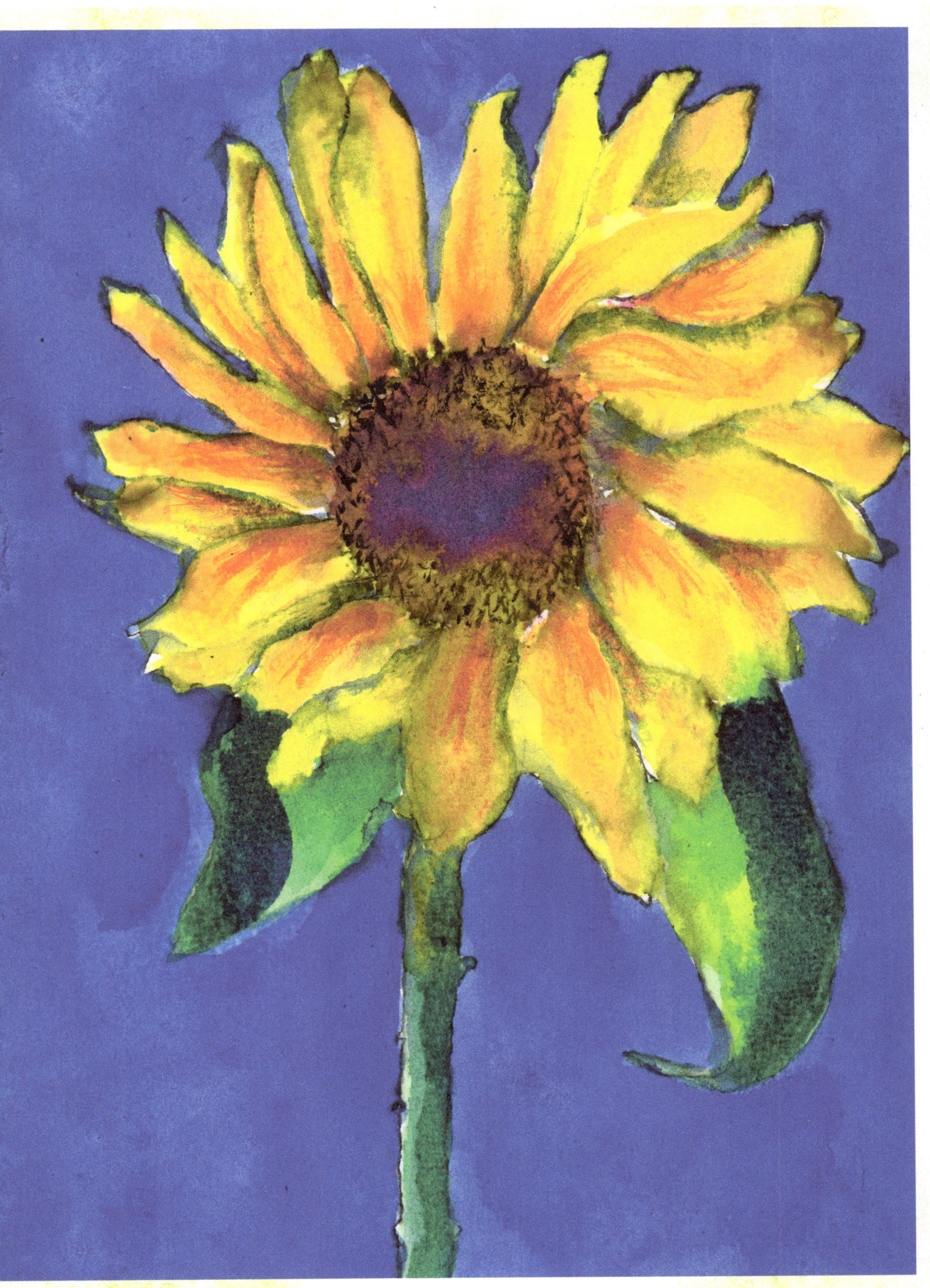

Foods that contain saturated fats include meat, eggs, lard and dairy (including milk, cheese, yoghurt, butter and cream).

Trans Fats - These are formed when vegetable oils are processed in a method called hydrogenation. The oil is changed into a form that the body does not recognise or know what to do with. Trans fats stay in your body and do it harm.

Foods containing trans fats - include processed foods such as packet cakes/biscuits, pies, donuts, chips, and margarines. If you want to avoid trans fats, do not eat anything in a packet that has "hydrogenated oil" in the ingredients.

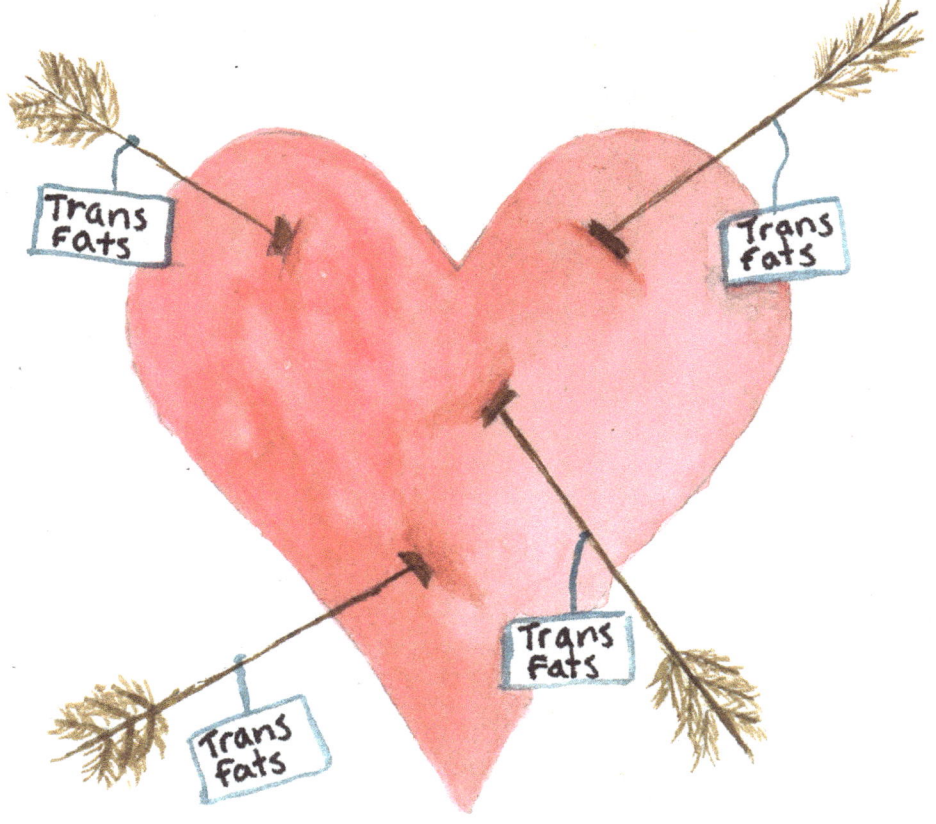

Interesting fact: Introducing enzyme-rich vegetable juices into your diet, such as carrot juice, will aid your body to release trans fats, according to the article, *"Fat/Cellulite Detox,"* written by Dr. Linda Page and published by Healthy Healing Publications.

What Is Wrong With Eating Too Much Junk Food?

Remember all that good stuff and what it does for you? Every time you eat food that contains no healthy building blocks, your body has missed out on it's next meal. It may feel like you have eaten a proper meal because your tummy is full, but the cells in your body are still starving.
That is why sometimes you need to eat more of the bad stuff to feel satisfied. Junk foods are empty. They contain nothing good, but plenty of junk that is not good for your body.

Too much bad fat will stay in your body and clog up all those important veins and arteries that carry your blood around your body. Foods that have lots of bad fat are chips, shop bought cakes and pastries and take away foods. People who eat too much fat for too long end up carrying it on their body and are in danger of having problems with their heart.

Too much sugar will make your body's army weak, will make you tired after a short burst of energy (this is called a sugar low), and will make it very hard for your body to control how much of that sugar is in your blood. People who eat too much sugar for too long can get a disease called diabetes. Too much sugar will also lead to obesity and heart disease as the fructose in sugar turns into fat. When you are having sugar regularly, your body is creating large amounts of fat.

Many foods that are in packets at the shop have things added to them to make them last longer on the shelf, or to make them more colourful, sweeter and to taste like things that they aren't. These things are called additives. They are not food and they are also not good for you. They can affect your brain, making you sad, angry or frustrated. They can make your body unhealthy and they can make you want to eat more even when you have had enough.

RAW-Some Food

Cooking is lots of fun, but sometimes it is just as much fun to prepare foods that do not involve heat. Salads, bliss balls, raw fudge, brownies and smoothies can all be made without cooking the ingredients. Fresh, organic fruits, vegetables, nuts and seeds that have not been heated actually contain more nutritional value than those that have been cooked. This is because the cooking process destroys some of the nutrients.

Also, there is an important balance that needs to be maintained in our bodies. It is called the **pH balance**. This balance refers to how acidic the blood is or how alkaline it is. The measurement is given a number. Lower numbers mean your blood is acidic and higher numbers mean it is alkaline. The perfect blood pH is around 7.4. It all sounds a bit technical but may be simplified using a straight-lined diagram. Here, the two extremes are illustrated.

1 2 3 4 5 6 7 8 9 10 11 12 13 14

Very acidic blood	**7.4 - perfect**	**Very alkaline blood**
Easier for disease to thrive.	**blood pH**	A rare problem.
Caused by junk foods	Achieved by eating	
and cooked foods.	more fresh, raw produce.	

As you can see, our blood can be very acidic, or alkaline. What it is meant to be is somewhere in the middle (pH of 7.4). The BEST ever alkaline food is sprouts. You can grow your own sprouts at home on the windowsill and they are so sweet and delicious when fresh.

> **Interesting fact:** You can measure your blood pH by buying some litmus paper test strips from the chemist. Put one on your tongue first thing in the morning and it will change colour. The colour will match a chart that comes with the papers and will tell you what the pH of your saliva is.

Most people have quite acidic blood because they do not eat enough fresh, raw produce. Disease thrives in an acidic environment, but finds it very hard to exist in an alkaline environment. Through changing what you eat, there is something you can do about acidic blood.

To help your body become more alkaline try any of the following:
- Once a day have a raw smoothie - see recipes in this book.
- Drink more fresh, raw vegetable juices.
- Include a raw salad with each meal.
- Instead of crackers, eat raw vegetable sticks with your dips.
- Try some of the raw food treats in this book.

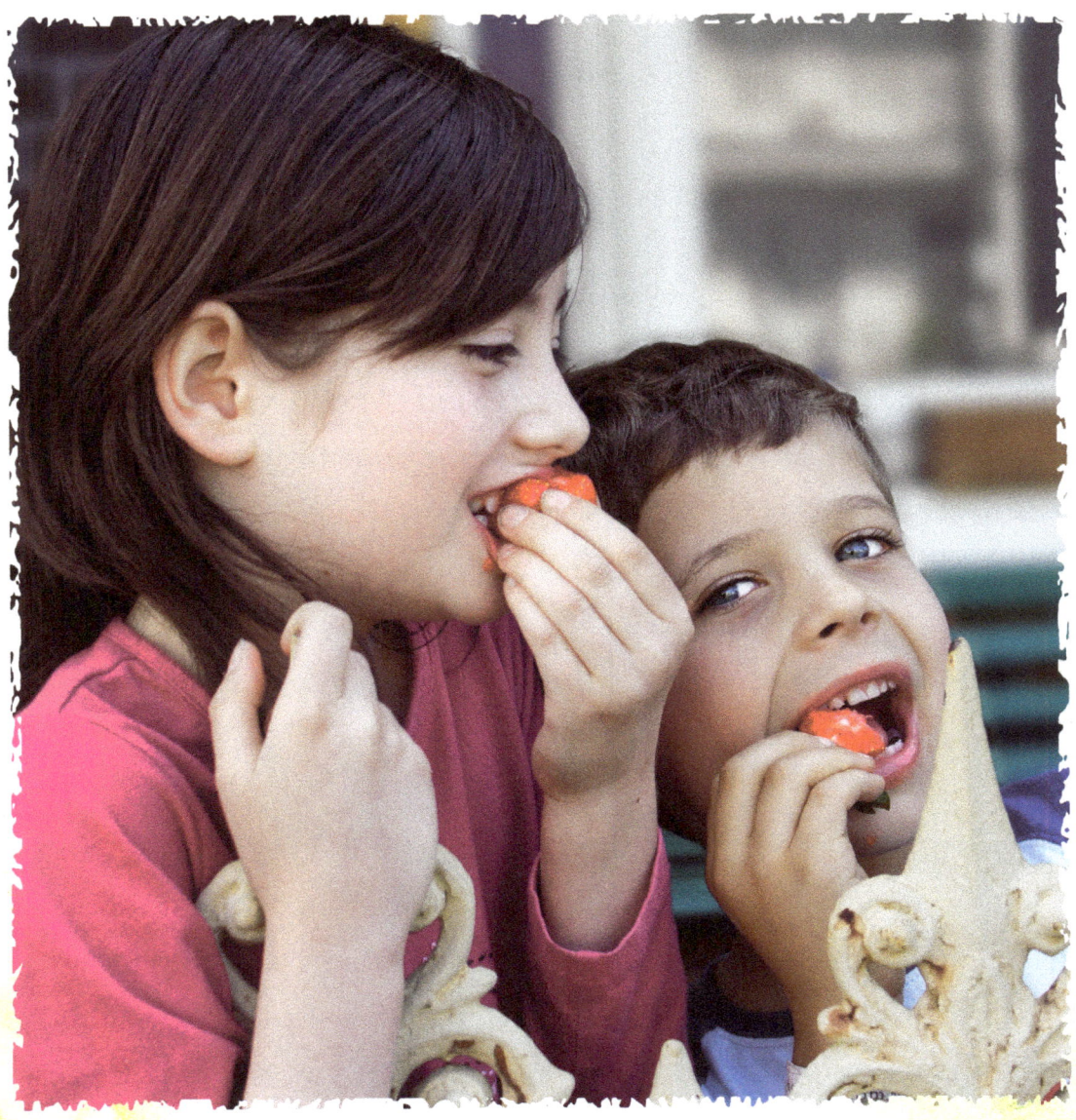

How Do Your Taste Buds Work?

Taste buds are the tiny dots on our tongue and roof of our mouths that are responsible for allowing us to taste food. Most people already know something about that, but a secret a lot of people do not know is that you can train your taste buds. You know how there are some foods that just don't taste good when you put them into your mouth? If they are foods that aren't good for you then it doesn't really matter, but if it is a food that is very high in nutrients, then it is such a shame for our bodies to miss out just because we cannot get the food past our taste buds. Sometimes taste buds can be a little stubborn, but try training them and you will like the taste of a whole range of foods you didn't like before. See, taste buds get used to eating what they have always eaten. Sometimes they decide that they don't like new foods. So here is how to do it - step by step!

Taste Bud Training

1. **Choose a food that is very good for your body, one that you don't really like the taste of.**
2. **Once a day, have a small piece of that food. At first you may just chew it up and spit it out. That is okay. As long as your taste buds get to try it.**
3. **Continue giving your taste buds a try. Sometimes, instead of spitting the food out, put it onto your fork with a food you like and try the two tastes together.**
4. **Persist. Be firm with your taste buds and guess what. Eventually they will be wanting more!**

There are some situations where our taste buds and our bodies do not want a certain food because we have an allergy or intolerance to that food.
You need to decide when this is the case. It is all about listening to our bodies and working with them rather than against them. Just remember that using this as an excuse not to try new foods will not help you, so do your best to be honest with yourself and your Mum and Dad.

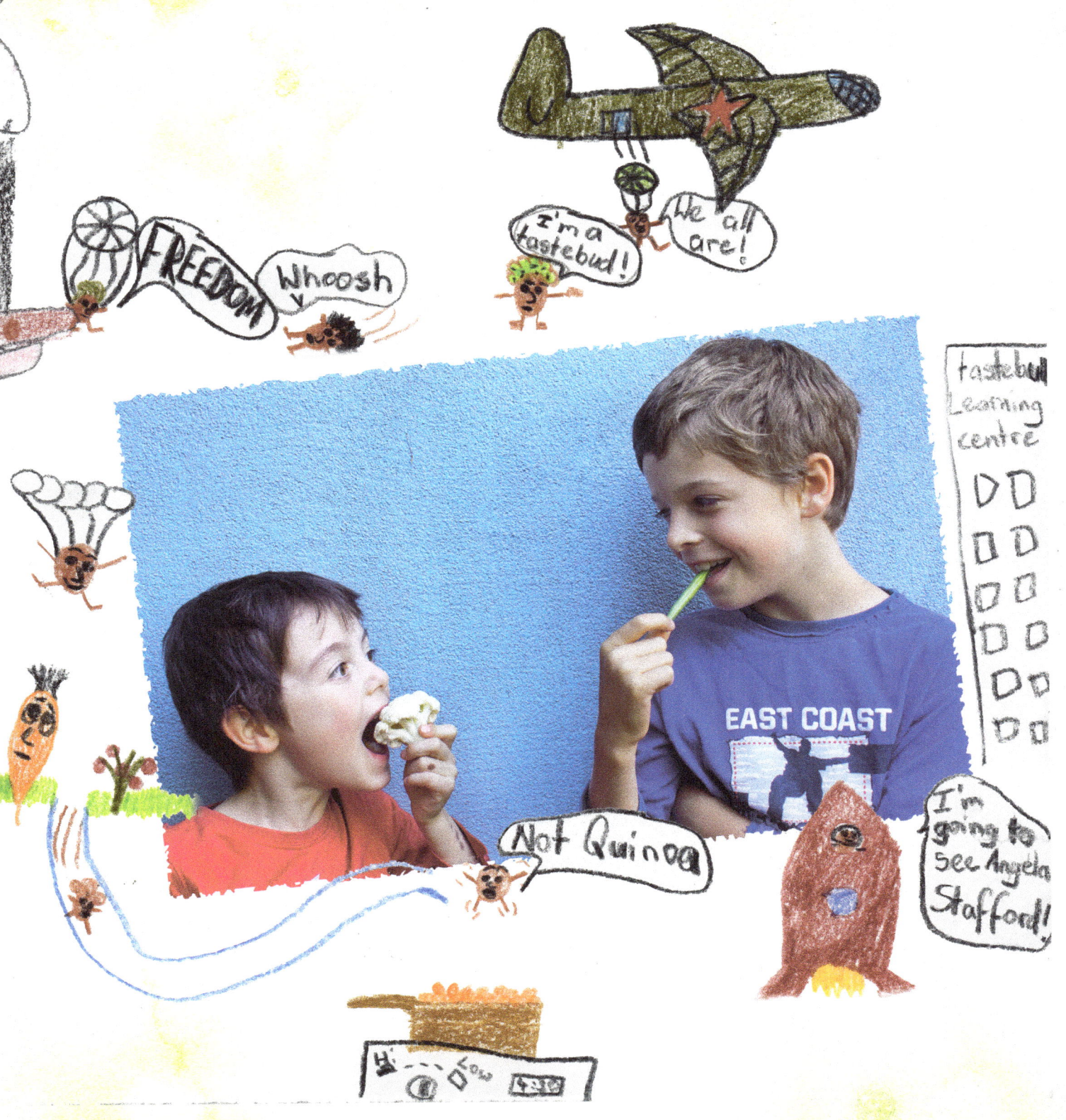

Where Does Your Food Come From?

We have already discussed the difference between a whole food diet and one of processed foods. Here we will look at where all of those lovely whole foods start off. There is a difference between organic and non-organic farms just as there are factory and free range eggs.

Organic farming

An organic farm is one that works in harmony with nature rather than against it. What this means is that the farmer uses natural ways to control pests and grow the yummiest most nutritious fruits and vegetables possible.

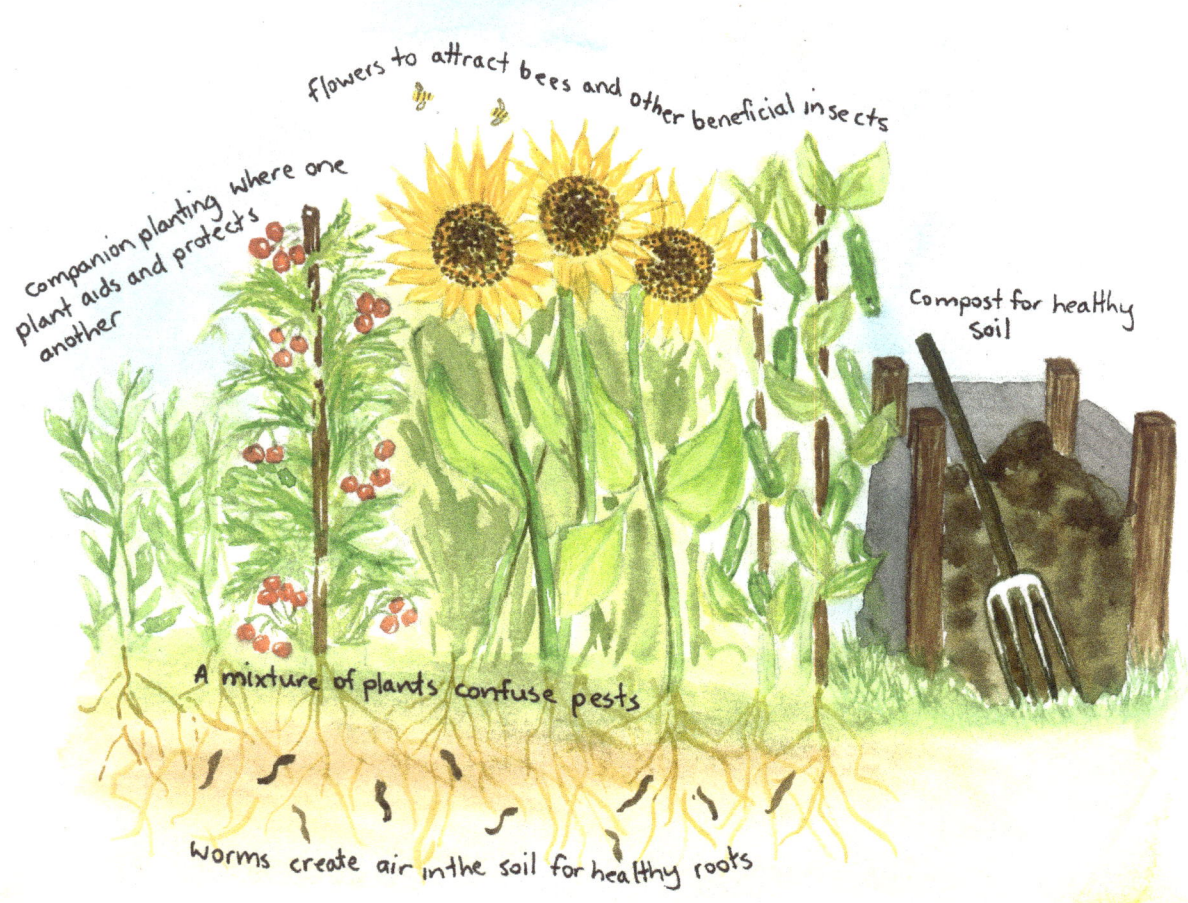

Non-Organic Farming

Many farms do not use natural methods to control pests and not as much importance is placed on the nutrients in the soil. In place of the methods described in organic farming, these farmers spray their crops with poisons, (called pesticides) that kill the bugs trying to eat the food.

This way of farming requires less preparation and allows farmers to grow large quantities of the same foods. Unfortunately the result is food containing less vitamins and minerals due to over farming in poor soil. The crops also contain poisons that don't always wash off. These fruits and vegetables cost less money to produce and therefore less money to buy. The long term effect on a person eating these foods is a less healthy body and may end up costing you more in medical bills. Non-organic fruits and vegetables do not taste as good, are not as nutritious and may still contain some of the pesticides that have been sprayed on them.

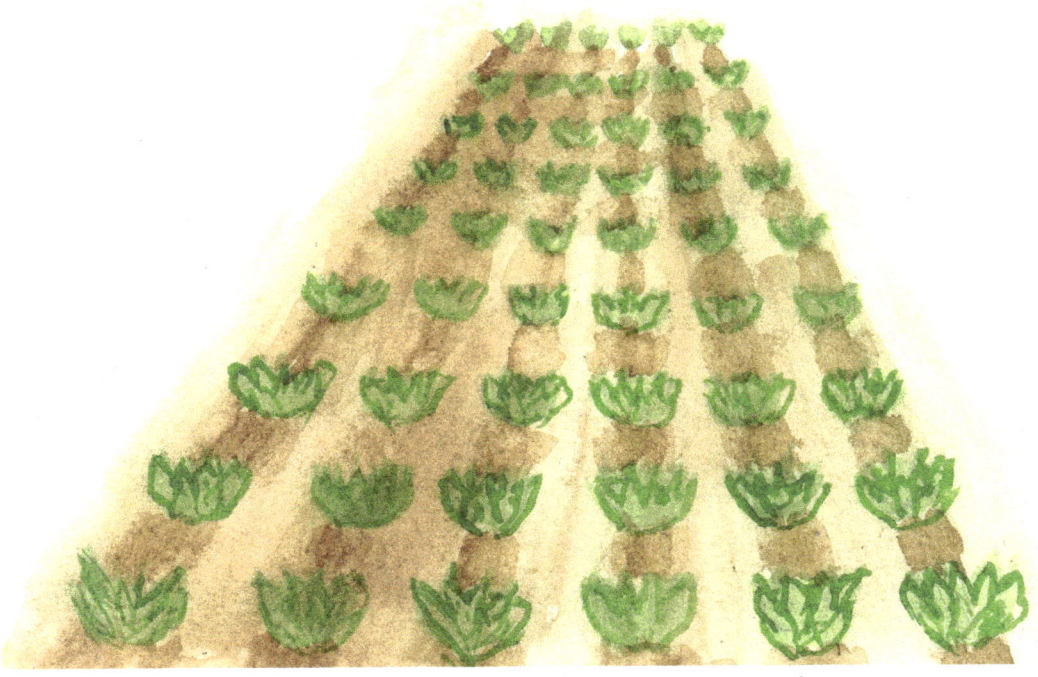

Crops planted in rows need more protection from pests.
Without the aid of other plants and healthy soil,
crops are often sprayed with pesticides.

Free-Range Animal Farms

These farms allow the animals that are raised for meat, milk and eggs to go outside and play. They breathe fresh air, eat fresh grass and run around. This kind of farming costs the farmers more money because they need more land for the animals. This means the price of their meat, eggs and milk is higher.

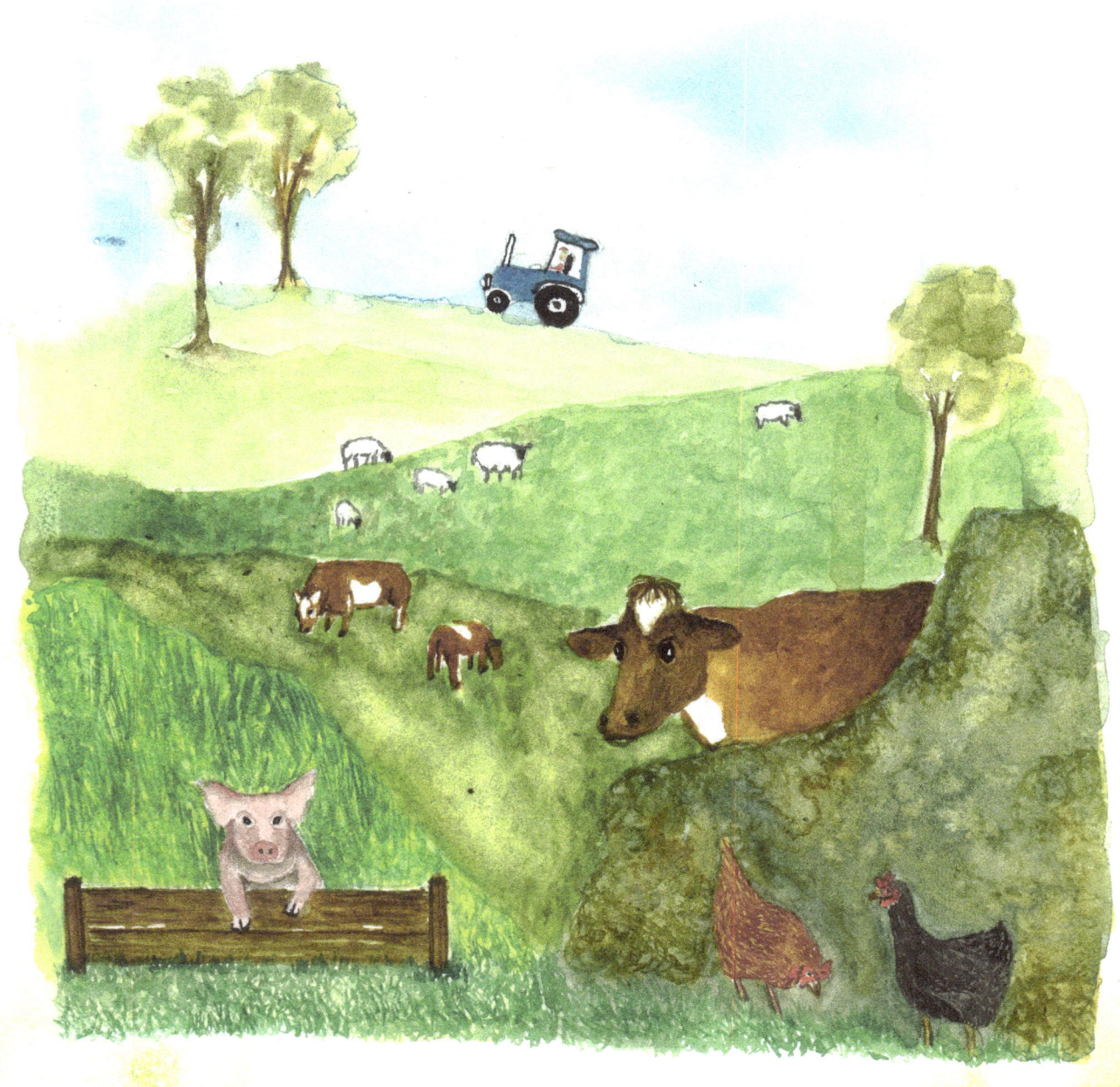

Factory Farms

These farms keep the animals in barns, stalls and cages so that the farmers do not have to buy as much land. It is cheaper for the farmer and cheaper to buy the eggs, milk and meat that come from these farms. However, the animals spend their lives in small spaces, do not get much fresh air and no time to go outside and play.

In Australia, most of the cows and sheep raised for meat are kept in large pastures. Pigs, chickens and turkeys are often not. When you buy your meat and eggs do some research into where they have come from and what the farms are like where they lived. The butcher or packaging will usually say if the product is free-range.

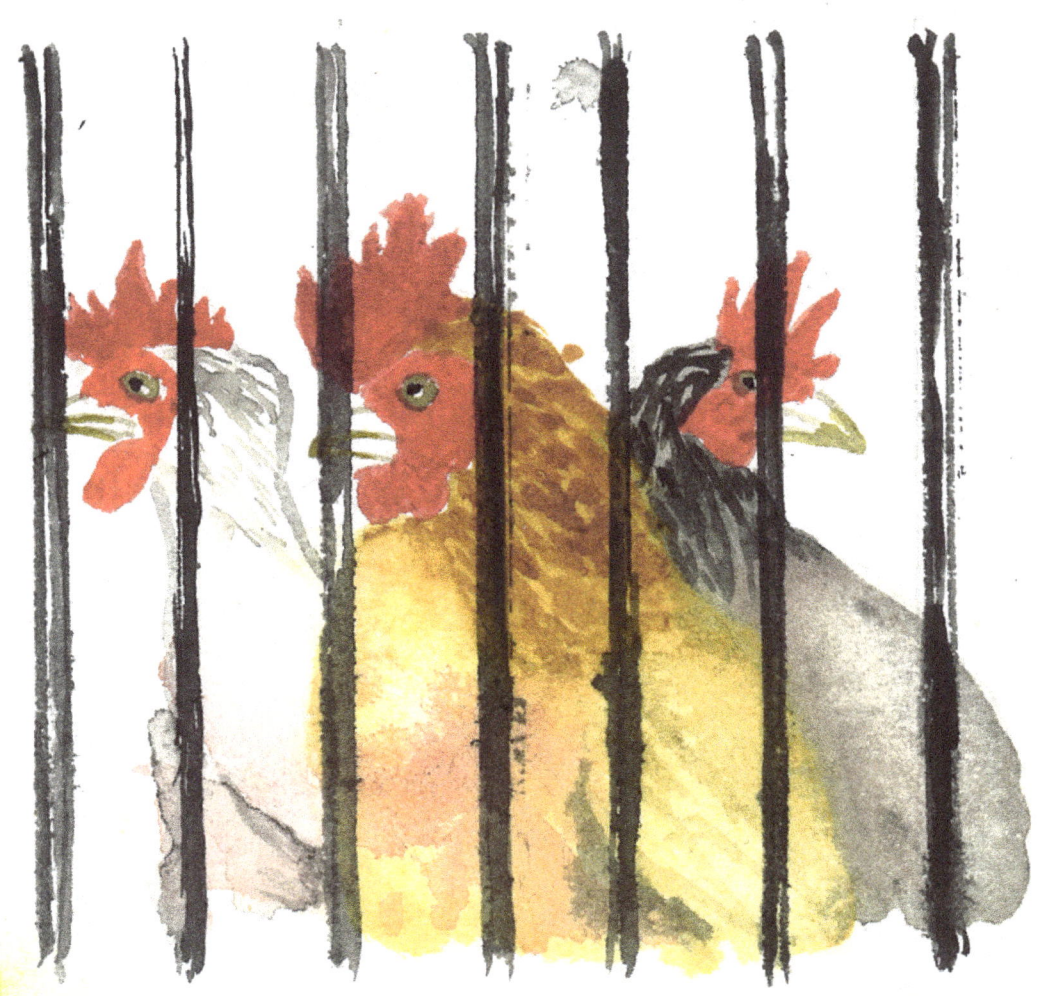

Organic, Free-Range Farms

These farms are a mixture of the free range and organic farms. They are often known as biodynamic or permaculture farms. They use organic farming methods to grow the fruits and vegetables and they give their animals space to run around in. They also feed the animals with organic foods so that the meat, eggs and milk is free from poisons. On these farms, the relationship between the earth and its cycles, the animals and sometimes even the moon (when planting using a lunar calendar) is part of the farming practice. Waste is recycled so that farmers work in harmony with the earth and lunar energies to maintain healthy soils, plants and animals.

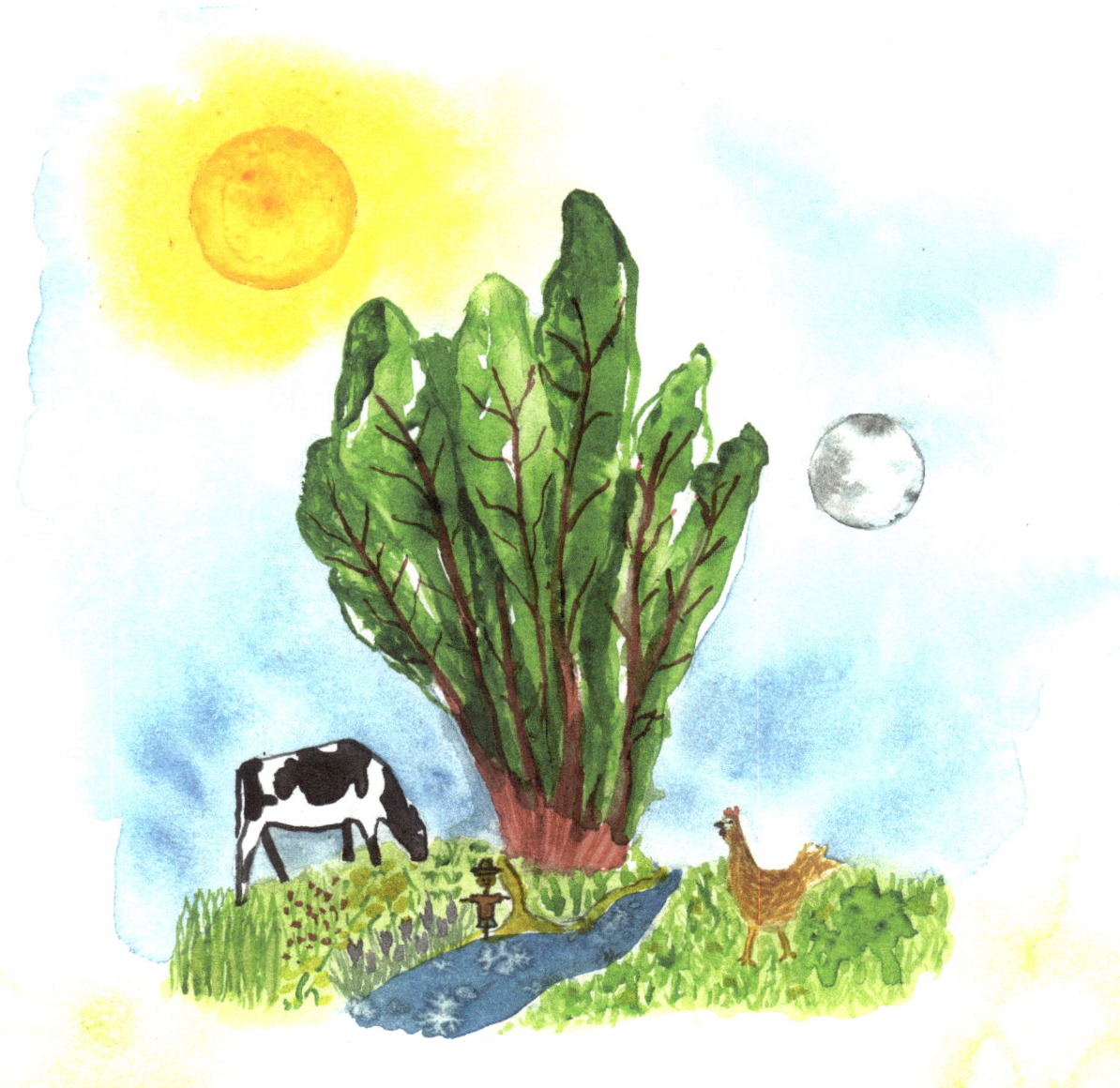

Eating For a Happier Earth

Choosing to eat foods produced with love and in harmony with nature contributes to a healthier, happier and cleaner Earth.

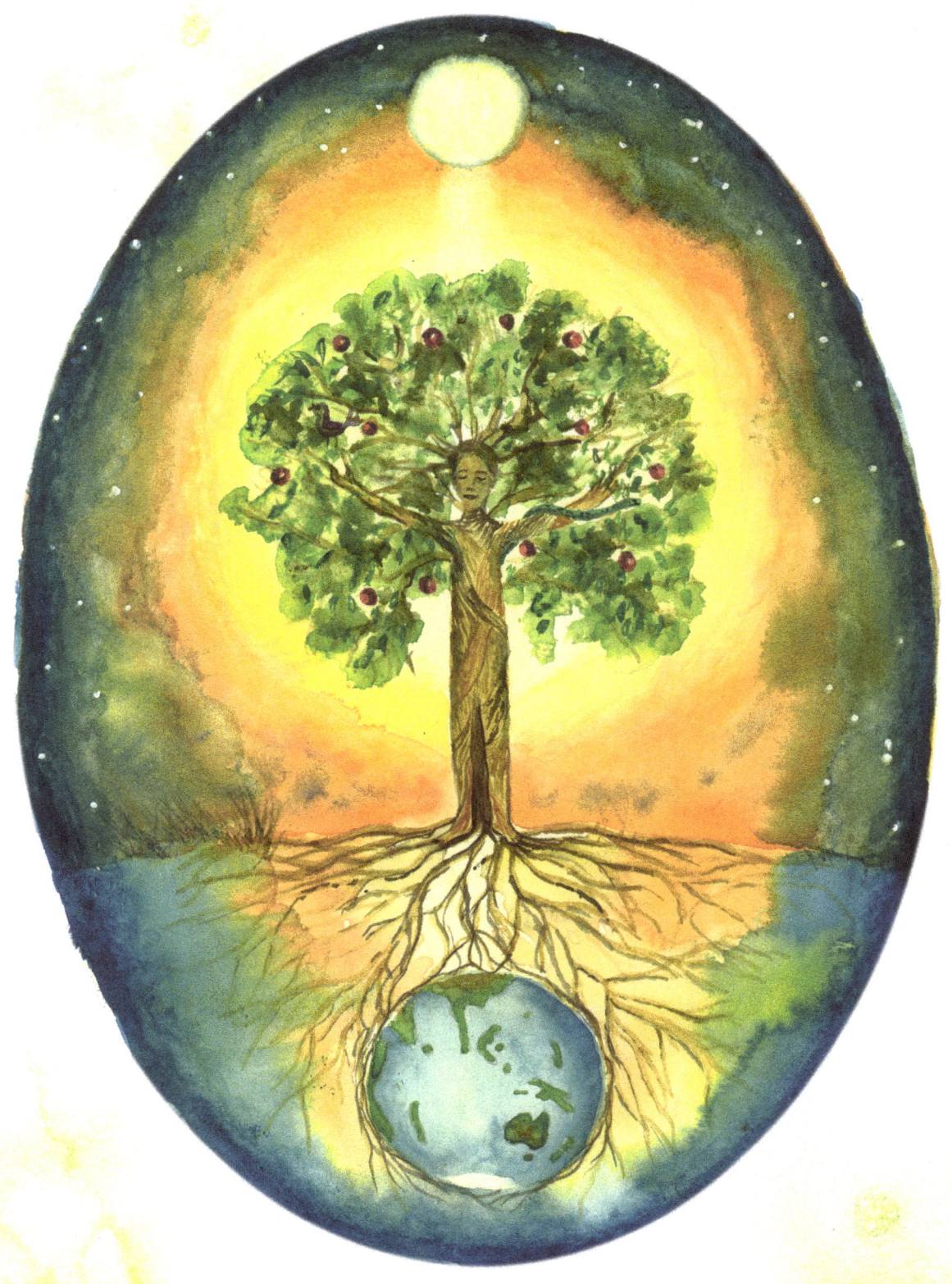

Your Own Fresh Eggs

One way to make sure your eggs have been produced by happy chooks is to have your own. They make lovely companions in the garden (as long as you keep them out of the vegetable patch) and despite popular opinion, that these creatures are a little lacking in the brains department, they do have their own unique personalities. Yes, they often behave in a way that shows they didn't really think things through, but this is always good entertainment.
Our white chook, Daisy, likes to sit on our windowsill and watch me cook!
She is pictured here with our son, Ryan.

Not only do our chickens provide us with fresh eggs but they make plenty of fertiliser too. Last year our mulberry trees produced next to no fruit. This year, with the help of the chook poo, they were leaden with fruit!

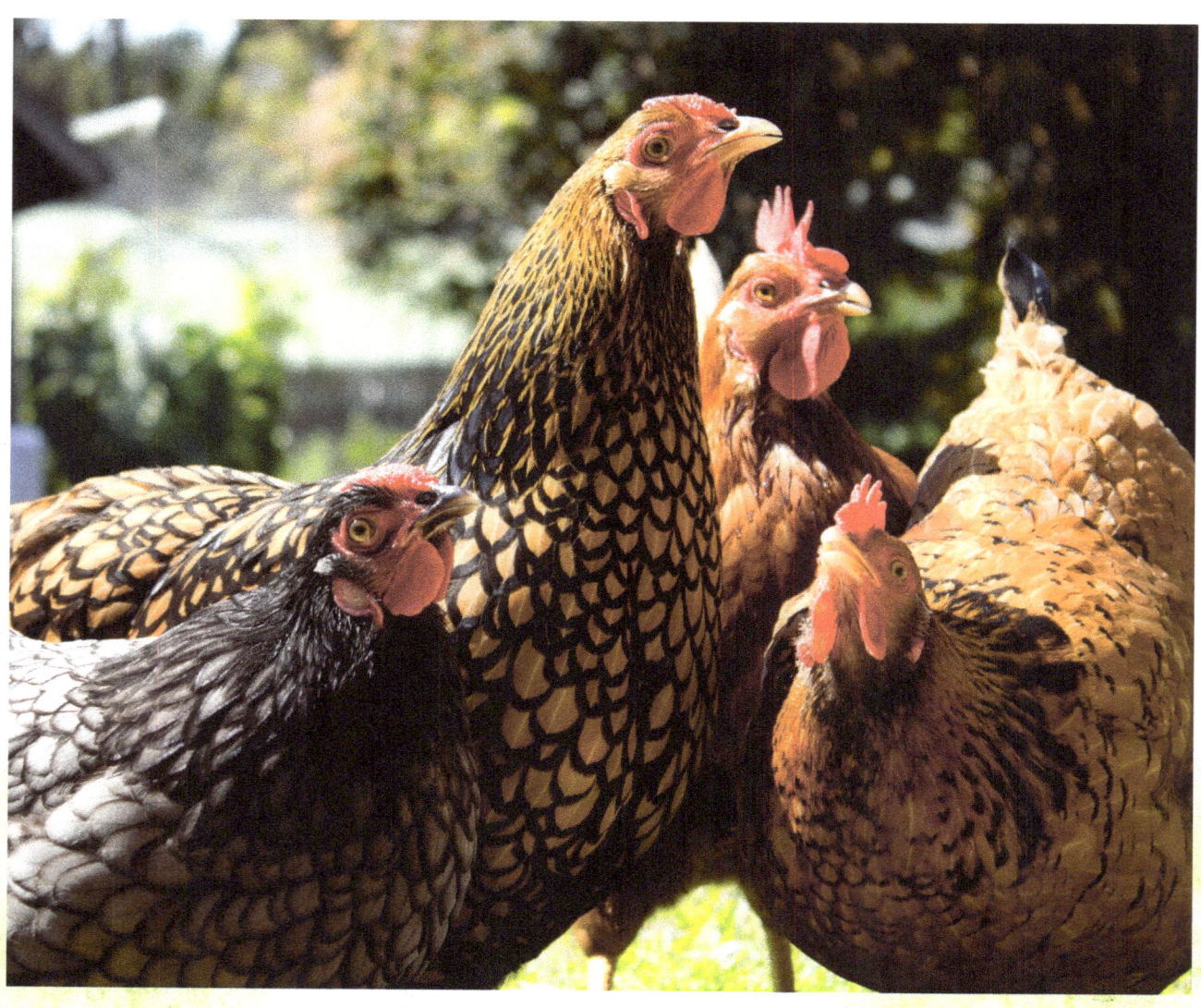

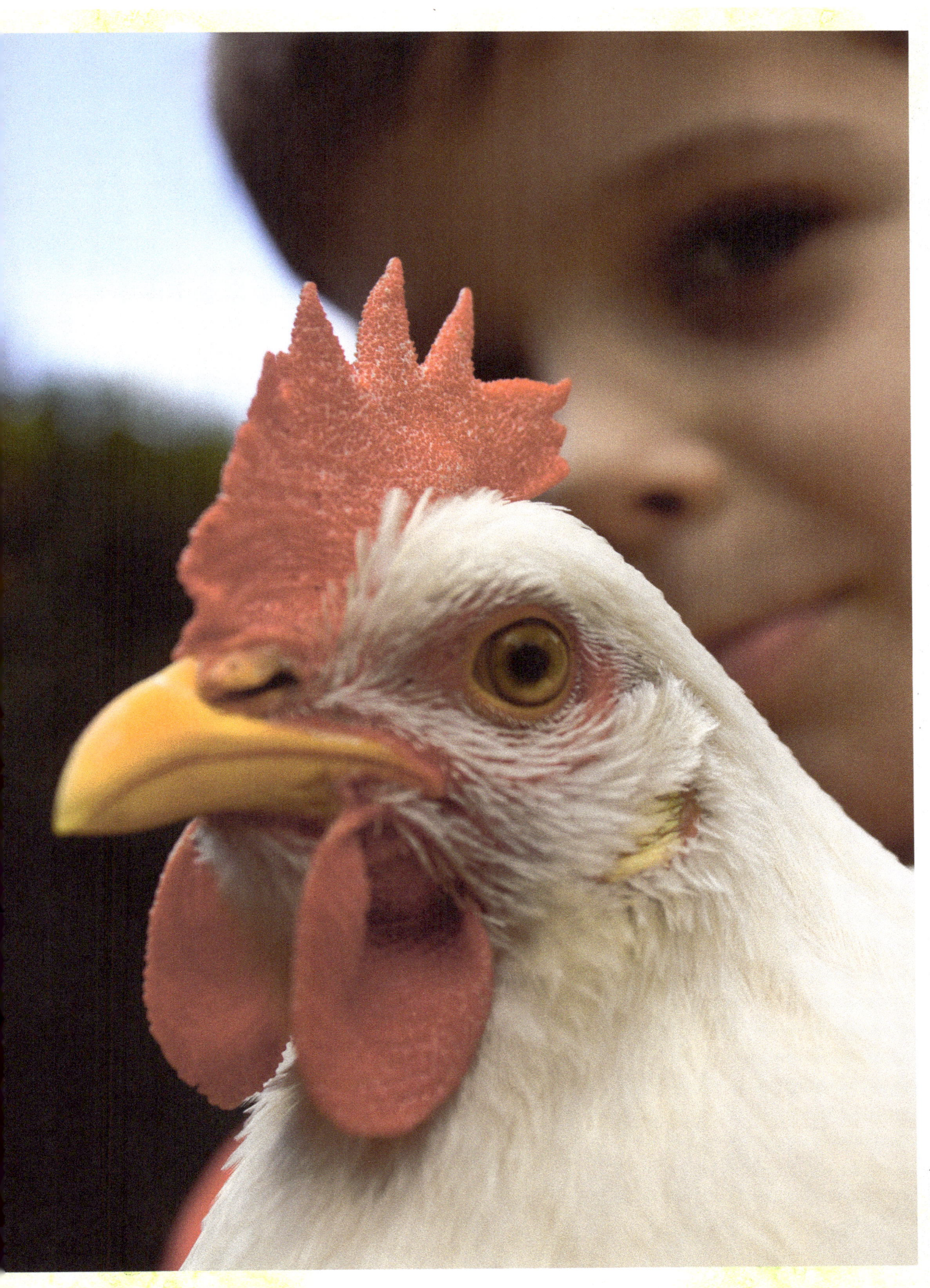

Lets Get Started!

Now that we know what our bodies need to be strong and healthy, lets get started in the kitchen.

Deciding what to cook

Before we start cooking we need to decide what it is we are going to cook. You may already have an idea in mind or you may have no idea. The best place to start is by looking through your recipes. When you are first learning, it is good to always follow a recipe exactly as it is written. This way you know that the dish will turn out right. By following the recipe you will see how the different foods go together, so in the future you will know which combinations work well.

When you are choosing a recipe consider the following points:
- What ingredients do I have to work with?
- What equipment do I have to work with? (Read through potential recipes to find out what you need).
- Do I need to start with something very easy or am I ready to try something harder?
- How much help do I need and is that help available?
- Will this food be eaten soon and if not can it be stored for later?
- How many people am I preparing food for?
- Am I ready to also clean up after myself?

Before beginning there are some important steps to take:
- Get permission from a responsible adult.
- Make sure you are wearing covered shoes to protect your feet.
- Wash your hands well with soap.
- If you have an apron, put it on, or change out of your good clothes.
- Make your work space comfortable. (For more information, see page 42).
- Measure out your ingredients.

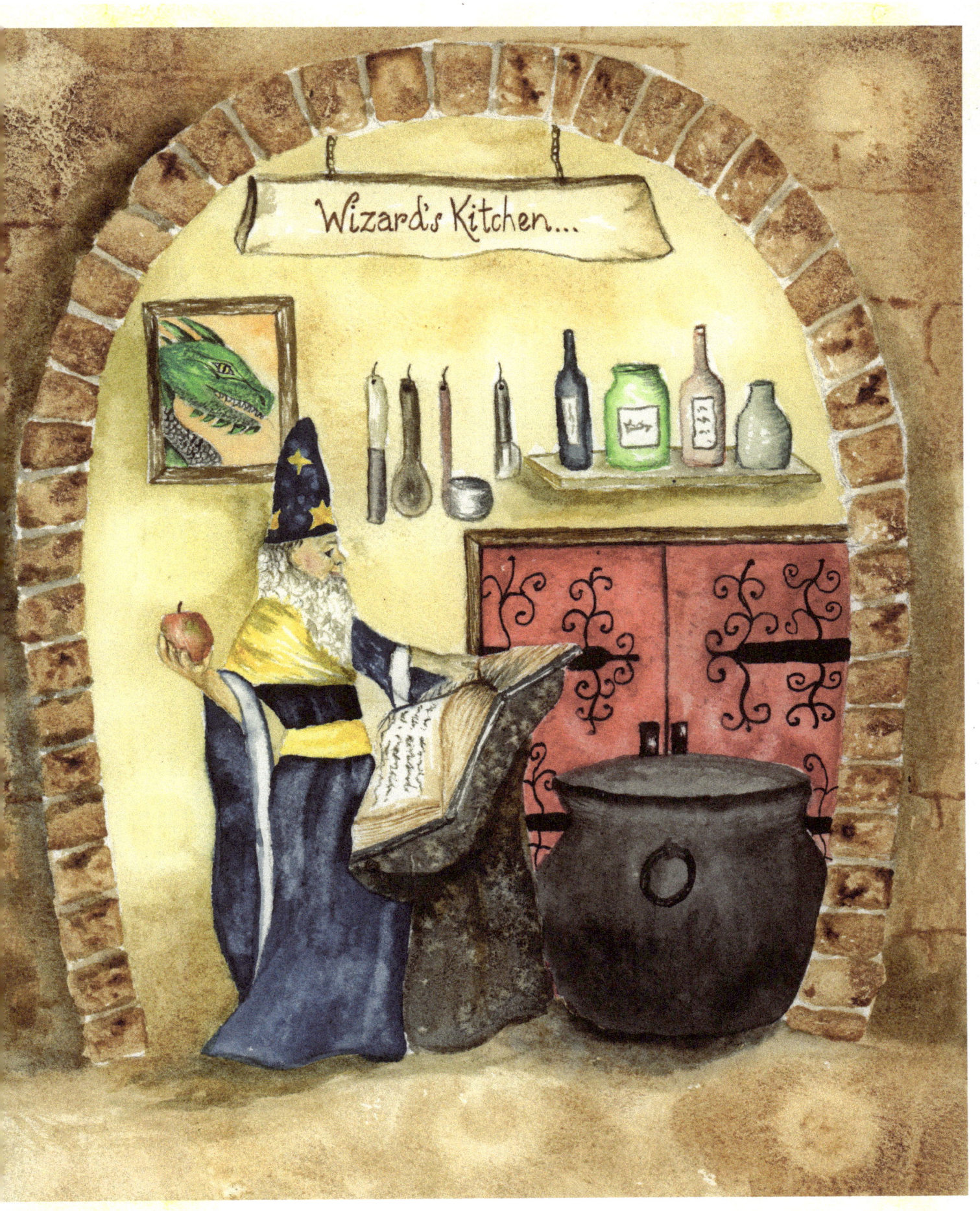

Read through your recipe from start to finish so that you know exactly what you need.

Cooking Equipment

I am not going to list every piece of equipment you could be using in the kitchen because if you have ever visited a kitchen shop, you will know that the possibilities are endless. However there are a few items that I consider either essential or very helpful in the kitchen.

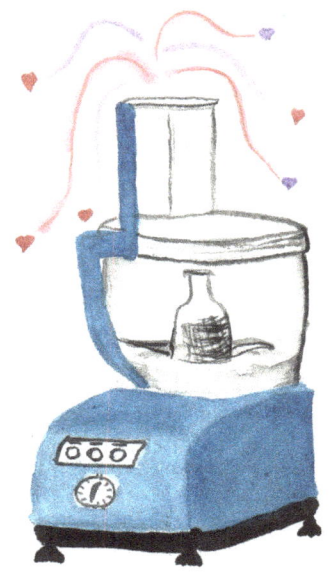

A food processor - This would be one of my champions in the kitchen. If you buy a decent one, you can make fantastic dips, smoothies, bliss balls, nut flours and purees. You can also reduce your cutting time significantly by throwing your onion, garlic, ginger and chillis into the food processor at the start of a recipe. It will pulverise your vegetables, finely chop your herbs, knead bread mix and whisk egg whites. Some even juice citrus.
A worthy investment in any kitchen!

A pressure cooker - I love this piece of equipment because it cuts down on cooking time in a big way. Beans, such as kidney, canellini, borlotti etc. take less than an hour as opposed to many hours and soups are done in 15 minutes. I do not like waiting and I do not like being hungry, so for me, this is the answer!

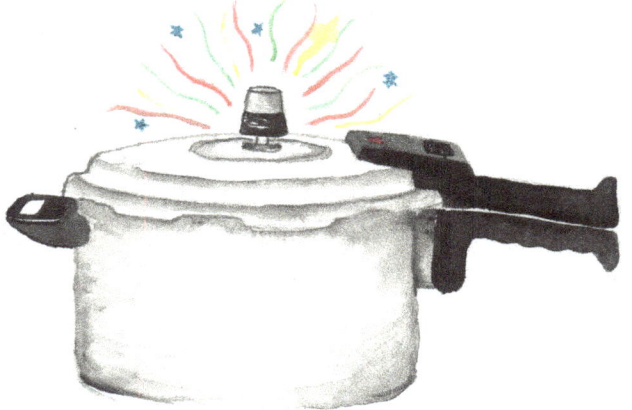

> **Personal note:** Our kitchen does not contain a microwave as after wading through the information available on their safety and effect on foods, I am not comfortable with using one. For this reason, none of my recipes have microwave instructions.

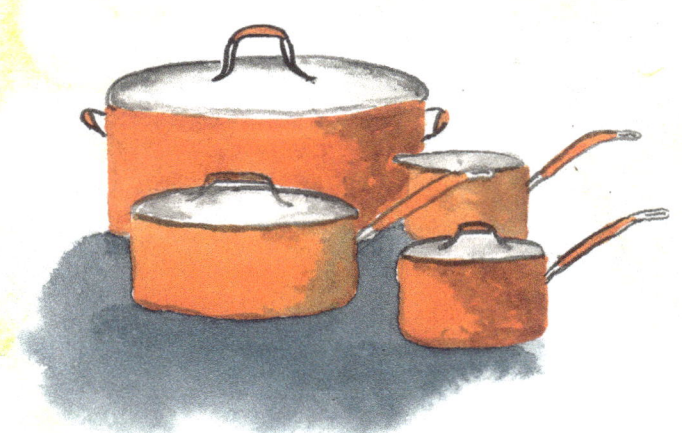

A good set of saucepans - For me, the metal of choice in saucepans is stainless steel including a good heavy based one for large meals. A heavy base will distribute the heat evenly, reducing the chance of burning the food. Stay away from aluminium which will eventually break down and go into your food. Teflon also raises questions in regards to health and safety. Unfortunately, many people have eaten their Teflon coatings and the long term affects of this are not yet understood.

A salad spinner - This is a very inexpensive item but can make your green salads infinitely better. There is nothing worse than soggy salad greens and a spinner will dry them perfectly. At the same time you will build up your arm muscles!

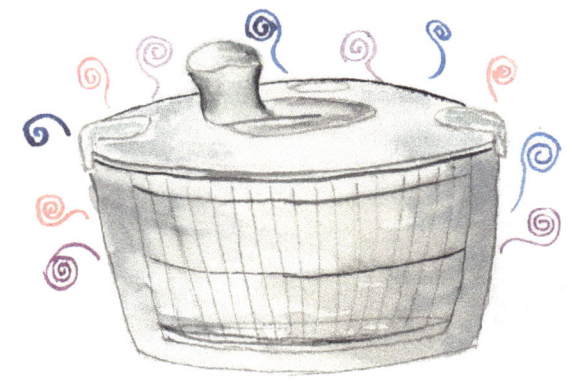

A safe, non-stick frying pan - There are now non-stick frying pans available that are Teflon free and safer to use. Lets face it, pancakes and eggs are so much easier to cook in a non-stick pan and they come out looking a lot nicer.

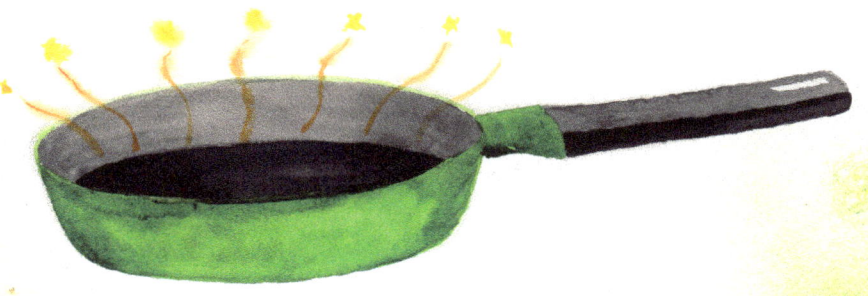

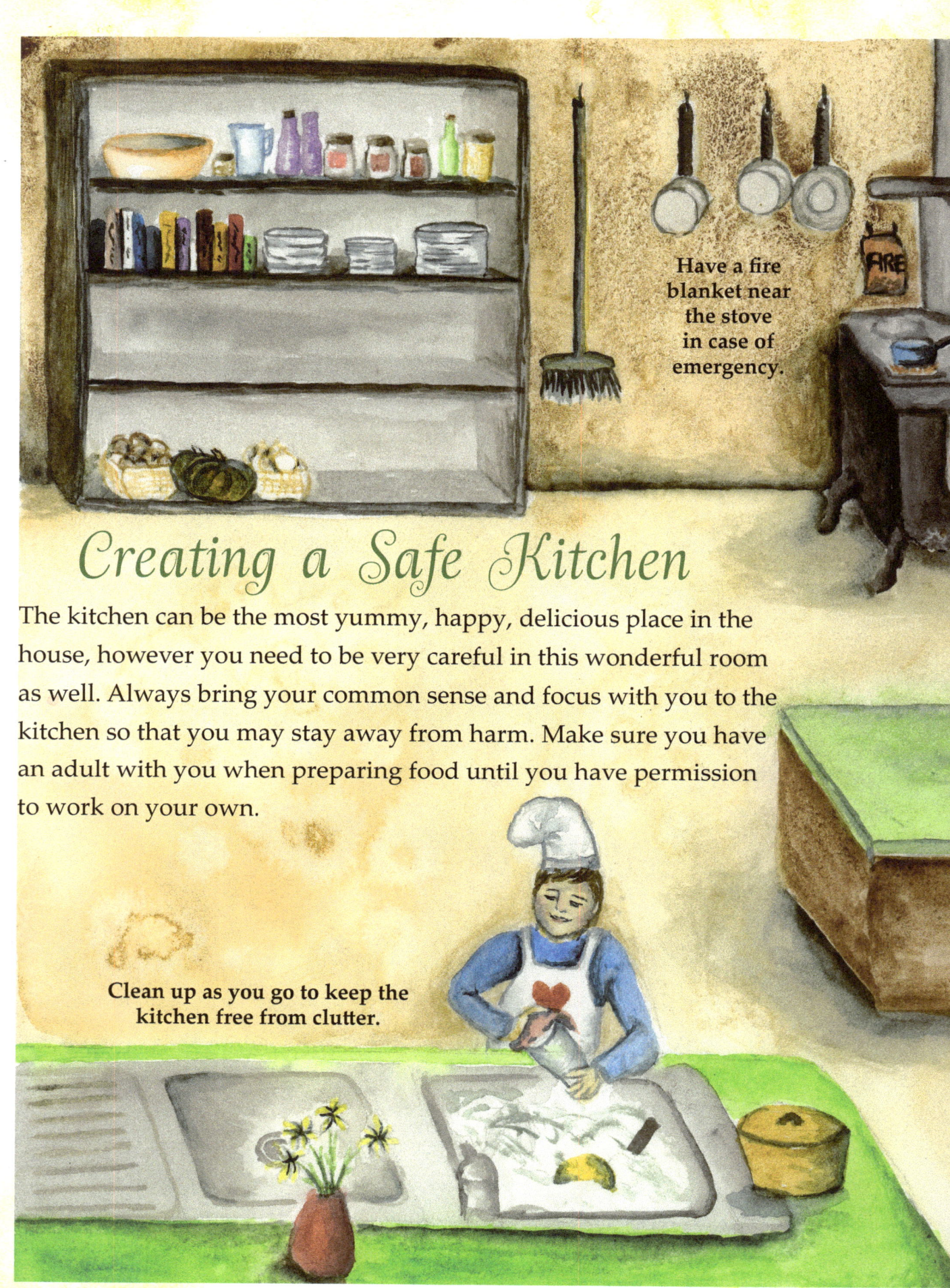

Have a fire blanket near the stove in case of emergency.

Creating a Safe Kitchen

The kitchen can be the most yummy, happy, delicious place in the house, however you need to be very careful in this wonderful room as well. Always bring your common sense and focus with you to the kitchen so that you may stay away from harm. Make sure you have an adult with you when preparing food until you have permission to work on your own.

Clean up as you go to keep the kitchen free from clutter.

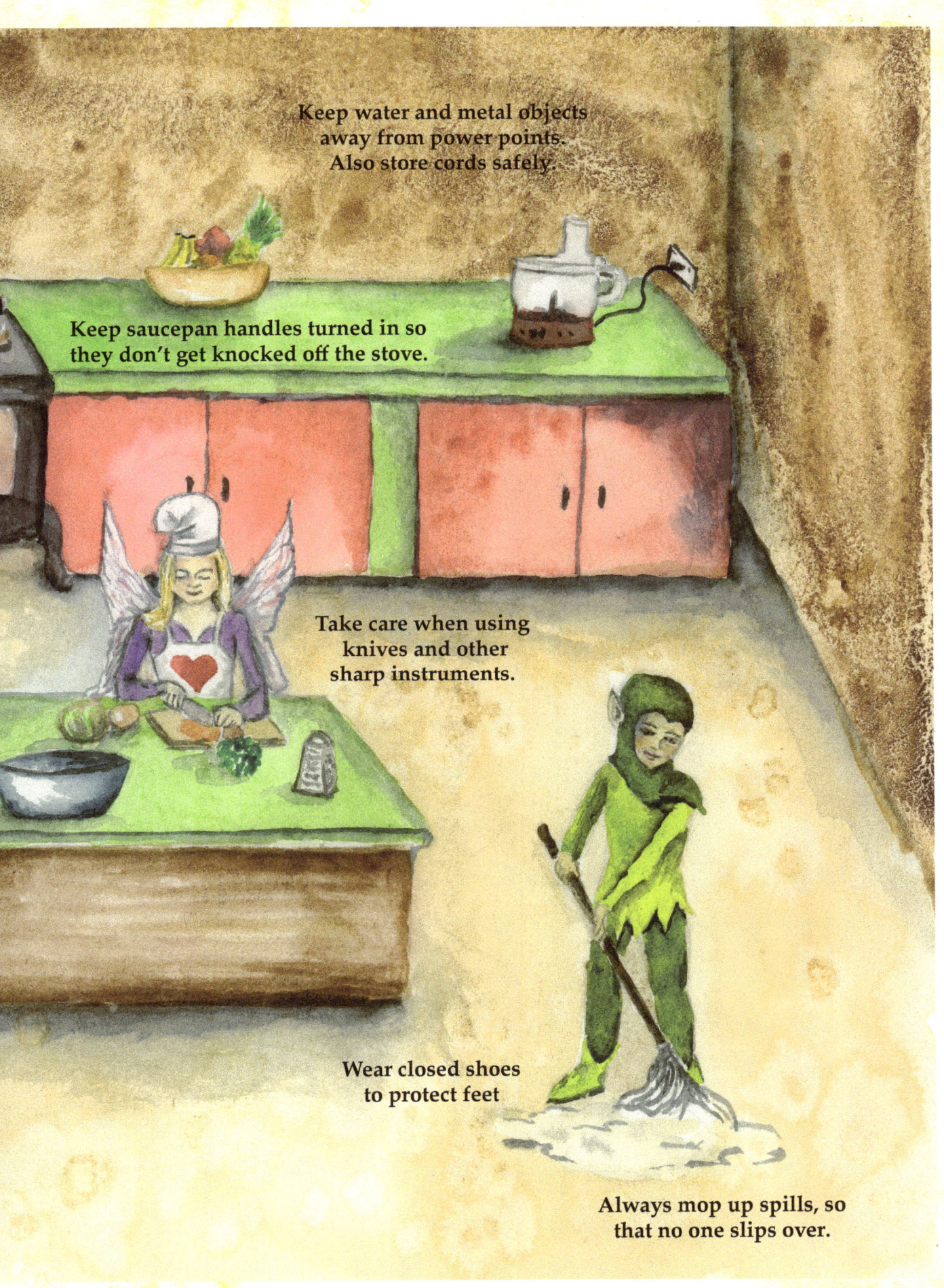

Ambience in the Kitchen

The word **"ambience"** refers to how a place feels. When you are preparing food for yourself or someone else, it is a creative process. You are not just adding ingredients to the bowl, you are also adding the energy of how you feel. If you put love and happiness into your food, the people who eat it will feel better than if you put frustration, anger and sadness in there.
You may not be able to see emotions but they are energy that become a part of all that you do.

To help you to feel relaxed and loving in the kitchen, make sure it is a place that you feel good in. Here are some ideas to help you out:

- Start in a clean kitchen.
- Have lots of fresh air circulating by opening windows.
- Put some music on that you enjoy.
- Wear comfortable clothes.
- If there is anyone around who you find distracting or annoying, organise for them to either leave or sit quietly.
- Remain patient with yourself while you are learning and do not always expect to do a perfect job.
- Work at your own pace, being careful not to rush anything.
- If you are working with an adult, find a patient one whom you can trust to support you.

> *"Music gives a soul to the universe,*
> *wings to the mind,*
> *flight to the imagination*
> *and life to everything."*
> *~ Plato*

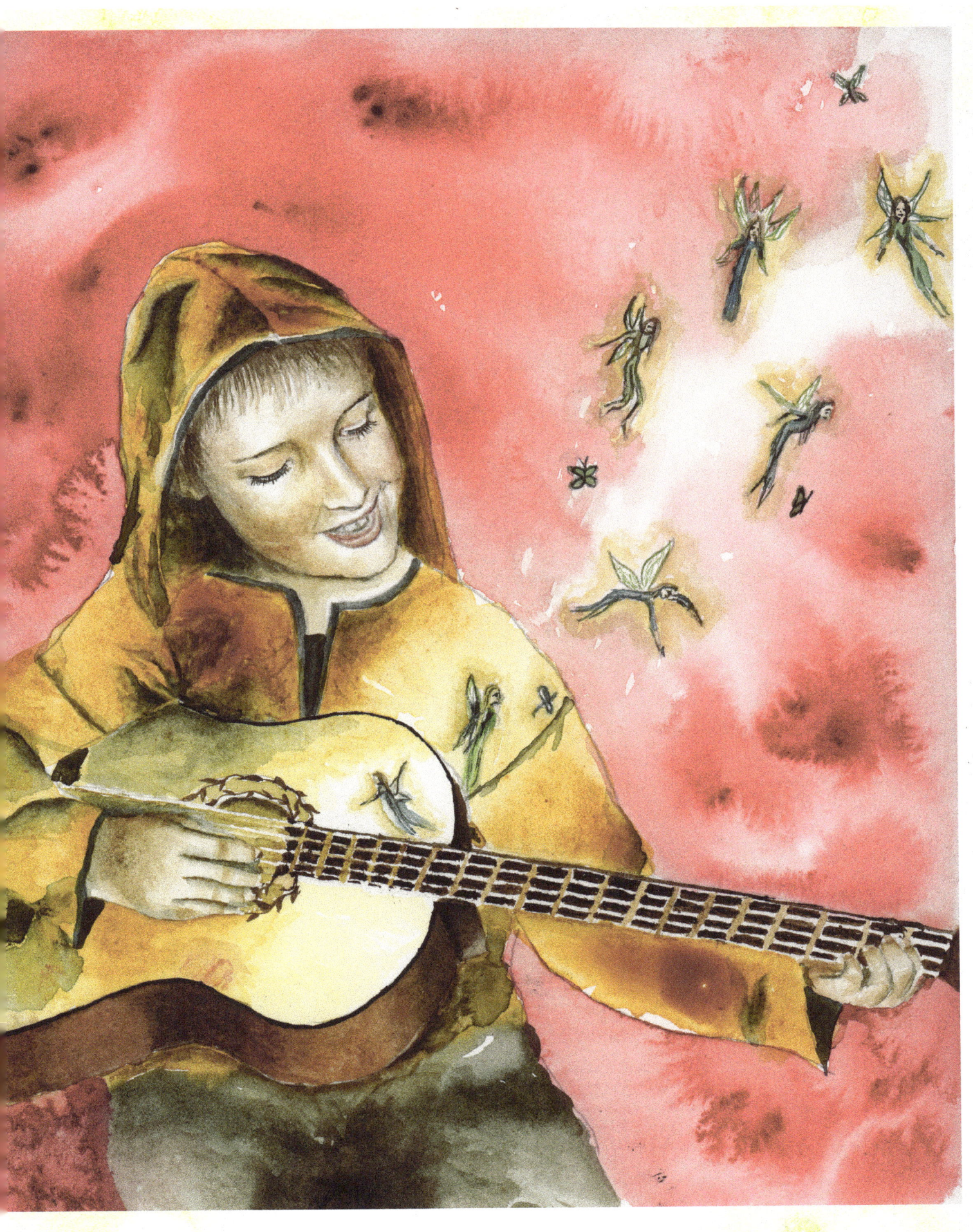

Cooking Terms

You may not understand all of the terms used in recipes. Have a look through this list so that you may become familiar with them.

Term	Definition
preheat	Refers to heating the oven to the correct temperature before putting the food in to cook.
fan forced	An oven setting where a fan blows the heat through the oven.
convection	An oven setting using an element (or hot bar) at the top and an element at the bottom.
whisk	Mixing ingredients with a fork or whisk tool to put air through.
grill	Toasting food with the top element in the oven or a separate grilling element.
bake	Cooking inside the oven.
steam	Cooking with steam. Water is boiled in a saucepan underneath another saucepan containing the food. The saucepan on the top has holes to allow the steam to cook the food. This is a very healthy way of cooking.
dice	Cutting food into cubes.
pulverise	Chopping an ingredient so finely it goes mushy.

Conversion Tables		
Unit	Metric	Imperial
1 teaspoon	5ml	1 teaspoon
1 tablespoon	15ml	½ fluid oz.
3 teaspoons	1 tablespoon	1 tablespoon
1 cup*	250ml	8.45 fluid oz.
Grams (g)	1g	.035 oz
	225g	8 oz
	500g	1.1 pounds
	1kg	2.2 pounds

*Note: when I created my last book, Wild Vegan (A.K.A. Wild Morsels) the standard measuring cup was 240ml. However it seems that now a 250ml cup is more common.
Also, check your measuring spoons as sometimes tablespoons are 15ml and sometimes 20ml. I have used a 15ml spoon throughout this book.

There are two different ways of measuring temperature. The table below gives equivalent measures of both Celsius and Fahrenheit.

Celsius	Fahrenheit
0°	32°
100°	212°
150°	300°
175°	350°
180°	356°
200°	400°
220°	425°

Name Variations

Some food names vary between Australia, the United Kingdom and the United States. I have provided a list of the ones relevant to this book.

Australia	USA	UK
coriander	cilantro	coriander
capsicum	bell pepper	pepper
zucchini	zucchini	courgette
eggplant	eggplant	aubergine
pumpkin	butternut squash (pumpkin)	butternut squash
chickpeas	garbanzo beans	chickpeas
biscuits	cookies	cookies
beetroot	beet	beetroot
cornflour	cornstarch	cornflour
polenta	cornmeal	polenta
muesli	granola	muesli
wholemeal	whole wheat	wholemeal

Alternative Ingredients

Sometimes it is appropriate to use an alternative ingredient: that is, a different ingredient that will perform the same job in a recipe. There are times when we need to do this because someone who is going to eat the food may have an allergy to one of the ingredients. Examples of this may be allergies to dairy, eggs or nuts. Another reason to substitute a food would be if a person has chosen not to eat a food for ethical reasons. Vegans do not eat any animal products, including meat, dairy, eggs or honey.

I have also presented alternatives here that are healthier than those most often used. For example instead of using white sugar in a recipe, you could use rapadura sugar (see over the page).

Following is a list of ingredients that are considered "normal" and next to them are alternatives.

Meat - The majority of people are brought up on meat.
It is usually considered the main source of iron and protein in a meal and forms the staple for many recipes. For this reason, many people depend on its use to create what is considered to be a healthy and/or delicious meal. Even if you are not a vegetarian, you sometimes may need to cook for someone who is. Beans, lentils, nuts, grains and seeds can provide plenty of protein within a vegetarian or vegan diet.
Iron is obtained through any of the following: sea vegetables, fortified bran flakes, oats, soybeans, chickpeas, blackstrap molasses, lentils, pumpkin seeds (or pepitas), tempeh, tofu, black beans, soy milk, dried apricots, kidney beans, beet greens, wheat germ, sunflower seeds, cashews, raisins.

Milk - *When I list "milk" as an ingredient in any of my recipes, I do not mean cow's milk, I mean the milk of your choosing.* You may use soy, rice, oat, almond, cow or goats milk. It is the one ingredient that is quite easy to substitute. When cooking with alternative milks, substitution requires some discretion according to the taste the milk will add to your recipe, e.g. some milks are particularly nutty or grainy in flavour.

I find the best overall substitutes to be almond milk and rice milk, but try out a few for yourself to see which suits you.

A major concern with a non-dairy diet is the maintenance of the body's calcium levels. There are actually very few whole foods that do not contain calcium. The following foods will provide you with high levels of this mineral: sesame seeds, leafy greens, almonds, beans, molasses, figs and tofu.

Eggs - The purpose of eggs in cooking is to bind the ingredients together. At first it may seem impossible to cook things like cakes and burgers without eggs, but on the contrary, there are many alternative binders.

Below is a list of alternatives as well as the purpose for which they are best used. Throughout this book I have used eggs in some recipes however there are many without.

Egg replacer - There are a number of commercially-produced egg replacers on the market, most of which are made from potato starch and tapioca flour. The directions on the box will give a guide as to how much of the product will replace one egg. In this book, I have not used any commercial egg replacers in my recipes, not because they don't work, but because I prefer to use ingredients that I know will be available to everyone.

Mashed banana - A particularly good binder in cakes and puddings. Of course, there will also be the strong banana flavour. The amount of banana needed will depend on the recipe but I find that generally 1 banana = 1 egg.

Silken tofu - Tofu is a particularly good binder in cakes, brownies and puddings. 5 tablespoons of pureed tofu = 1 egg.

Soy flour - Add the following to the liquid in your recipe.
1 tablespoon = 1 egg

Sugars - The word "sugar" does not only refer to the white table sugar produced from sugarcane. There are natural sugars in fruit, honey, grains and various other plants. These other sweeteners contain more nutrients than white sugar, which has been stripped of its vitamins and minerals. The only sugar I have used in my recipes that comes from sugarcane is rapadura sugar. It is the least processed of all the sugars and still contains the molasses which is high in nutrients. It is a much better alternative to white sugar and I have found it adds a richer, deeper flavour to the recipes. I have also used honey, agave and maple syrups to provide variety.
It is important to remember though, that sugar is sugar. Whether it is more natural or more processed it is still not good for you in large quantities. In excess, it has been linked to obesity, diabetes and heart disease and therefore, foods that have been sweetened need to make up only a small portion of your diet.

Liquid Sweeteners - Include honey, rice syrup, maple syrup, barley malt, black strap molasses, agave syrup/nectar and fruit juices. These include not only normal fruit juice but concentrated fruit juices such as apple and pear. Each of these sweeteners adds their own unique flavour. Experiment to see what you like. Many of my sweet recipes use liquid sweeteners.
You don't have to stick to the ones I have used. Try varying them and see how they change the flavour of the recipe. *A note on agave syrup: it has recently come to my attention that this sweetener is very high in concentrated fructose, a substance that is hard for the body to process when it is not in its original form (as part of the plant). With this in mind, I now limit my use of agave syrup.*

Crystal Sweeteners - Include coconut sugar, rapadura sugar, date sugar, fructose, demerara, and many brown sugars. I have tried to vary the sweetening methods in my recipes so as not to be limited to one or two products. I have also chosen not to use products such as date sugar or coconut sugar specifically, in case they are not available to everyone. Therefore, when using a crystal sweetener, you may like to experiment.

Using Fruit as a Sweetener - Sometimes you may like to use a very sweet fruit to sweeten a recipe as I have done in some of my raw recipes. The "Chocolate Mint Balls" are sweetened only with dates. This is possible because dates are very, very sweet. You can also use other dried fruits as their sugar content is very concentrated. In other situations a banana or some pineapple is a good sweetener. Think of your smoothies. They need nothing more than the fruit to sweeten them.

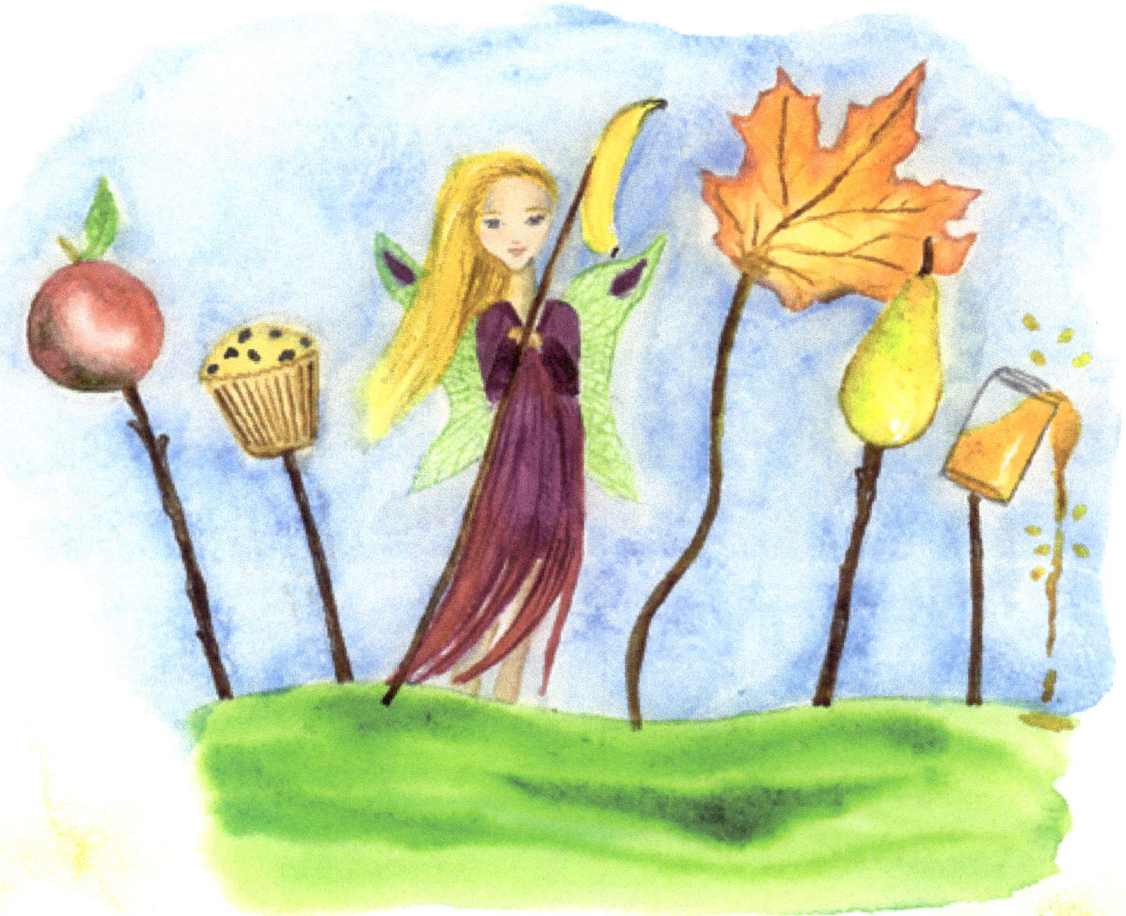

For more information on specific ingredients,
check out the Glossary on page 284

All About Flour

Something to consider when working with flour is that different flours behave in different ways. This does not just depend on the type of flour but also the way it is ground and how old it is. The most commonly used flour is made from wheat, however there are a host of other flours on the market now. Following is an outline of the most common ones.

Stone-ground wholemeal/whole-wheat flour - this is a coarsely ground flour made by milling whole wheat kernels through a stone mill. There is no white flour blended back into the mix, meaning that the flour still contains all the nutrients of the original grain. This type of flour will work well in breads and heavy pastry mixes however it can make a cake or biscuit quite dry.

Wholemeal/whole-wheat flour - Generally speaking, wholemeal flour is white flour with the bran added back in. This means that the flour still behaves itself in baked goods but does still contain the nutrients from the bran. Sometimes however, especially from bulk suppliers, the texture of a wholemeal flour can be courser than usual. You need to check this out before you use it to bake. I find that the wholemeal flour that I buy from a bulk food place near me is quite course compared to the ones in the supermarket. On the other hand, I often buy in bulk from a flour company whose wholemeal flour is beautifully fine but is still made without the addition of white flour. What I am illustrating with this point is that flour comes in many forms even when it is from the same grain! **Feel your flour, rubbing it between your fingers before you decide what to use it for.** If you only have stone-ground wholemeal flour as opposed to plain wholemeal flour, you can add some unbleached flour to it in order to make your own wholemeal flour for baking.

Unbleached wheat flour - This is flour without the bran. The goodness of the wheat shell has been removed and you are left with the silky softness of the ground grain. The unbleached flour is not bright white, however it tastes no different to the usual white flour and it has not been bleached with chemicals.

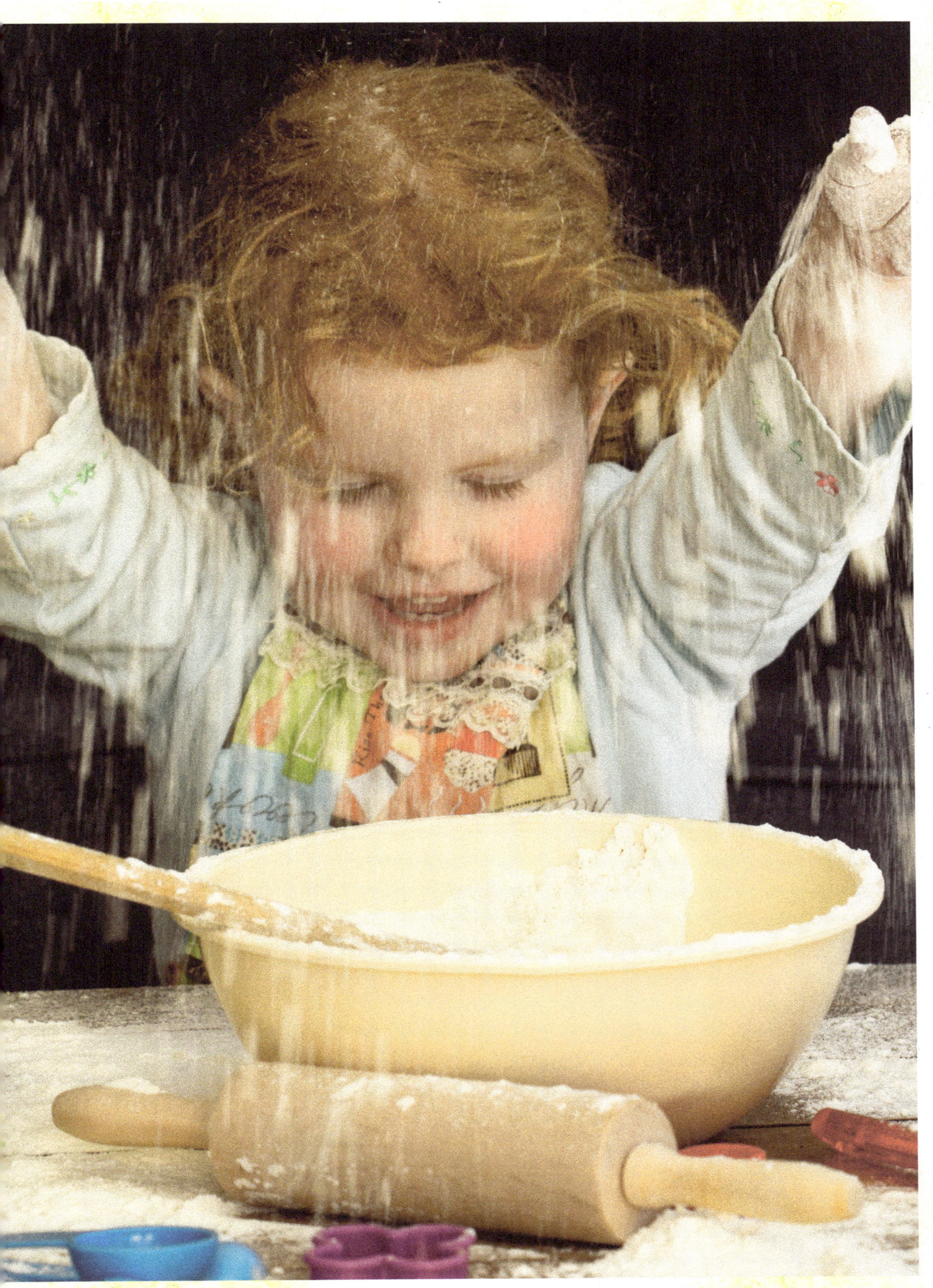

Join the Food Safari

White flour - White flour is at the bottom of the flour chain. It has not only had all of the goodness removed with the elimination of the bran but is also bleached with chemicals so that the cakes, biscuits and pastries it is used in are a whiter colour. These chemicals are harmful to our bodies and are totally unnecessary. Flour is only bleached to make foods look "prettier". The more you learn about food and nutrition, the less appealing these "white" foods will look.

Spelt flour - The spelt grain is related to the wheat grain and behaves the same way in cooking. The difference is that there is less gluten in spelt flour and so is easier to digest. People who have trouble with bloating and tummy upsets after eating wheat will sometimes tolerate spelt without affect. Spelt is available in unbleached and wholemeal varieties.

Gluten free flours - For those who cannot digest gluten, present in wheat, spelt, barley, rye and oats, there are gluten free flours available. They do not always produce the same result as regular flour as it is the gluten in flour that gives baked cakes, breads and muffins their bounce. I have not used gluten free flour in this cookbook as I prefer to create gluten free goods with the use of nuts and seeds.

The age of your flour - Flour quality decreases with age and also is dependant on how it is stored. It should always be kept in a dry cool place in an airtight container as heat and humidity will cause the flour to deteriorate.

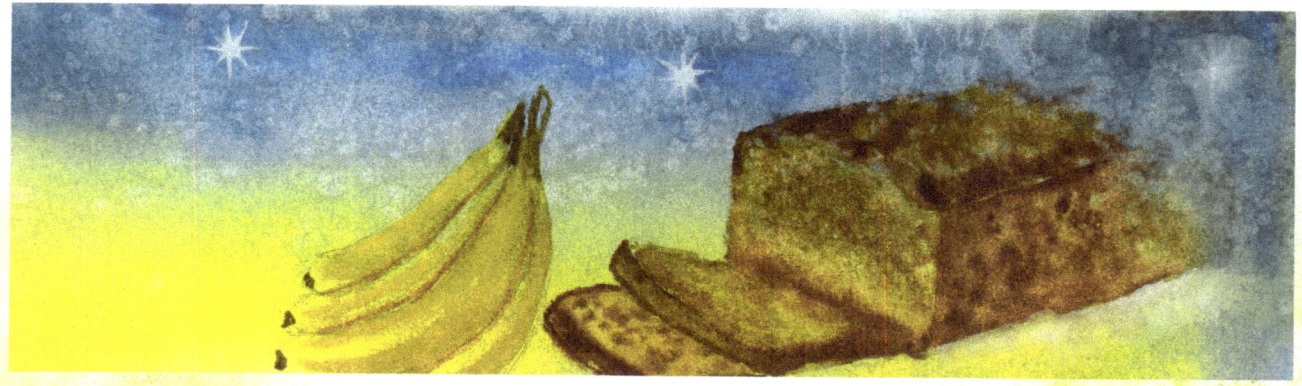

Which Milk?

In our house, we use homemade almond milk, but this is only one of many milks now available. You can choose between animal milks from a cow, goat or sheep, There are also plant based milks such as soy, rice, oat or almond. You can save money and have a more pure version of these plant-based milks by purchasing a soy-milk maker. It is with one of these that I make our almond milk. It is so quick and easy! All recipes in this book will work with whatever milk you choose. Some flavour variation may occur but they behave the same way in the recipes following. Remember, if you choose to use an animal milk, to check that animal has been raised in happy conditions.

Which Oil?

The recipes in this book that involve heating an oil, such as in baking or frying, do not specify the use of any particular oil. The choice is yours, based on affordability and taste. **Smoking point** refers to the point at which the oil will start to smoke. When this happens, the structure of the oil will be damaged and the flavour altered. Oils with a high smoking point are more suited to cooking. They include coconut, grapeseed, avocado, butter and olive oils.

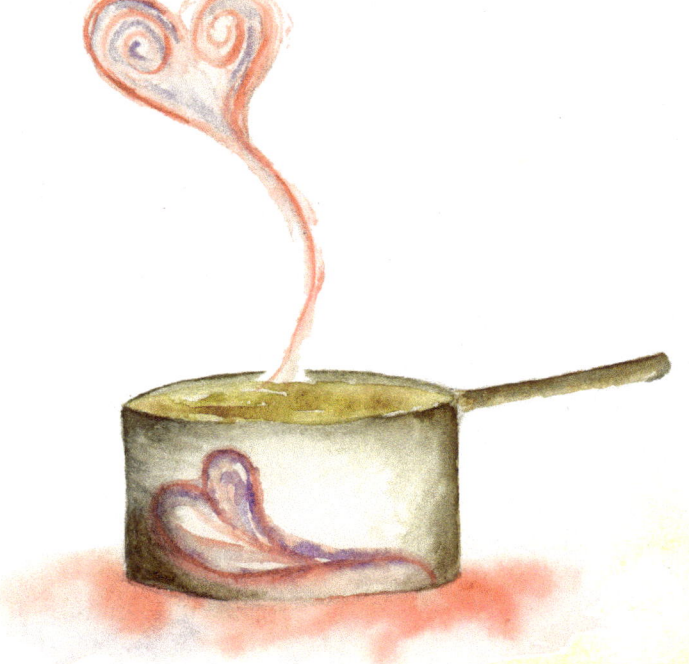

Use boutique oils, easily damaged by heat such as walnut and flaxseed in your dressings. Or add them to steamed vegetables after cooking.

Join the Food Safari

What Do Hormones Have To Do With Canned Food?

At the time of writing this book, I have been unable to find tinned tomatoes which do not contain a plastic lining inside the tin. Most of the time, this plastic contains BPA (BispHenol A), a chemical which interferes with the hormones in our bodies. It is very difficult to find information on which linings contain BPA and which don't.

What is a hormone?

Hormones are chemicals which are made by our body in order to perform specific functions. For example, there is a hormone called hGH (or Human Growth Hormone) which tells our bodies to grow. There is also a hormone named Parathyroid Hormone which controls how much calcium and magnesium we absorb. These minerals work together to make our bones, teeth and nails strong and also to ensure that the nervous system and heart tissue is healthy. hGH and Parathyroid Hormone are only two of the many hormones that affect the functions of our body. Hormones also tell us when to sleep and wake, how much weight to keep on our bodies and how much to convert to energy, they change a child's body into an adult's body and keep everything working together effectively.

Why BPA?

So if BPA is bad for our bodies, and plays horrible games with our hormones, why is it used in food packaging? Well the answer is cost. It is a lot cheaper to make plastic containing BPA than without. It is a binder for the plastic molecules. The trouble is, when it is holding food, and even worse, when it is heated with food (as in a plastic container), some of that BPA enters the food and we eat it, causing disruptions in our hormones.

As people have learnt of the dangers of BPA, it has become easier to buy plastic containers and drink bottles that do not contain this poison.

Unfortunately, canned foods are still on the thumbs down list. Maybe soon this will not be the case.

My Solution

After finding that I could not buy canned tomatoes and canned beans without the BPA lining, I made some changes. The canned beans were only ever emergency stores, as I prefer to cook them from scratch if I have time. Now I cook large batches of beans and chickpeas and store them into 2 cups portions in the freezer. It is so much cheaper too, so what a bonus!

As for canned tomatoes, they were a bit trickier as fresh tomatoes are not always in season. My solution has been to replace the cans with bottles of passata which is tomato puree. Passata is also available organically.

Coconut cream/milk was another hurdle. I found you can buy it powdered and mix with water as an alternative. Where coconut milk/cream is used in this book, I have put measurements for both.

Hopefully it will not be too long before manufacturers of canned goods catch up with the new trend of producing BPA-free plastic. We all have a right to know that the products we consume are safe for our long term health.

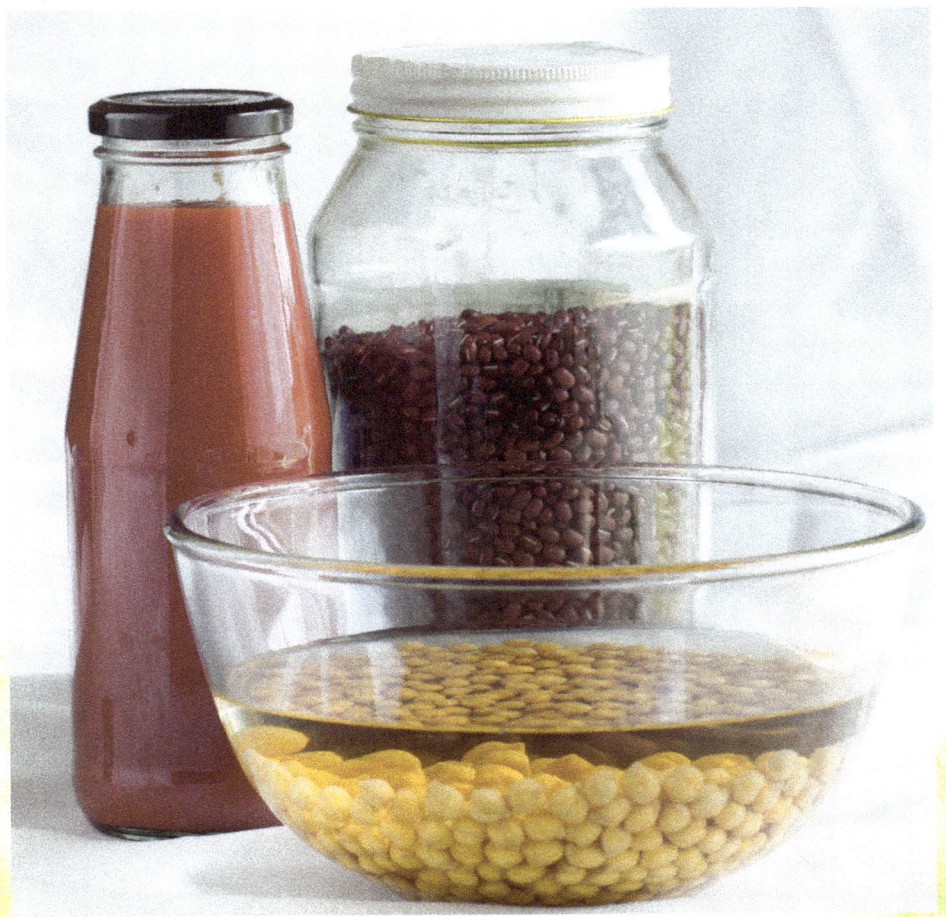

Cooking With Herbs

What is a herb? Herbs are plants that are used to provide flavour in cooking. Not only that, herbs provide the body with many vitamins and minerals and can actually be used as natural medicines.

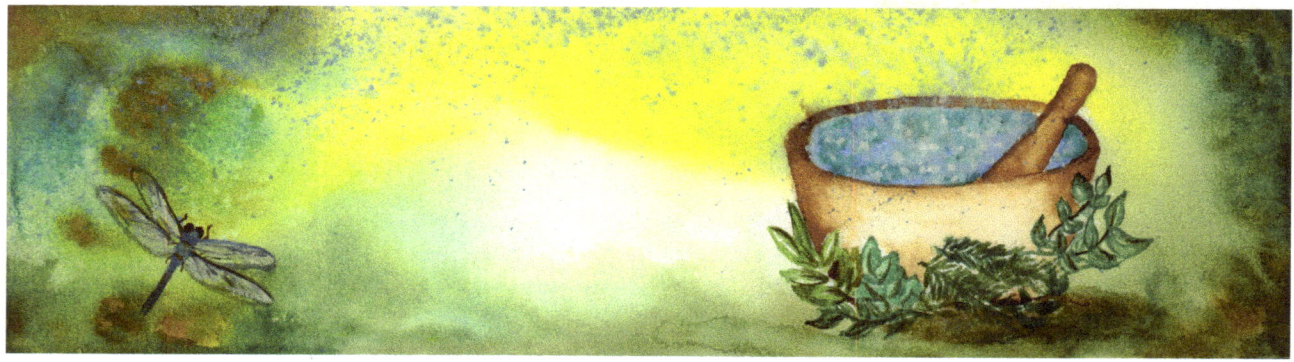

Using herbs in your cooking adds fresh and unique flavours to your dishes. There are a wide variety of herbs that I use in my recipes and they provide a great deal of flavour in the meals. Herbs including parsley, mint, coriander, dill, basil, thyme, rosemary, oregano and sage. There are many, many more and it is fun to experiment with them in both sweet and savoury dishes.

It may surprise you to know that herbs are often used in sweet biscuits, cakes and scones. Examples are lavender, lemon myrtle, lemon balm, peppermint and pineapple sage. Herbs are one of those ingredients that you can add to dishes without too much risk. As long as you know that you like the taste of that herb then you will have some idea of how it will affect the meal. More woody herbs such as rosemary and thyme should be added earlier in the cooking process and lighter herbs such as dill, parsley, basil and coriander are best added once a dish has been removed from heat.

For ideas on which specific herbs to use with other ingredients, look at the information on **Regional Flavours** *on page 58*

Growing your own herbs maybe a good introduction to backyard gardening. Herbs will grow well in pots and if grown close to the house, are easy to water. Small potted herbs are widely available at markets and nurseries and are such a great addition to your kitchen garden. It is so satisfying to be able to duck outside to gather fresh ingredients for your cooking.

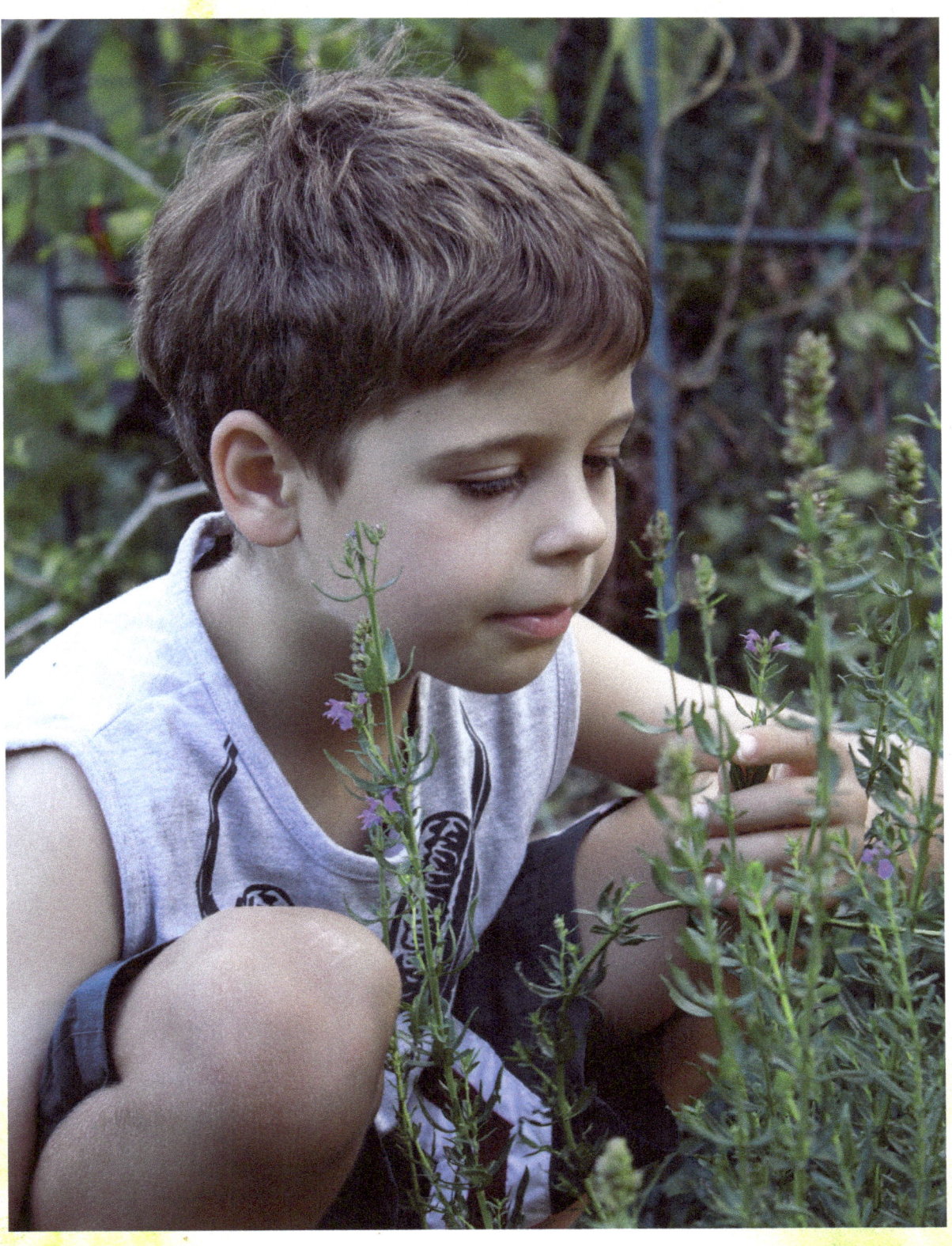

Regional Flavours

Multi-cultural countries such as Australia, New Zealand, England, USA, and Canada have a rich culture of different foods because there are so many influences from around the world. We are so lucky to have access to such a fountain of knowledge. Part of your Food Safari involves learning about these regional flavours and what tastes go well together. A good way to do this is by looking at different cultures' food combinations for inspiration.

These are some of the main ingredients and dishes particular to the regions listed. They are not the only foods used but are key to the flavours of that region. As your confidence in the kitchen increases, you will be able to create your own recipes, or alter recipes you know to suit the flavours from a particular region.

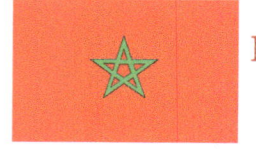 **Morocco**

The flavours of Morrocco are also common in other parts of Africa.

Ingredients include:

couscous
chickpeas
lemons - fresh and preserved
paprika, cumin, saffron, cinnamon
harissa - chilli paste
orange blossom water
rose water

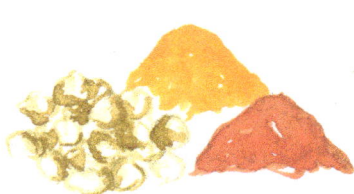

Examples of Dishes:

- harrira - soup of lentils, vegetables and chickpeas
- tagines
- couscous, seasoned
- meat kebabs
- flatbread

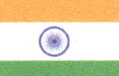 ## India

Ingredients include:

tomatoes

garlic

onions

ginger

chillis

spices such as cumin, ground coriander, fennel seeds, cardamon, turmeric, fenugreek seeds, cloves, nigella seeds

yoghurt

lentils

chickpeas

rice and papadums

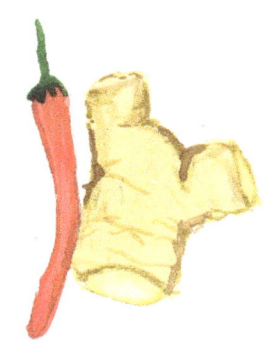

Examples of Dishes:

- appetisers such as samosas, marinated meat, fried vegetable pakoras and fritters.
- curry, curry and more curry
- dahls - curries made with lentils
- naan breads with butter, garlic or stuffed with vegetables or meat.
- biriyani - curry and vegetable rice
- pilaf - rice with spices, yoghurt and coconut

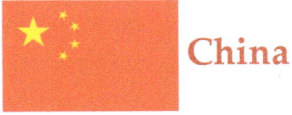 ## China

Ingredients include:

onions

garlic

ginger

chilli

soy sauce

oyster sauce

sesame oil

rice vinegar

Chinese five spice

rice and noodles

tofu

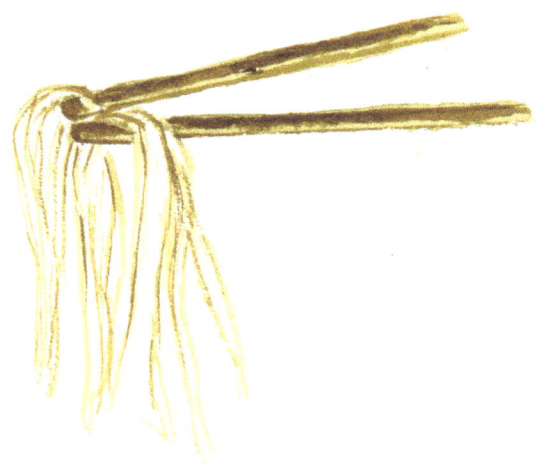

Examples of Dishes:

- appetisers such as spring rolls, prawn cutlets, dumplings, dim sims
- curries
- stir-fries
- watery broths filled with meat, vegetables, noodles, won-tons.
- rice and fried rice
- fried noodles
- steamed greens

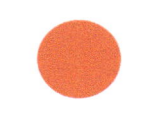 Japan

Ingredients include:

ginger
chilli
shoyu- Japanese soy sauce
sesame oil
rice mirin
dashi - stock
wasabi - horseradish
mayonaise
pickled ginger and daikon
nori and other seaweeds
rice and noodles
seafood
shitake mushrooms
tofu
sesame seeds and sesame oil

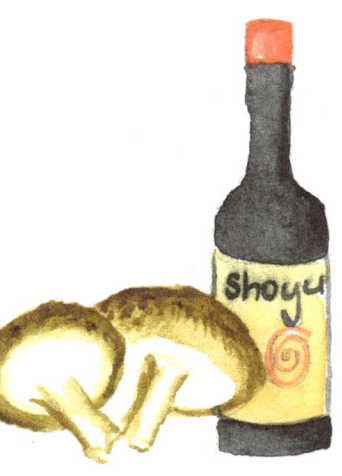

Examples of Dishes:

- sushi and sashimi
- bento boxes - containing small portions of different ingredients
- crumbed meat or vegetables with rice and a curry sauce
- stir-fries
- curries
- fried noodles
- watery broth soups containing vegetables, meat, noodles

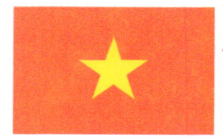 Vietnam

Ingredients include:

fish sauce
hoi-sin sauce
lemongrass
chilli
star anise
sesame seeds
Vietnamese mint, chives, dill and coriander
rice and noodles
bean sprouts and bamboo shoots
jackfruit, lychee and dragonfruit

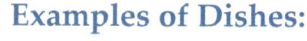

Examples of Dishes:

- pho- noodle soup
- rice paper rolls
- dumplings
- savoury rice pancakes
- stir-fries
- fresh salads made with vegetables, herbs and fruits
- fried noodles

Join the Food Safari

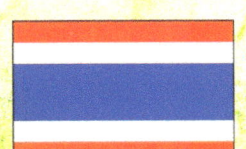 ## Thailand

Ingredients include:

onion
garlic
galangal and ginger
chilli
fish sauce
shrimp paste
soy sauce
coriander, thai basil, kaffir
lime leaves, lemongrass
lime
palm sugar
tamarind
coconut milk
rice and noodles

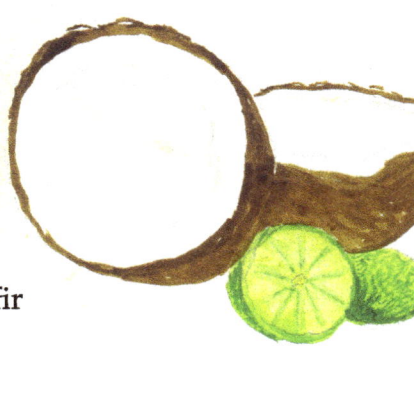

Examples of Dishes:

- spring rolls and curry puffs
- stir-fried vegetables or meat with rice
- stir fried noodles with meat, vegetables, egg, tofu
- curries made with coconut milk
- salads made with fresh vegetables, herbs and meat

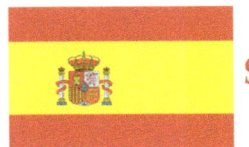 ## Spain

Ingredients include:

bread
olive oil
garlic
cheese
rice
paprika, turmeric and saffron
quince paste

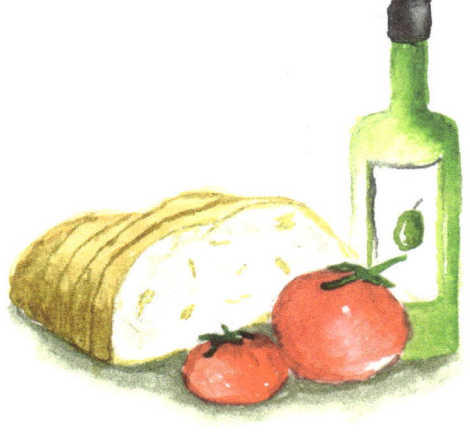

Examples of Dishes:

- tapas - small serves of appetisers including fried potatoes, olives, croquettes, chorizo sausage, prawns, octopus, cured cheese
- paella
- stews made from beans meat and vegetables

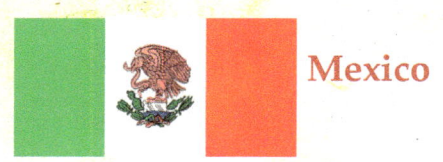 **Mexico**

Ingredients include:

chillis - jalepeno, habenero, ancho, guajillo, pasilla
garlic
onions
pinto beans
tomatoes
capsicum
avocado
jicama or yam bean
limes
coriander
cheese
corn
tortillas
chocolate (dark - for drinks)

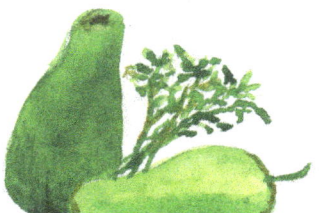

Examples of Dishes:

- guacamole
- quesadillas
- burritos
- tacos
- enchiladas
- frijoles - refried beans
- Mexican rice
- stews made with meat and beans

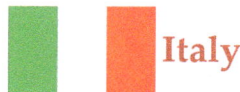 **Italy**

Ingredients include:

tomatoes
garlic
capsicum
basil, oregano, thyme and parsley
balsamic vinegar
cheeses such as mozzerella, bocconcini, parmesan and ricotta
dried and fresh pasta
olives and olive oil

Examples of Dishes:

- pizza
- pasta
- anti-pasta
- bruschetta
- risotto
- minestrone soup
- breads dipped in olive oil
- meat, bean and vegetable stews

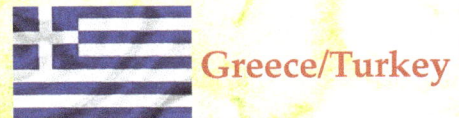 **Greece/Turkey**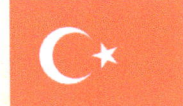

Ingredients include:
olive oil
lemons
cinnamon
dill, parsley and mint
feta cheese
tomatoes, zucchini and eggplant
garlic
wild greens
vine leaves
rice
capers
figs

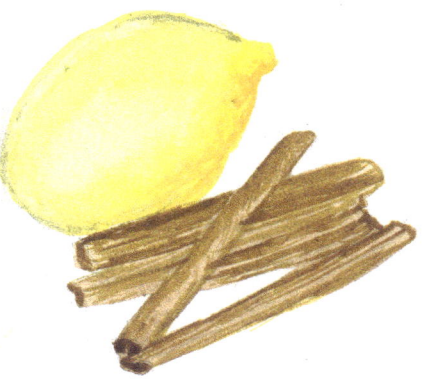

Examples of Dishes:
- lentil and bean soups
- mezze plates which include dips, rice stuffed vine leaves, cheeses, sliced tomatoes and cucumbers
- stuffed tomatoes and capsicums
- moussaka
- pide (turkish pizza)
- claypot casseroles made with chickpeas, vegetables and/or meat

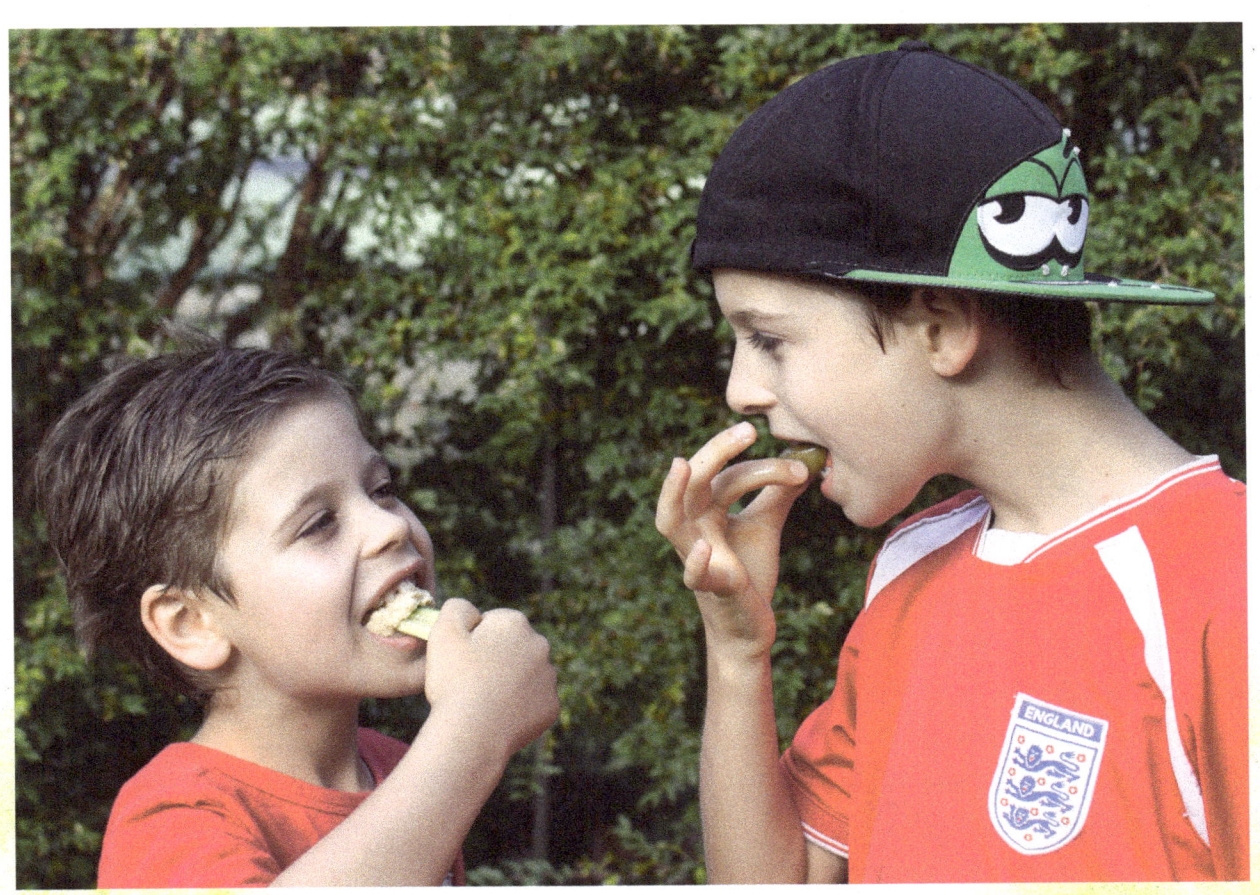

Cooking and Sprouting Techniques

Beans and Lentils - Soaking and cooking times for different beans and lentils vary. Consult the table below for detailed information. The soaking aspect is actually very important not only in order to soften the bean/pulse and shorten the cooking time but also because it changes the bean/pulse's structure. Soaking neutralises phytic acid, which is a substance that inhibits the absorption of important minerals. Sprouting also neutralises enzyme inhibitors which interfere with normal digestion.

- All soaking times are minimum, therefore overnight or all day soaking will only increase the benefit.
- Wash all beans and lentils thoroughly before and after soaking, discarding the soaking water.
- Use soft water for soaking as the heavy metals in hard water will prevent the beans from softening. Add baking soda to hard water.
- When cooking, cover well with water, bring to the boil and then simmer until soft.
- Refrigerate beans after cooking if they are not to be used right away.
- Cooked beans and lentils freeze well. Frozen portions will save time later.
- Adding a strip of Kombu seaweed to the soaking or cooking water will aid the release of gas producing enzymes.

* Fast cooking, therefore soaking time is only for health benefits.

Dried Bean/Lentil	1 cup dried equals	Soaking Time (hours)	Cooking Time (minutes)
Red Lentils*	3 cups cooked	6	10
Puy/Green/Brown Lentils	3 cups cooked	6	10
Split Peas	3 cups cooked	6	15
Chickpeas	2 1/2 cups cooked	10	60
Blackeye Beans*	2 1/2 cups cooked	6	25
Canellini Beans	2 1/2 cups cooked	6	25
Pinto/Borlotti Beans	3 cups cooked	6	35
Adzuki Beans	3 cups cooked	8	25
Kidney Beans	3 cups cooked	8	30

Sprouting Menagerie - As mentioned previously in the information on raw food, sprouting is a great way to create alkalising foods to help maintain a healthy blood pH. It is beneficial to sprout beans, lentils, seeds and many nuts. See the table below for specific times.

	Soaking time (hours)	Sprouting time (days)
Almonds	8	They won't sprout shoots
Lentils	7	3
Chickpeas	10	3
Mung Beans	8	2-3
Alfalfa	6	2-3
Adzuki Beans	8	3-4
Buckwheat	6	2
Barley/spelt/wheat	7	2-3
Quinoa	2	1-2
Sesame Seeds	6	2
Fenugreek Seeds	8	2

- All ingredients must be soaked before you begin the sprouting process.
- To sprout, use a glass jar with a netted top or covered in a stocking, to allow the water to drain.
- During the sprouting process, rinse the nut/seed/legume at least twice per day (rinsing more frequently in humid climates and hot weather).
- Sprouts need to be kept damp but without pools of water. Leave the jar tilted on an angle or upside down to allow excess water to drain freely.
- Climate will affect sprouting time.
- Refrigerate sprouts for up to 3 days after they are ready.
- Add to salads, dips, as a side for meals, onto your breakfast cereal and porridge, or with avocado on toast.

Interesting fact: If you eat fenugreek sprouts, for lunch, by bedtime your armpits will smell like fenugreek. Go on, try it!

Varieties of Rice

White Rice

There are a number of different types of white rice. Below are the ones widely available in Australia. All white rices are low in nutrients as the nutritious husk has been removed. Apart from basmati rice, white rices are high in natural sugar.

Basmati - Indian/Pakistani rice which is low GI and has a distinct flavour and scent. In fact, the Hindi translation of the word "basmati" is "queen of scents". It is not sticky at all and when cooked correctly, has seperate, fluffy grains. It is considered the most gourmet of all the rices and is therefore, higher in price.

Jasmine - Thai rice, high in natural sugar and has a slight jasmine scent when cooked. It is only slightly sticky and is lower in price than basmati.

Short grain - include arborio and sushi rices which are sticky and soft. These rices are used in dishes which require a certain texture.

For example sushi and nori rolls need the rice to stick together well in order to hold their shape. Risotto is made with arborio rice as the dish has a porridgy consistency.

Long grain - is blander tasting and therefore lower in price. It is a slightly off-white colour and is not sticky.

Medium grain - like the long grain, is blander tasting and therefore lower in price. It is a slightly off-white colour and is stickier than the long grain.

Brown Rice

Brown rice comes in short or medium grain and is not particularly sticky unless over-cooked. It is very high in nutrients, has a nutty flavour and is more filling than white rice. Brown rice also requires a longer cooking time and more water.

Other Varieties of Rice

Wild Rice - A different type of rice as it is actually the seed of a grass plant. Its grains are long, dark and chewy in texture and they have a nutty flavour. Wild rice is usually used sparingly with other rices as it is very expensive and is mostly used only to compliment other flavours.

Black Rice - This rice has a nutty flavour and a dark colour. It is non-glutinous and soft when cooked. It is usually used in place of brown rice and so requires the same amount of cooking time and water.

Red Rice - A Himalayan version of brown rice where the hull is red instead of brown. Like black rice, red rice requires the same amount of cooking time and water as brown rice.

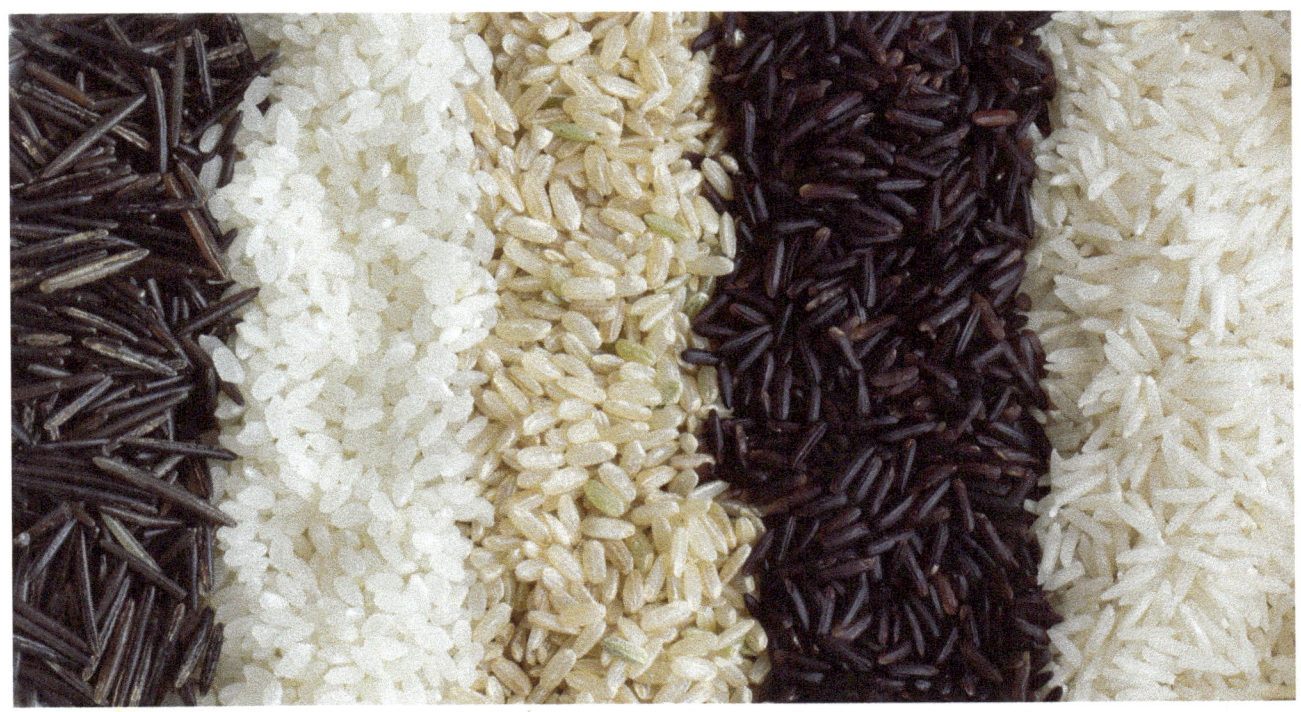

From left to right: wild rice, sushi rice, brown rice, black rice, basmati rice

Cooking Great Rice

Basic cooking instructions for white rice

(excluding the short grain varieties which are prepared according to specific recipes)

1. Measure the rice so that you know how much water to use. 1 cup of rice requires 1½ cups of water. You will soon know by sight and this step will become unecessary. I add water to the rice until it measures from the tip of my pointer finger to the first line.
2. Rinse rice several times, stirring it with your hand to release the starch. Drain rice in a seive and leave to stand for 5 minutes.
3. Place rice into a saucepan and cover with measured water and a lid.
4. Place over medium heat and bring to boil, then reduce to a simmer until most of the water has been absorbed. This will take approximately 10 minutes. Do NOT stir the rice during cooking time.
5. Remove from heat and leave to stand with the lid on for a further 10 minutes. This will steam the remaining moisture into the rice without burning it, giving a perfect texture. Fluff with a fork and serve.

Basic cooking instructions for brown rice

1. Measure the rice so that you know how much water to use. 1 cup of rice requires 1 ¾ cups of water. You will soon know by sight and this step will become unecessary.
2. Rinse rice only once, as there is very little starch. Drain in a seive.
3. Place rice into a saucepan and cover with measured water and a lid.
4. Place over medium heat and bring to boil, then reduce to a simmer until most of the water has been absorbed. This will take approximately 25 minutes. Do NOT stir the rice during cooking time.
5. Remove from heat and leave to stand with the lid on for a further 10 minutes. This will steam the remaining moisture into the rice without burning it, giving a perfect texture. Fluff with a fork and serve.

Another way to cook brown rice is to add three or four cups of water to every cup of rice, boil until the rice is tender and then strain it. Put it back into the saucepan with the lid on to steam in the remaining moisture on the rice.

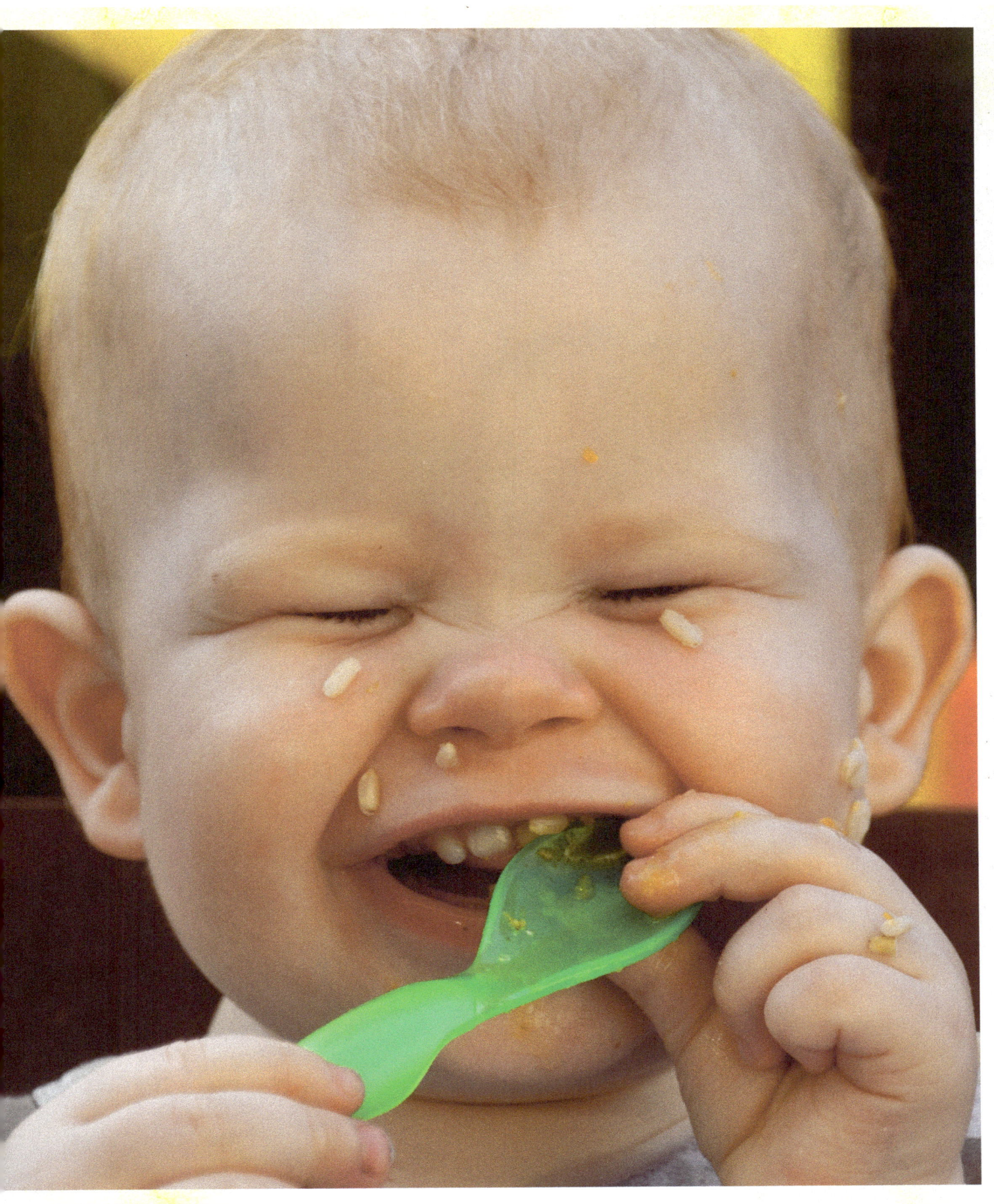

"There is no love sincerer than the love of food."
~George Bernard Shaw

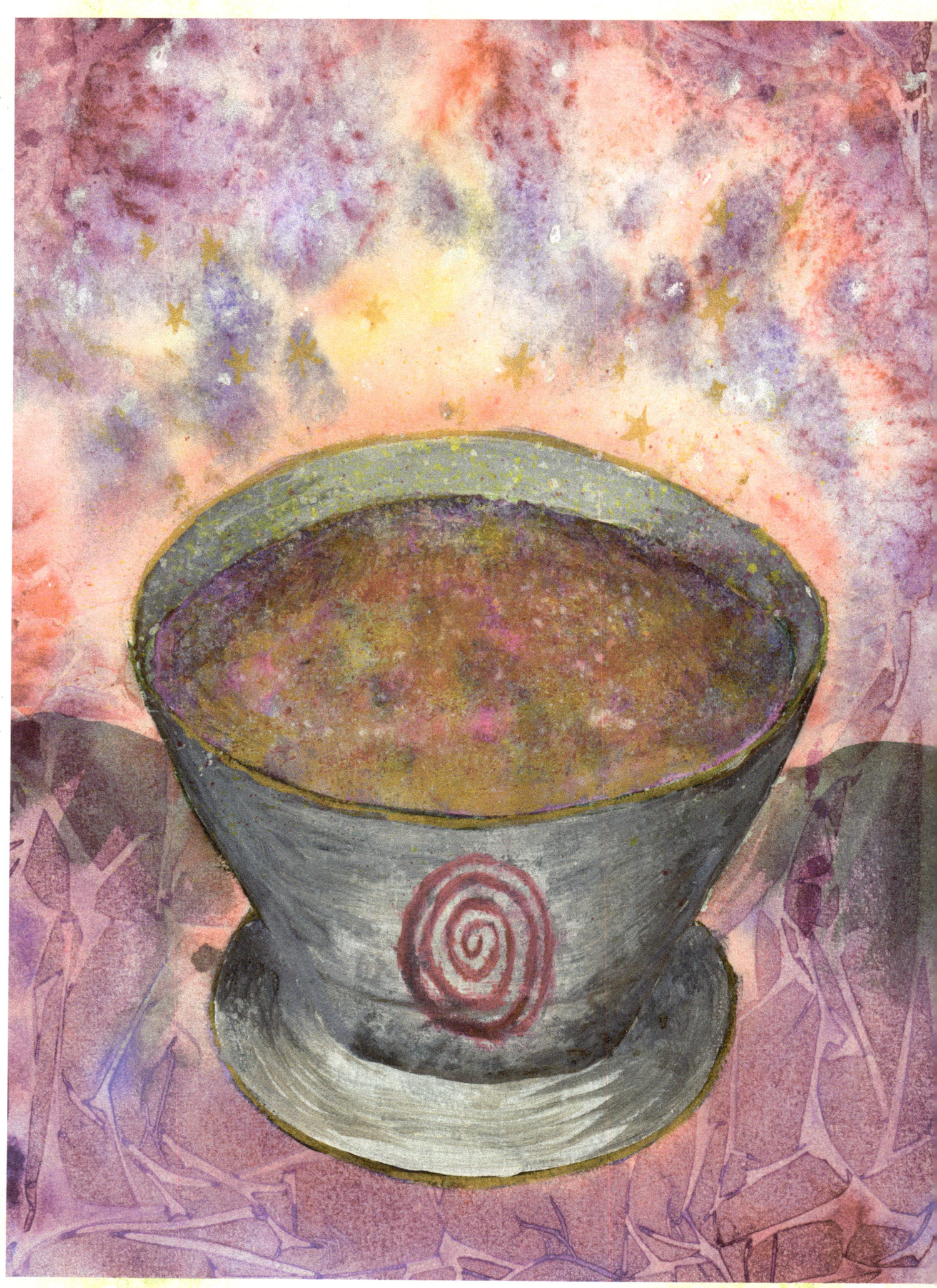

Getting Creative and Expanding Your Knowledge

Once you have practiced the recipes in this book and feel confident with food and using different ingredients, there will be a whole world of possibility available to you.

I have been cooking ever since I can remember and yet I still learn about new ways to combine food from books, the internet, restaurants and cooking shows. I never tire of it! The kitchen can be your studio, a place to express your creativity and then enjoy the tastes afterwards. So go forth and explore, create, be gentle with yourself and above all, HAVE FUN!

A Word Before You Begin....

All information within this section has been researched to the best of my ability. I have read from many different sources and done my best to present a balanced and well supported view of nutrition and whole food eating. Remember though, that new discoveries are constantly being made, more research being done and new information comes from this. So do your own research as you grow, just remember to look at both sides of an argument and ALWAYS look at who is arguing and whether they have a vested interest in the outcome of a study.

Apart from the research you can do out there in the big, wide world, one place you can always come back to for accurate information is your own body. Listen to it and you will know what is right for you...

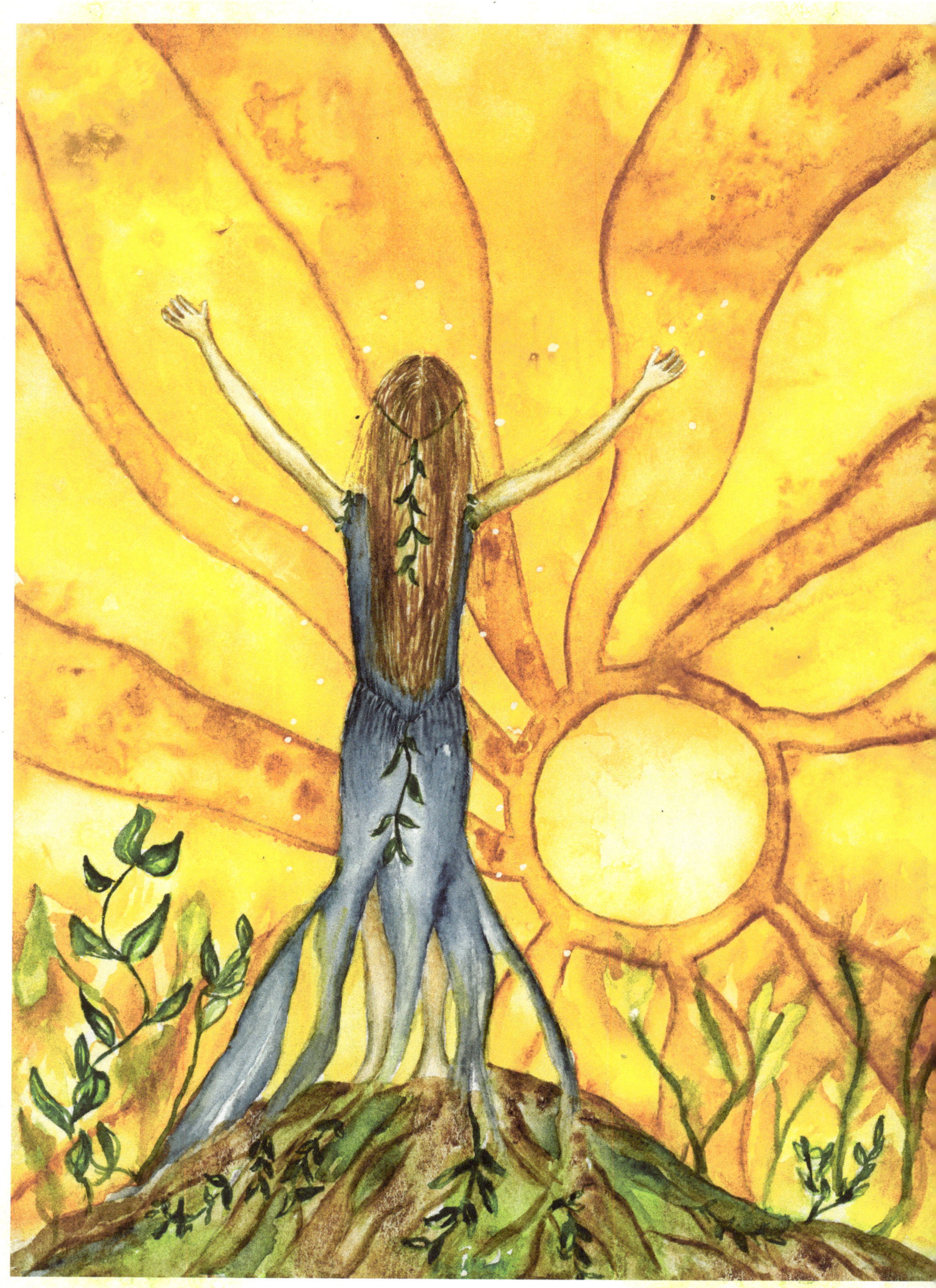

Beautiful Beginnings

After rising from your peaceful slumber, the first thing you need more than anything, is water....It is essential for almost every process that happens in the body. After a night of breathing, possibly sweating and going to the toilet, you are in desperate need of rehydrating. With this in mind, before eating anything, treat yourself to a glass of pure, clean, water and your body will thank you for it. It is one of the best preventative medicines you can take.

This brings you to what many consider the most important meal of the day. **Breakfast is made up of two words, "break" and "fast"**. The food you eat at this time literally breaks the fast after a night's sleep. To nourish and nurture yourself, eat a meal that will give you the nutrition, energy and concentration you need to get through the morning. There are many fresh and delicious foods you can use to prepare a wonderful breakfast that will provide you with a great start to the day .

Do this for yourself. You deserve it!

"Let food be thy medicine, and medicine be thy food."
~Hippocrates

Marvelous Toasted Muesli

This muesli is a gourmet treat that is full of goodness. The recipe is a guideline to start you off. Involve the children by getting them to come up with their own designs or try one of the creative variations below. This version has a cranberry, cinnamon and apple flavour.

500g rolled oats

½ cup of apple juice concentrate

1 tablespoon of honey or rice syrup

¼ cup of water

½ teaspoon of cinnamon

½ cup of unsweetened dried cranberries

½ cup of crushed pecans (or extra seeds to make it nut-free)

½ cup of pepitas (pumpkins seeds)

½ cup of sunflower seeds

½ cup of shredded coconut

1. Pre-heat the oven to 180°C convection or 160°C fan-forced.
2. Place oats into a mixing bowl.
3. In a small saucepan, warm the apple juice concentrate, honey, water and cinnamon. Stir until smooth and then pour over the oats.
4. Mix until oats are well coated and place onto a baking tray lined with baking paper. Make sure the layer is thin so that all of the oats will be toasted. You may need two trays.
5. Bake for 20 minutes or until most of the mixture is crunchy and brown. (Note that part of the hardening will happen as the mixture cools.) Leave to cool on the trays.
6. In a large container, combine oats with the remaining muesli ingredients.
7. Serve with your choice of milk and fresh fruit.

Play Time!

- Instead of cranberry, cinnamon and apple flavour, try apricot and almond or walnut and raisin.
- Add other flavours such as mixed spice, nutmeg or vanilla.
- Try a sweetener such as maple syrup instead of the apple juice concentrate and honey.
- Vary the nuts and seeds you use. For example, almonds, walnuts, hazelnuts, brazil nuts, cashews, macadamia nuts, linseeds, puffed amaranth, puffed quinoa, and puffed rice.
- To make it nut free leave out nuts and use more seeds and dried fruit.
- Use any variety of dried fruit to add sweetness. Even banana chips can add a nice crunch (find the ones that aren't loaded with sugar).

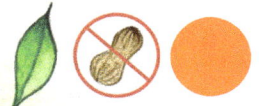

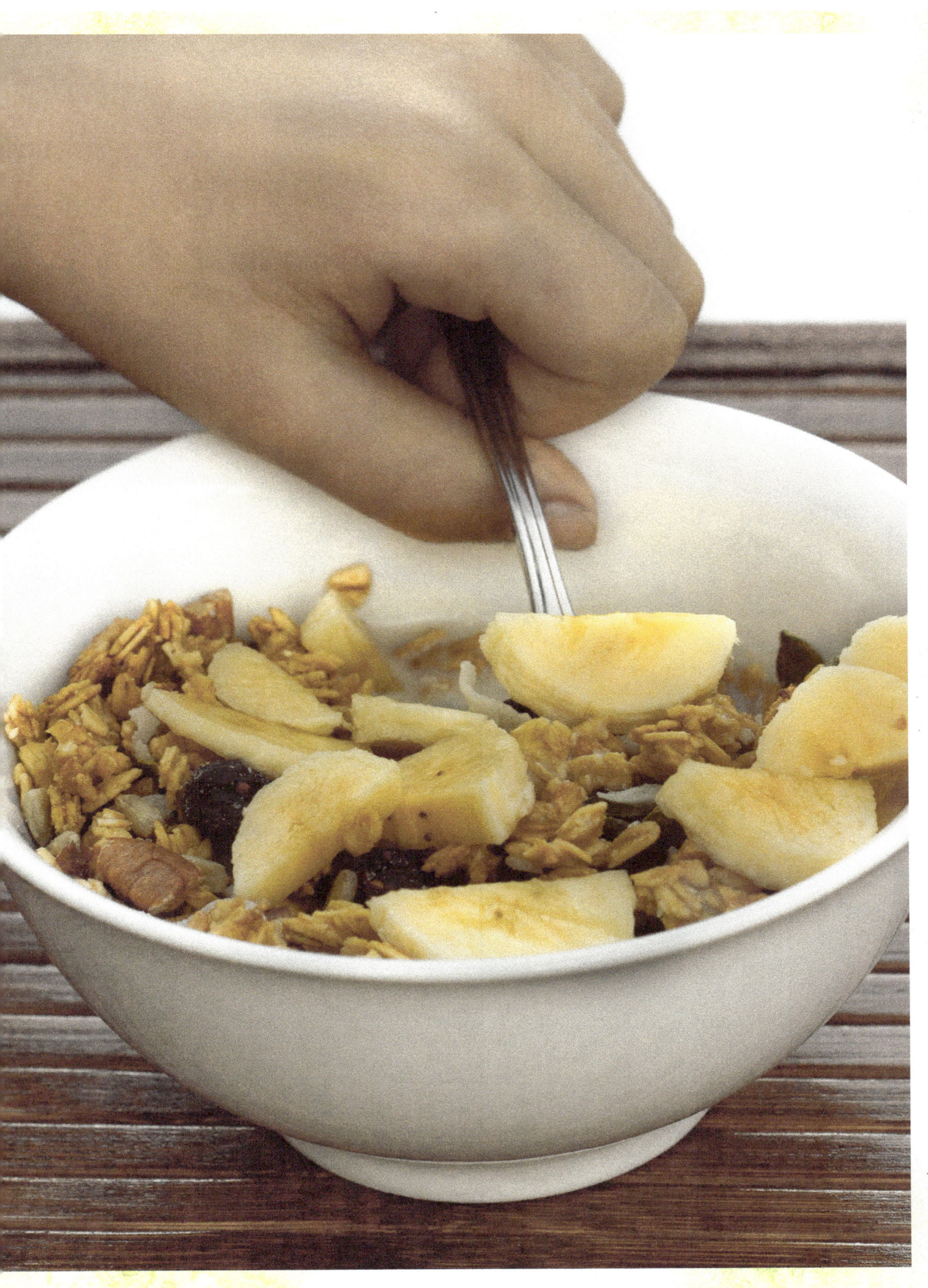

Swiss Muesli

For this recipe, you need to make up a batch of raw muesli: recipe below. The quantities of each ingredient in a serving of Swiss muesli are a personal preference, as it depends on how much you like to eat and how sweet your tooth is. We use unsweetened yoghurt, allowing the apple and honey to provide the sugar. It is a great one for children too, as sometimes they may like to add their own ingredients to the top such as extra nuts, dried fruit or coconut.

Please note this needs to be prepared the night before.

Raw muesli base - batch quantity
500g rolled oats
½ cup of sultanas
½ cup of crushed almonds (use extra seeds to make it nut-free)
½ cup of pepitas (pumpkins seeds)
½ cup of sunflower seeds
½ cup of shredded coconut

Combine all ingredients in a large, airtight storage container.

Individual serve
one serving of muesli
milk, enough to cover the muesli
1 grated apple
dollop of yoghurt (plain or vanilla)*
honey or maple syrup to sweeten

*If you are avoiding dairy, it is now possible to buy soy or coconut milk yoghurts.

1. Spoon one serving of muesli into a breakfast, bowl keeping in mind that this makes up only half of the quantity of the meal.
2. Soak your muesli in milk so that it is just covered, and leave overnight in the fridge.
3. When you are ready to eat, top the muesli with the grated apple and yoghurt, then drizzle with honey or maple syrup and serve.

Play Time!

- Vary the type of nuts, seeds and/or dried fruit used in the muesli base.
- Use pear instead of apple for the top.
- Add extras such as fresh berries, mango or passionfruit.
- Throw in some superfoods such as soaked chia seeds, goji berries or hemp seeds.

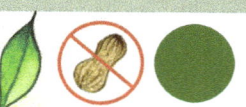

Gluten Free Toasted Muesli

Gluten free muesli is often expensive, especially if you like the gourmet ones. This recipe can be varied in a hundred different ways and is not full of air as is common with shop bought ones. The buckwheat, seeds and nuts give it the bulk you need to stay satisfied until morning tea or lunch.

250g buckwheat (soaked for 6 hours or overnight)
3 cups of puffed quinoa
½ cup of apple juice concentrate
¼ cup of water
2 tablespoons of honey or rice syrup
1 teaspoon of mixed spice
½ cup of finely chopped dried apricots
½ cup of crushed almonds
½ cup of pepitas (pumpkins seeds)
½ cup of sunflower seeds
½ cup of shredded coconut

1. Preheat the oven to 180°C convection or 160°C fan-forced.
2. Drain and rinse the buckwheat.
3. Place buckwheat and quinoa into a mixing bowl and combine.
4. In a small saucepan, warm the apple juice concentrate, honey, water and mixed spice. Stir until smooth and then pour over the buckwheat mixture.
5. Mix until buckwheat and quinoa are well coated and place onto a baking tray lined with baking paper. Make sure the layer is thin so that it all has a chance to bake. You may need two trays.
6. Bake for 20 minutes or until most of the mixture is crunchy and brown. (Note that part of the hardening will happen as the mixture cools.) Leave to cool on the trays.
7. In a large container, combine baked mix with the remaining muesli ingredients.
8. Serve with your choice of milk and fresh fruit.

Play Time!

- See the suggestions for Marvelous Toasted Muesli on page 74.

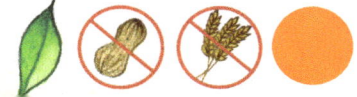

Berry Apple Porridge

Not everyone feels good after eating oats but this does not rule out a porridge breakfast. Apart from rolled oats, there is also rolled spelt and barley, flaked quinoa and flaked rice. Any of these may be used in this recipe, although you may need to adjust the milk content. Note it is only the rolled quinoa and flaked rice that are gluten free. Porridge is an easy meal for children to make at the stove with supervision and guidance. My sons make their own and love to try different flavours using a mixture of fruit and, nuts and spices such as cinnamon, mixed spice and nutmeg.

Serves 2

1 cup of rolled oats, spelt, flaked quinoa or flaked rice.
Note that quick oats do not need as much liquid.
1 ½ cups of water
½ teaspoon of cinnamon
1 large apple (cored and pulverised or grated)
1 ½ cups of milk (guideline only)
½ cup of fresh or frozen blueberries
maple syrup or honey to top

1. If using oats or spelt, it is best to soak your grain in the water overnight for easier digestion and a faster cooking time.
2. Combine water, grain, cinnamon, apple and a little of the milk, in a medium-sized saucepan and bring to the boil.
3. Immediately turn the heat to low and stir often to prevent your porridge sticking to the bottom of the pan. Gradually add more milk as needed.
4. If you are using oats or spelt and it was soaked, the porridge will take about 5 minutes to cook as will quinoa and rice porridge. If not, give it a good 10 minutes. Once done, the consistency will be creamy and the grains soft.
5. If your blueberries are frozen, add them before you remove the porridge from the heat so that they defrost, otherwise add at serving time.
6. Serve in bowls topped with a drizzle of maple syrup or honey.

Play Time!

- Try other flavours of porridge. Substitute the apple and blueberry for finely chopped dried apricots and top with honey. Leave the cinnamon in too, as it is a good complement.
- Try walnut and pear, raspberry and flaked coconut or sultana and banana.
- Top with a dollop of yoghurt.

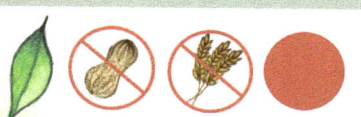

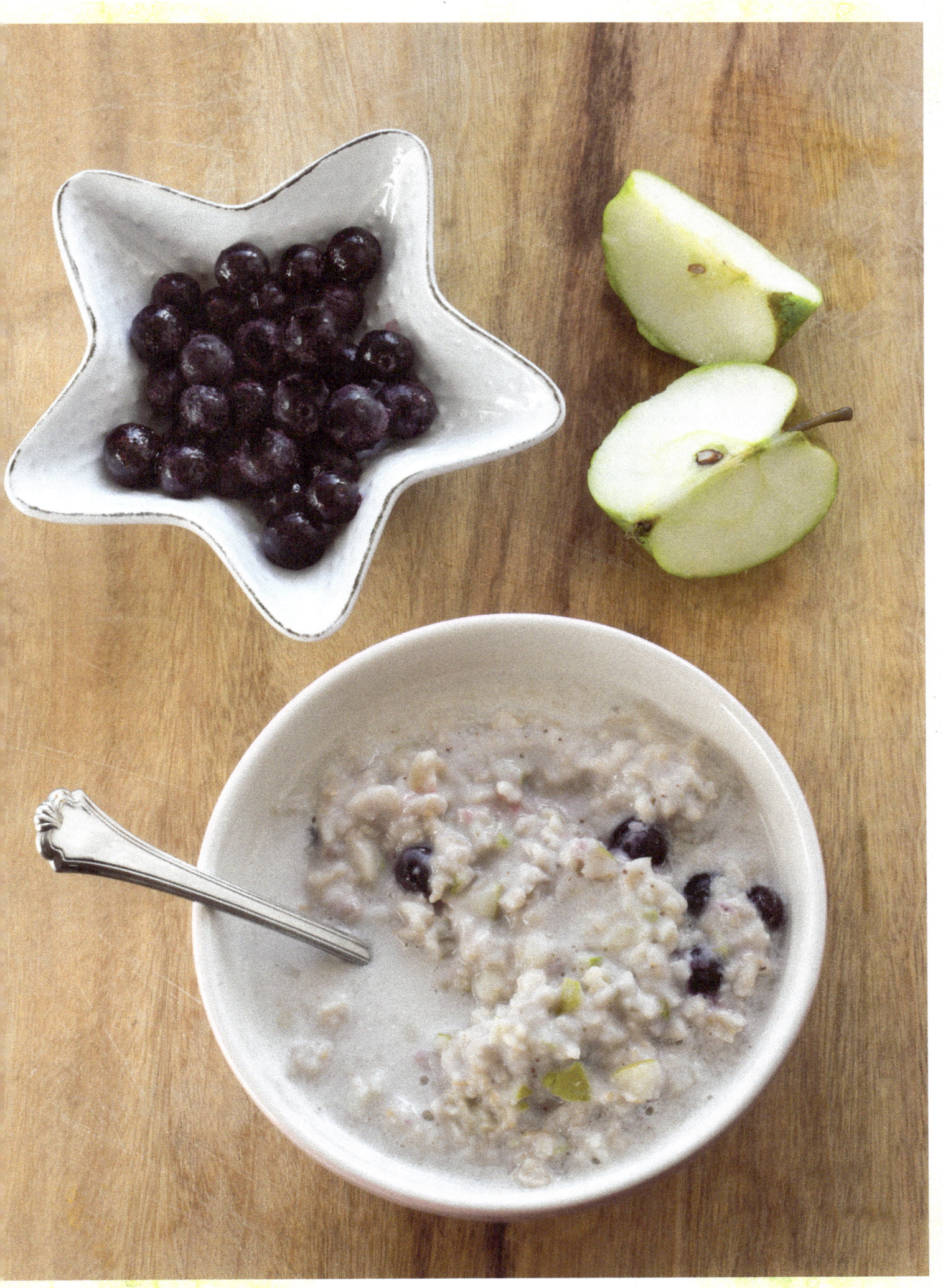

Omelettes

Omelettes are a great breakfast as they contain the protein from the eggs and they can be adapted to different tastes by changing the filling ingredients. Children can assist with the choice and preparation of the fillings, beat the eggs and pour ingredients into the pan. Below is a list of suggestions for fillings, but there are endless combinations. There is no playtime for this recipe because as you can see, the variations are in the recipe.

For every omelette
2 eggs
1 tablespoon of water
freshly ground pepper (optional)
butter or oil to grease

Filling ingredients (suggestions)
grated cheese
corn kernels
finely chopped mushrooms
sliced olives
finely chopped semi-dried tomatoes
finely chopped herbs such as chives, basil, dill or parsley

diced tomatoes
finely chopped red onion
diced capsicum
leftover roast vegetables (diced)

1. Prepare your filling ingredients and have them ready to go.
2. Beat together the omelette ingredients, making sure you add the water as this makes a fluffier omelette.
3. Heat your pan until it is hot to touch and grease with a little butter or oil.
4. Pour the omelette ingredients into the pan and as it cooks, gently bring some of the egg from the outside into the middle and move the pan around so that the uncooked egg in the middle moves to the outside.. You want it all to cook evenly and if you don't move the underneath layer around, the middle will cook last and the edges will be rubbery. You will end up with a crinkled look underneath but that only adds to the omelette's charm.
5. When the omelette is mostly cooked, spread your filling ingredients over one half of the omelette.
6. Flip half the omelette over onto the filling to make a big semi-circle and slide onto your plate.

Fruit Salad with Coconut Snow Cream

This cream is sweet and soft. It is a great alternative to dairy cream and it contains the goodness of coconut, cashews and chia seeds (high in protein and omega oils).

Fruit Salad
4 cups of diced, seasonal fruit

Snow cream
½ cup of raw cashews
1 ⅓ cups of coconut water or filtered water
1 teaspoon of vanilla extract
2 tablespoons of maple syrup
100g of coconut meat
2 tablespoons of white chia seeds

1. Puree the nuts, water, vanilla, maple syrup and coconut until smooth and creamy.
2. Stir in the chia seeds and leave to stand for 15 minutes. It will thicken even more if refrigerated.
3. Meanwhile, make your fruit salad by combining the diced fruit. Serve into bowls.
4. Spoon the snow cream over the fruit salad.

Play Time!

- You can use this snow cream as a side to many other dishes. Serve with pancakes, waffles, cake or pudding.
- Use other sweeteners such as honey, rice syrup or a couple of dates in the snow cream to change its flavour. Of course dates will change the colour as well.
- Add cinnamon, nutmeg or mixed spice to the snow cream.
- Use macadamia nuts instead of cashews.
- For a nut free version, just add another 100g of coconut to the recipe to make a nut free version. (Coconut is not technically a nut).

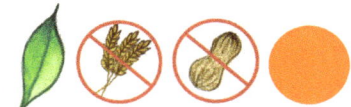

Beautiful Beginnings

Waffles

Waffles are usually a treat that do not include much nutritional value. However these waffles are full of fibre and taste. They are light, sweet, moist and delicious. I have included them in the breakfast section of this book as they are traditionally a breakfast meal, however they are also a great after school treat or dessert at night dressed up with strawberries, and a little ice cream. The mixture is easy for children to make and some waffle makers are also very child friendly.

Makes 4 large waffles

1 x 250g pear or apple
2 eggs
½ cup of milk
1 teaspoon of vanilla extract
¼ cup of oil
¾ cup of unbleached wheat or spelt flour
¾ cup of wholemeal wheat or spelt flour
½ cup of flaxseed meal
2 teaspoons of baking powder

1. Core the apple or pear and grate or pulverise the fruit in a food processor.
2. In a mixing bowl, whisk the fruit into the remaining wet ingredients.
3. Add dry ingredients and whisk until well combined. Leave to sit for 20-30 minutes. The mix will end up being quite thick.
4. Pour into a preheated waffle iron and cook until ready.*
5. Serve with fruit and maple syrup.

*Note: Waffle irons come with instructions. They also come coated in Teflon or made of cast iron. The latter is the safer option given that the safety of Teflon is unconfirmed.

Play Time!

- Try adding blueberries to the waffle mix to sweeten and provide bursting bubbles of flavour.
- Instead of serving with only maple syrup, make a fruit sauce from pureed fruit, cinnamon, vanilla and maple syrup or honey.
- Turn it into a dessert by serving with a chocolate sauce made from warmed coconut oil, raw cacao and maple syrup or honey.

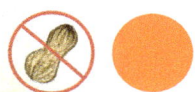

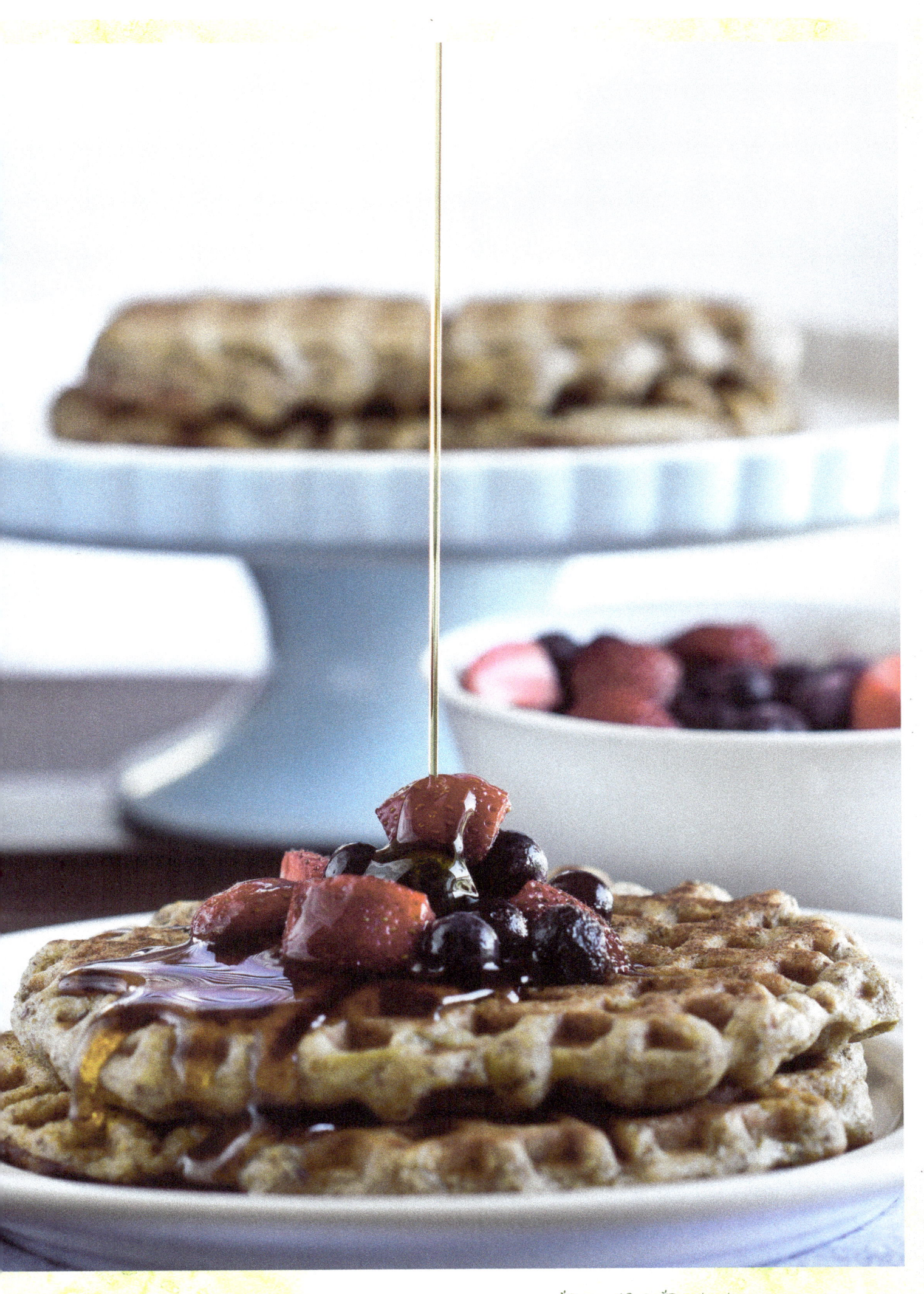

Perfect Pikelets

Pancakes and pikelets are made with the same mixture, therefore either can be made with this recipe. They are a great snack for children to make as they are simple to mix and easy to flip in the frying pan. Many recipes contain sugar, however it is not needed as the sweetness comes from sweet toppings. They can be served as a special breakfast with yummy fruit and maple syrup, or as a morning or afternoon tea with butter or jam. In this picture I have served them with mango, banana and coconut snow cream: recipe page 81

Makes 20-23 pikelets

2 eggs
1 ½ cups of milk
1 cup of unbleached wheat or spelt flour
1 cup of wholemeal wheat or spelt flour
2 teaspoons of baking powder

1. Whisk wet ingredients together.
2. Add the flour and baking powder and whisk until there are no lumps and the mix is bubbly.
3. Leave mixture to sit for 15-20 minutes (this resting time makes the pancakes fluffier).
4. Warm your frying pan and grease with a little oil or butter.
5. Pour mix in to make the desired size of your pancake or pikelet.
6. When bubbles appear on the surface, lift gently to see if the underside is cooked. It should be a golden to brown colour.
7. Flip your pikelet over quickly when ready and allow to cook on the other side. Make sure you don't have the pan too hot or the outside of your pikelets will burn and the middle will be gooey. You must cook them gently.
8. Serve as suggested in the recipe description.

Play Time!

- To make a fruity version, add berries, (fresh or frozen), sliced banana, grated apple or grated pear to the mixture before cooking.
- Instead of serving with only maple syrup, make a fruit sauce from pureed fruit, cinnamon, vanilla and maple syrup or honey.
- Turn it into a dessert by serving with a chocolate sauce made from warmed coconut oil, raw cacao and maple syrup or honey.

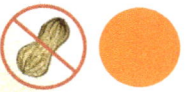

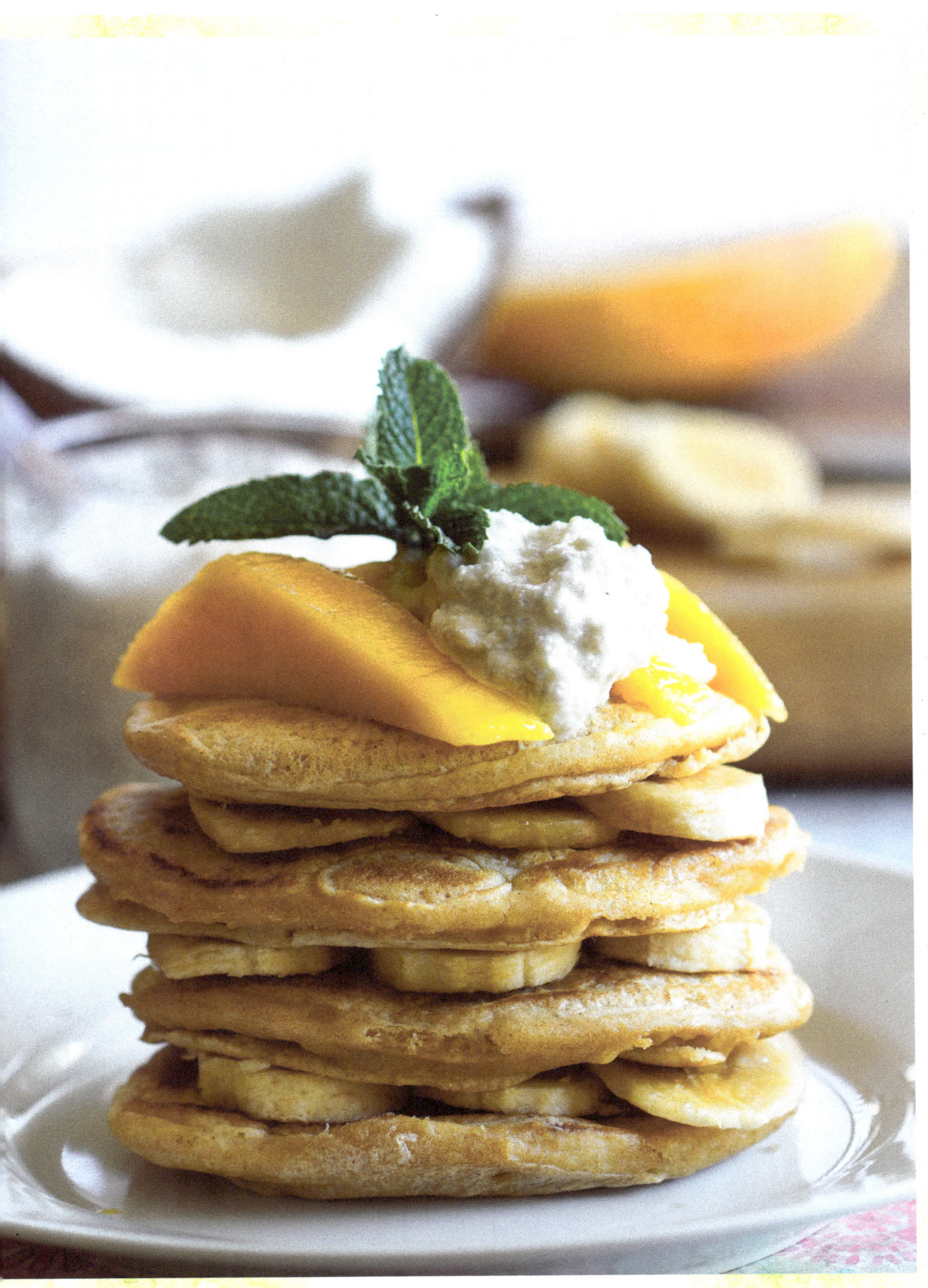

Pikelets with Coconut Snow Cream

Beautiful Beginnings

LSA

LSA, which is the acronym for linseeds, sunflower seeds and almonds, is a mix that tastes great added to muesli, porridge and smoothies. It provides the body with protein, omega oils and minerals. Linseeds do not grind well in the average food processor as they are so small. A coffee grinder will do the job nicely.

2 cups of linseeds (also known as flaxseeds)
1 cup of sunflower seeds
1 cup of raw almonds

1. Grind linseeds in a coffee grinder (unless you have a powerful food processor).
2. In a food processor, combine remaining ingredients with the linseeds, grinding to a fine crumb.
3. Store in the refrigerator to prevent the linseed oils from going rancid.*

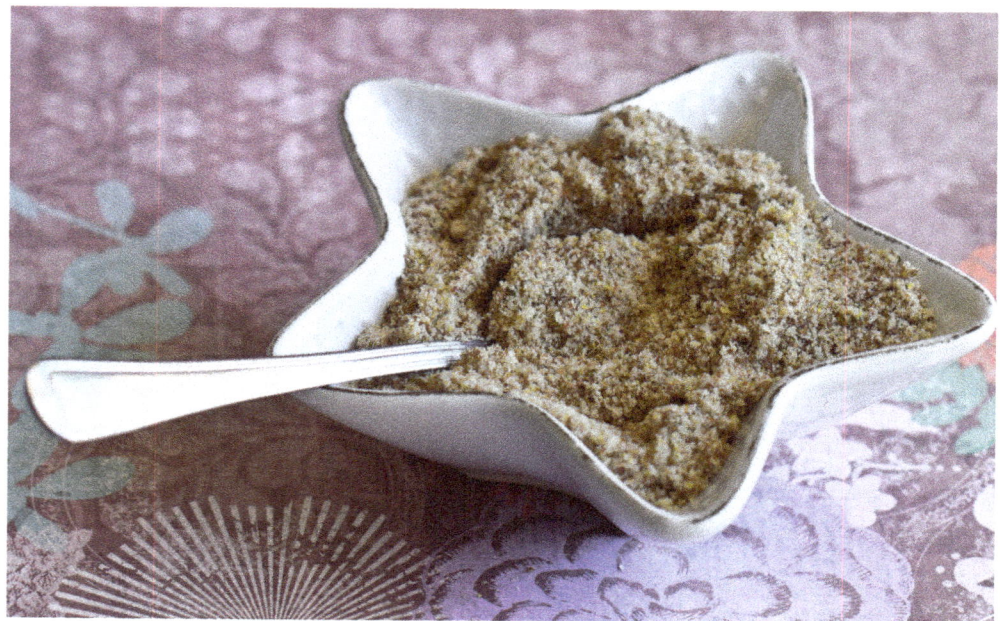

*Note: LSA or ground linseeds (flaxseeds) are often found for sale in bulk food stores. However be careful buying them already ground as if they have not been stored in a refrigerator, the oils will be rancid. The same applies for flaxseed oil.

Play Time!

- I often add pepitas (pumpkin seeds) into the mix because they are a great source of zinc: essential for healthy immune function. In the case of those with nut allergies, you could use the pepitas in place of the almonds. Hemp seeds are also a great addition as they are sweet and nutty without actually being a nut.
- Add LSA to raw treats such as Bliss Balls, Brownies and Crispy Cashew Rice Treats (all featured in this book).

Powerful Banana Smoothie

*This smoothie is sweet and filling. It will give you the energy
you need to get through the morning.*

Serves 1

1 frozen banana, chopped

1 cup of milk

2 tablespoons of plain yoghurt (soy or coconut yoghurt for those avoiding dairy)

1 tablespoon of honey or rice syrup

sprinkle of cinnamon (optional)

1 tablespoon of LSA (recipe on facing page and for those with nut allergies, there is an option in the play time.)

Place all ingredients into a blender or food processor and blend until smooth.

General Smoothie Play Time!

- Making smoothies is a great activity for children. They can be creative with so many different ingredients and the only risk is mess...make sure they have the top in the blender or food processor, so that it doesn't spray all over the kitchen!
- The possibilities are endless! Pick your fruit, choose your base (water, coconut water or milk), add yoghurt if you like or a handful of greens and blend. It can be fun to experiment and write down your favourite flavours.
- Frozen fruit will thicken a smoothie and the more you put in, the closer it will come to ice cream!
- There are many nutritious ingredients you can add to a smoothie that do not alter the flavour. They include: LSA (see recipe on the facing page), soaked chia seeds, hemp seeds, sunflower or pepita seeds. If you do not have a powerful blender, it may be an idea to grind your seeds in a coffee grinder first, so that they blend into the smoothie seamlessly. You want the smoothie to be silky rather than gritty.
- Other ingredients that add nutrition and flavour are macca powder, raw cacao, goji berries, acai berries, ginger, lime and lemon juice.
- There are some herbs which will also add delicious flavours. They include pineapple sage, fruit salad sage, mint (there are many different flavoured mints), lemon balm and sorrel.

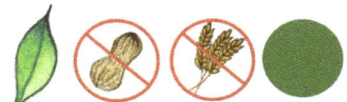

Beautiful Beginnings

Green Smoothie

Green smoothies are a great way to get your daily dose of greens without tasting them because the fruit provides the stronger flavour. For those who don't like the look of something green, a good handful of blueberries will do the trick!

Serves 1

1 frozen banana, chopped
1 chopped, fresh peach
handful of greens (use spinach, kale, or lettuce - avoiding peppery varieties)
1 cup of water or coconut water
squeeze of lime juice or small piece of ginger for extra zing!

Place all ingredients into a blender or food processor and blend until smooth.

Tropical Bliss Smoothie

A refreshing start to the morning, this smoothie uses tropical fruits. The ginger really adds something special.

Serves 1

½ cup of frozen mango, chopped
½ cup of chopped, fresh pineapple
1 cup of milk or coconut water
handful of fresh coconut
small slice of fresh ginger (optional)

Place all ingredients into a blender or food processor and blend until smooth.

"If you don't take care of your body, where are you going to live?"
~Unknown

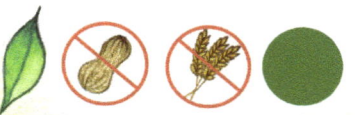

Beautiful Beginnings

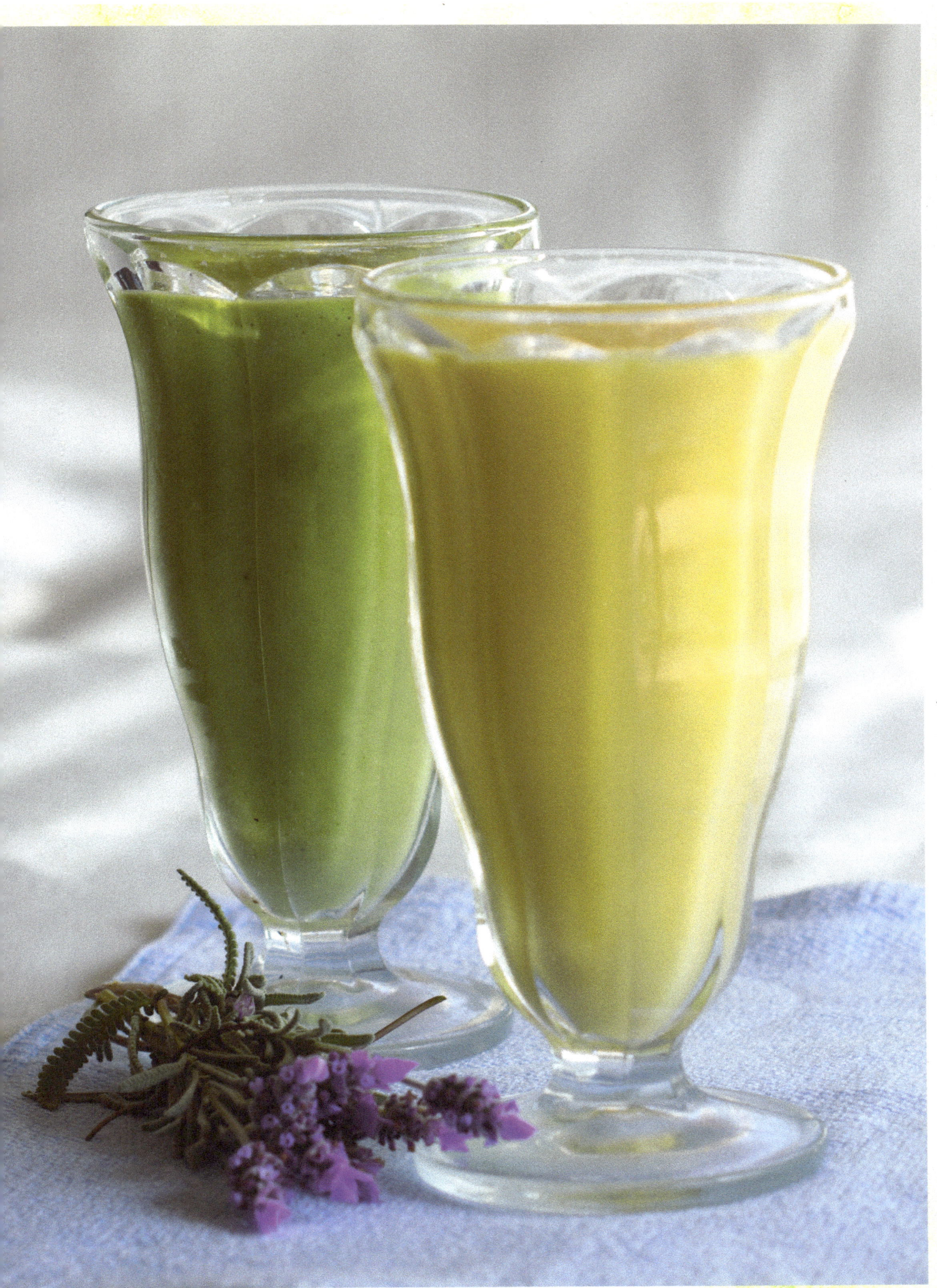

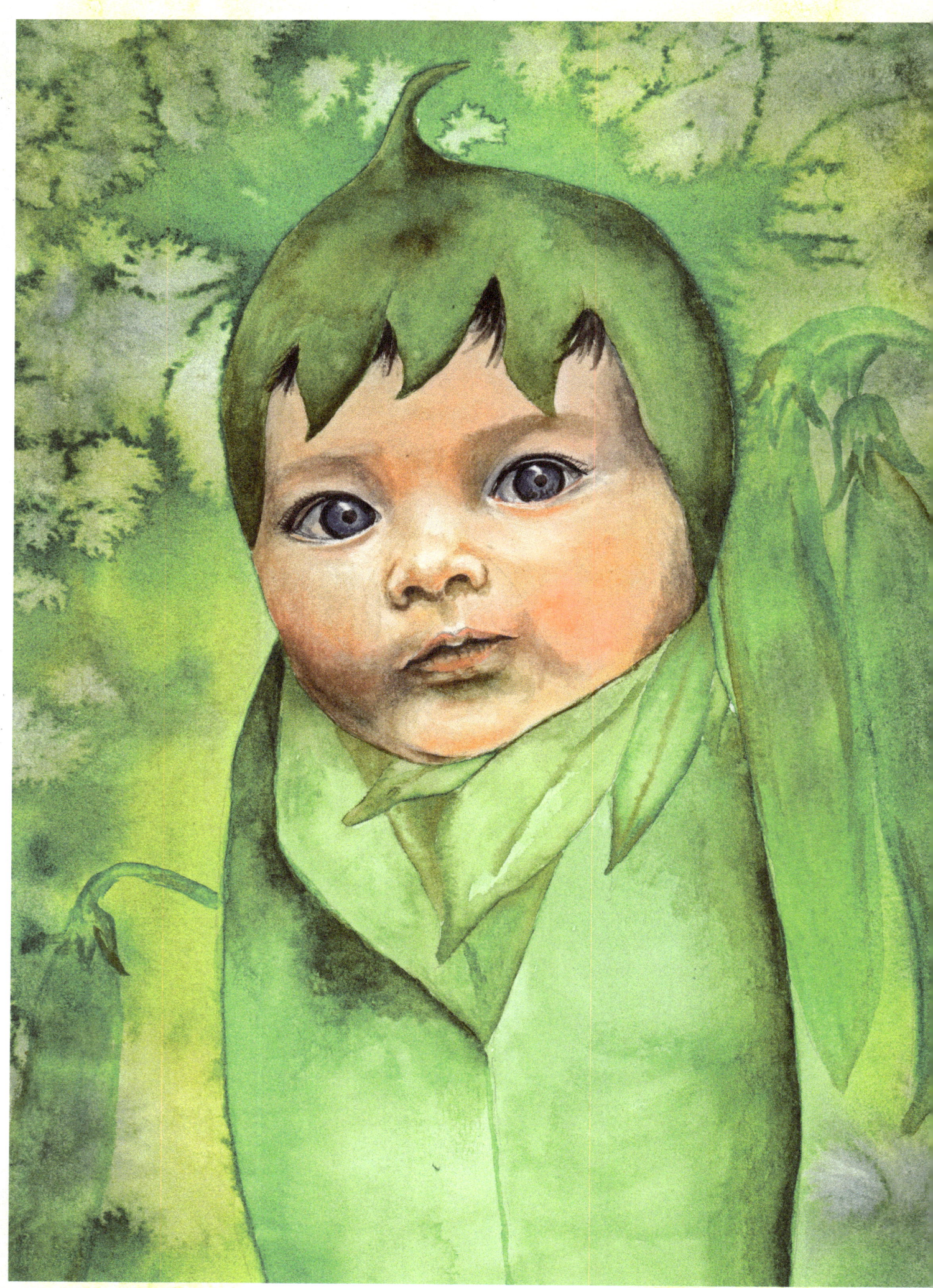

Little Morsels

Little Morsels

The recipes in this section cover three areas. First of all there are savoury snacks such as dips, crackers and h'orderves. They may be used for morning and afternoon tea or as appetisers. The second set of recipes are suitable as lunches or part of a meal. These include such items as sushi rolls, rice paper rolls and different types of burgers and patties. These recipes are very diverse as not only may they be used as lunches and dinners at home, but many of them are great to pack in the school lunch box.

Lastly, are the vegetable side dishes.

Bon Appetite!

"The first wealth is health."
~Ralph Waldo Emerson

Dips

Dips are great to make with children. Most of these recipes involve nothing hot or sharp and using the Play Time suggestions, there is ample room for creativity. Afterwards, organising the platter to present the dips can be lots of fun too. See the platter ideas on page 111. There are many dip recipes in this section for the simple reason that, in our family, we love dips!

Sunset Dip

This dip is smooth and sweet with a lemon tang. Serve with warm bread, crackers or raw vegetable pieces. A great after-school snack for the kids!

350g peeled and chopped pumpkin
1 tablespoon of oil
1 large red capsicum, seeded and halved
½ a head of garlic, unpeeled
1 cup of raw cashews
juice of ½ a lemon
1 small red chilli, seeds removed (optional)
½ teaspoon of sea salt
freshly ground black pepper to season

1. Preheat the oven to 180°C convection or 160°C fan-forced.
2. Coat pumpkin in oil and place on a baking tray with capsicum and garlic.
3. Roast in the oven until the garlic is soft and vegetables are slightly charred. You will probably need to take the garlic out earlier. Time will depend on the size of your pumpkin pieces. For small pieces I find half an hour is sufficient with the garlic taking only 20 minutes.
4. Once the vegetables are cooled, place in a food processor with all other ingredients and puree.
5. Taste test for seasoning and adjust salt, pepper and lemon juice to your liking.

Play Time!

- Vary the nuts: macadamias and almonds also work well.
- Add herbs such as parsley or basil.
- Use lime juice instead of lemon and add the grated zest for a stronger flavour.
- Use as a pasta sauce.

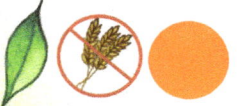

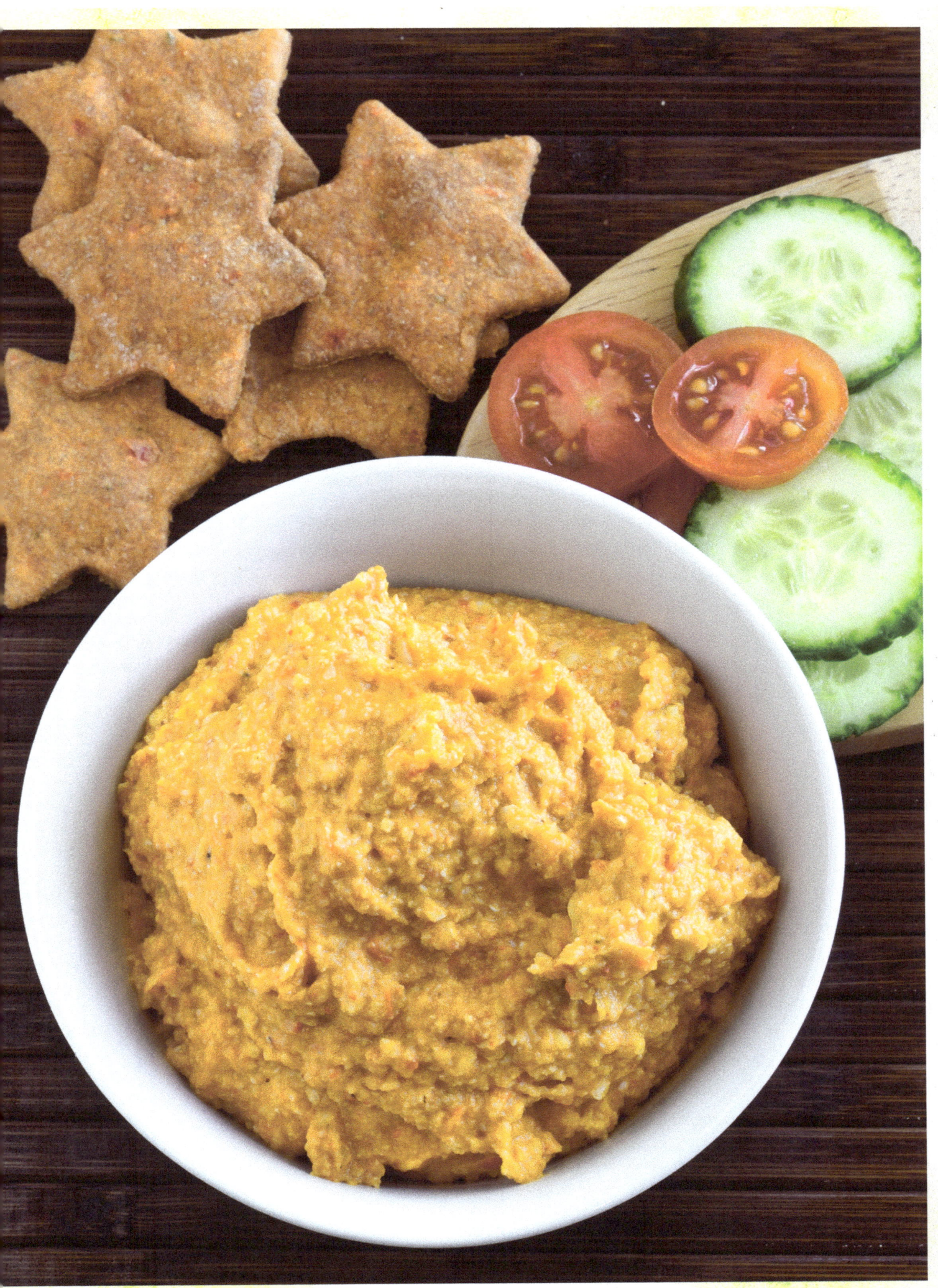

Smoky Baba Ghanoush

Baba Ghanoush is traditionally made over an open flame, giving the dip a smoky flavour. It is delicious with warm or toasted pita bread strips and other Middle Eastern h'orderves.

750g eggplant
juice of ½ a lemon
2 tablespoons of tahini
1 clove of garlic
¼ cup of cold pressed olive oil
½ teaspoon of sea salt
small handful of parsley (optional)

1. Preheat the oven to 180°C convection or 160°C fan-forced.
2. Lay the eggplant over a gas flame and leave for a couple of minutes until the skin starts to char. Turn regularly until mostly charred on the outside. The aim of this exercise is not to completely cook the eggplant but to impart a smoky flavour. Do not overdo it or the skin will flake and be hard to remove in large pieces.
3. Place the eggplant onto a tray and bake in the oven for approximately ½ an hour, or until soft.
4. Peel the eggplant and puree in a food processor with the remaining ingredients until smooth.
5. Adjust salt to taste.

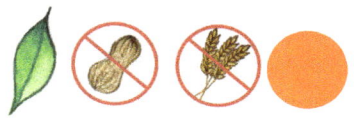

Enchanted Forest Dip

Resist the urge to throw the yoghurt into the food processor with the rest of the ingredients. If you do, you will have a drink instead of a dip! This is also great as an accompaniment to Greek salads and mains.

1 cup of tightly packed, chopped spinach
½ cup of loosely packed, roughly chopped dill leaves
1 small clove of garlic
½ teaspoon of sea salt
¼ teaspoon of mustard powder
1 cup of plain, pot set yoghurt. Those avoiding dairy can use plain soy yoghurt.

1. In a blender, combine all ingredients except the yoghurt, until pulverised.
2. Stir the yoghurt into the green mix and adjust seasonings to taste.

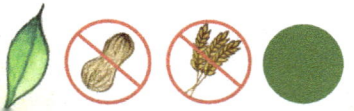

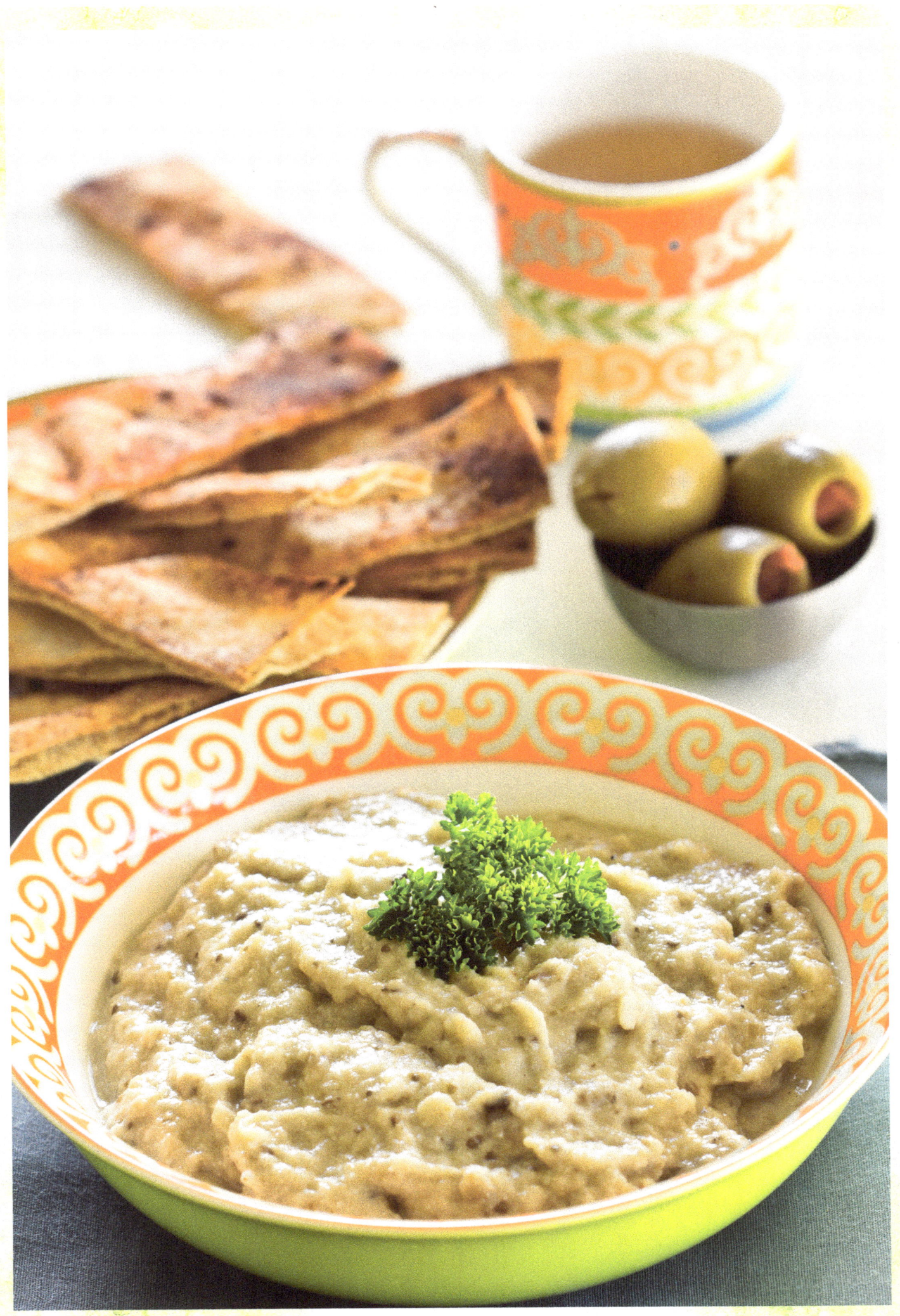

Stain-Your-Clothes Dip

This dip is sweet and refreshing. It tastes delicious with crackers and/or raw vegetable sticks. It is also good added to sandwiches or served as a side with burgers and patties. Your kids will love the bright colour, but check what they are wearing before serving. My boys usually eat this bare-chested.

350g peeled, fresh beetroot cut into bite-sized pieces or 310g drained, cooked beetroot (beetroot loses some weight after being cooked)
½ teaspoon of ground cumin
½ teaspoon of ground coriander
½ teaspoon of ground paprika
1 medium-sized clove of garlic
1 small bunch of fresh mint (leaves only)
½ cup of plain yoghurt (those avoiding dairy, see playtime notes)
1 tablespoon of lemon juice
sea salt and pepper to taste

1. If you are using raw beetroot, boil or steam until soft. This should take about 20 minutes (depending on the size of your pieces). Allow to cool.
2. Place all ingredients into a food processor and blend until smooth.

Play Time!

- Add salad oil to a portion of this dip to create a delicious dressing. Adjust lemon juice, pepper and salt to taste, as dressings are usually a little stronger in seasoning.
- You can leave the mint out of this recipe if it isn't to your liking and it is still just as tasty.
- For a dairy free version, leave the yoghurt out and double the lemon juice. Soy yoghurt does not work well in this recipe.

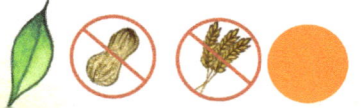

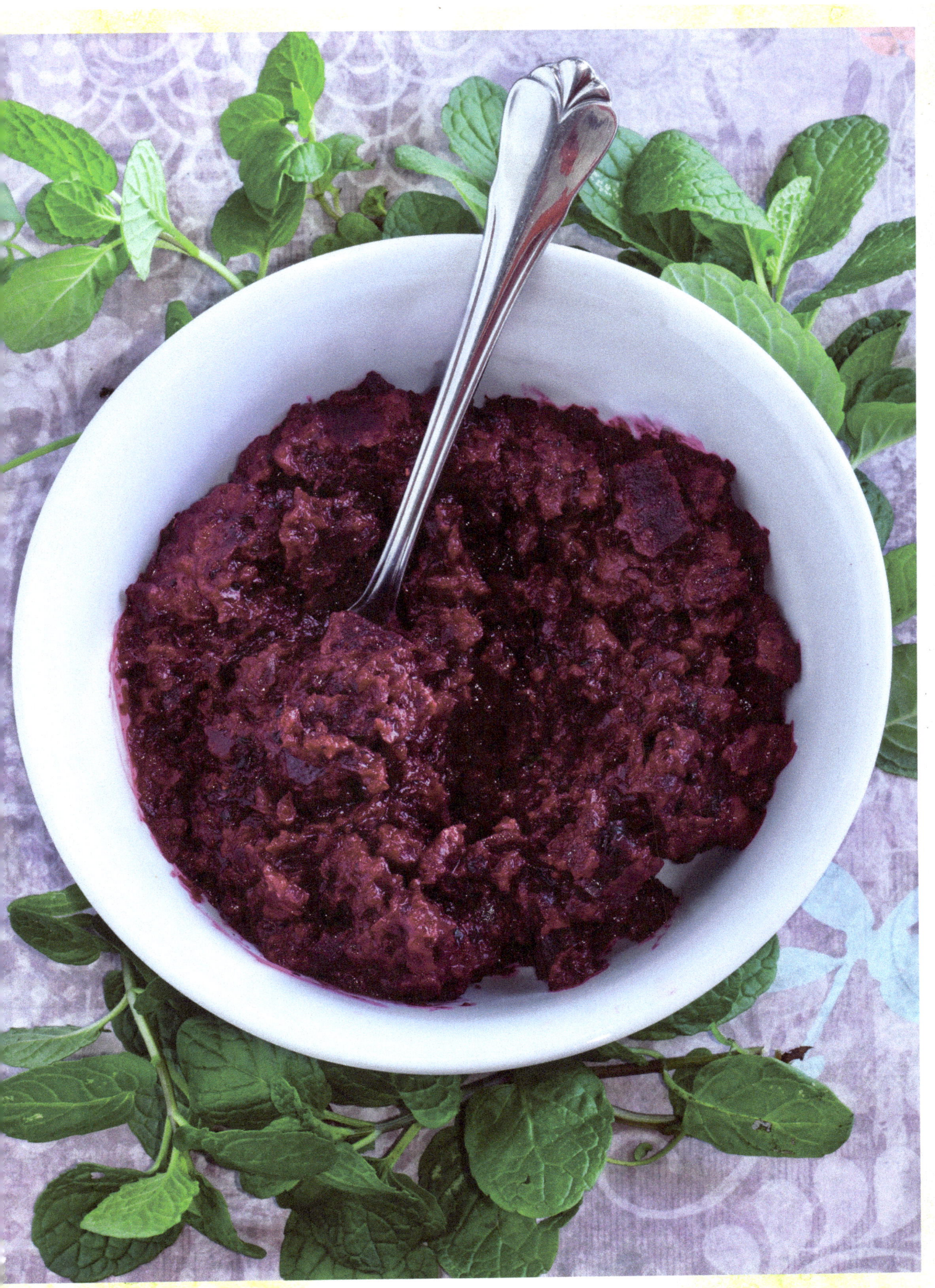

Guacamole

The quantity of my guacamole is quite large because we LOVE it and if there isn't enough, there are fights. "You have too much on your chip!", "Mum, he's eating it all!". So, to save arguments, we just make a big bowl of it. If you want to try it out first in a smaller quantity, simply halve the recipe.

3 large, ripe avocados
1 small clove of garlic
½ teaspoon of sea salt (or to taste)
small bunch of fresh coriander (approx. 25g)
juice of 1 small juicy lemon or lime (or to taste because some people like more of a zing than others)
1 large tomato, finely diced

1. Place all ingredients into a food processor, except tomato.
2. Combine on high until smooth.
3. Either stir the tomatoes in at the end or pulse in the food processor for a smoother dip.
4. Serve immediately with corn chips or use as a side in a Mexican meal.

Sassy Salsa

Another great Mexican treat. This, like Guacamole, is good with corn chips or served as a side with Mexican food. Children can do the food processing and hand mixing in this recipe.

1 small red onion
1 small bunch of fresh coriander (approx. 25g)
1 mild, green chilli, seeds removed
1 large capsicum (colour is optional), diced
5 medium-sized tomatoes (approx. 750g), diced
1 clove of garlic, crushed
2 teaspoons of ground cumin
2 tablespoons of lime juice
½ teaspoon of sea salt

1. Combine the onion, coriander and chilli and in a food processor or chop finely.
2. Mix the finely chopped ingredients with the remaining ingredients.
3. Serve at room temperature.

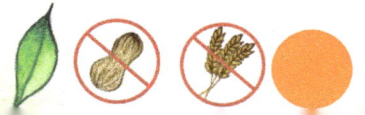

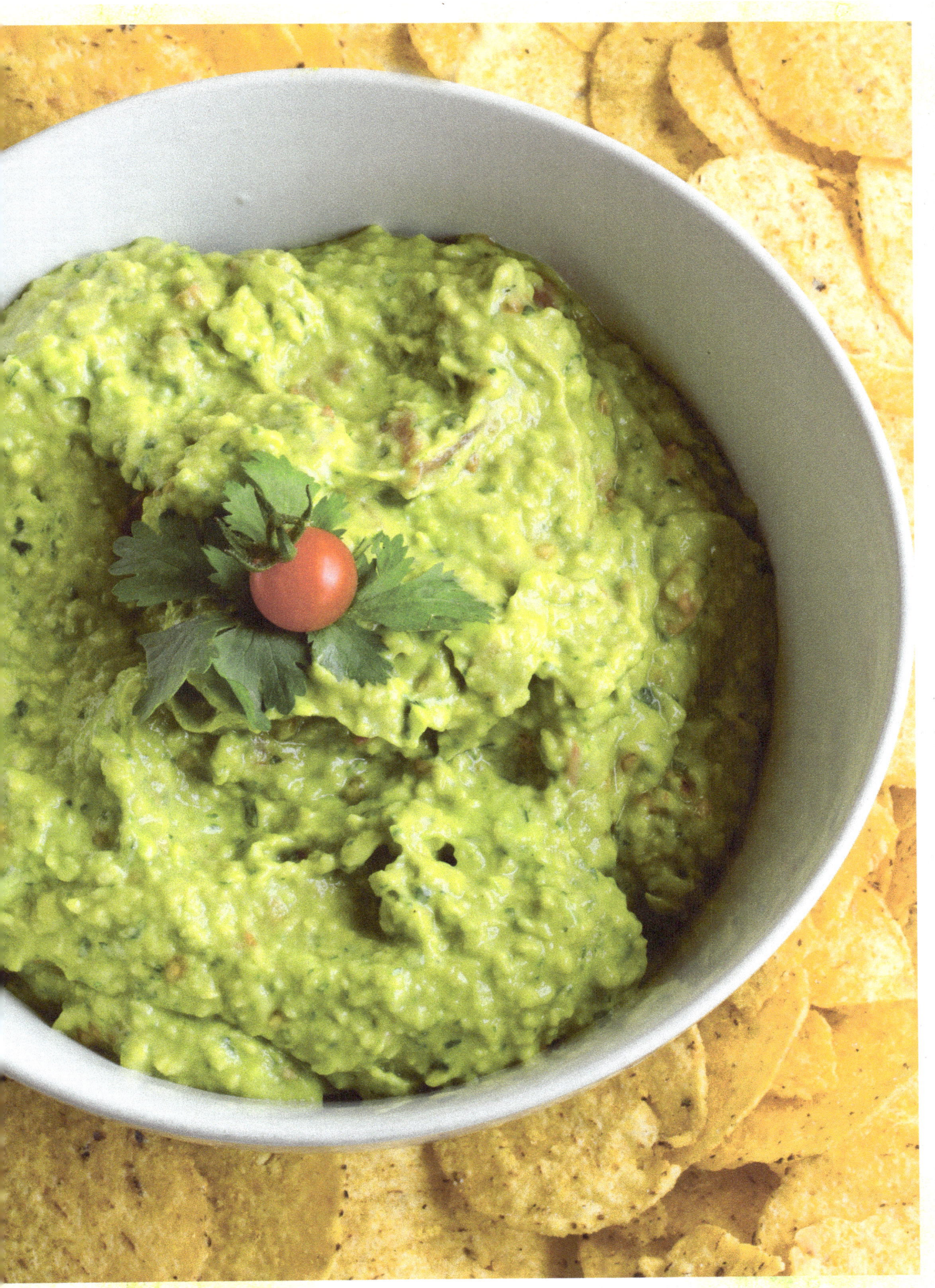

Hummus

Hummus is a Middle Eastern dip, which is so diverse and easy to make. You can adapt a hummus recipe to suit just about anyone. Below is my basic recipe as well as a host of other combinations. Try your own additions using the ingredients your family prefers. If you find chickpeas hard to digest or you are interested in including more raw food in your diet, then try the raw almond version on the page opposite.

Baby Bear Hummus

People differ in what they prefer as the dominant flavour in their hummus. Some like it very salty, others like the zing of lots of lemon. Then there are those who like all flavours to be equal. This particular recipe is one of balanced flavours, thus the name. If you like your hummus to be stronger in one flavour, adjust to taste.

2½ cups of cooked chickpeas (1 cup of dried)
½ cup of tahini
juice of 1 medium-sized lemon
½ cup of water
1 clove of garlic
3 tablespoons of cold-pressed olive oil
½ teaspoon of sea salt

1. If you are using dried chickpeas, cook according to directions on page 64.
2. Blend all ingredients in a food processor until smooth.
3. Serve with vegetable sticks, crackers or bread.

Play Time!

- The basic hummus is very tasty, but because of its mild flavour it can be used as a base for many other ingredients. I have included some of my own variations in the following pages. Try these or come up with your own.
- Use lime juice instead of lemon.
- Add herbs such as basil, parsley, dill or coriander.
- Throw in roasted or raw red capsicum (basil also goes well with the capsicum flavour).
- If you like spice, add a little chilli, cumin and sun-dried tomatoes.

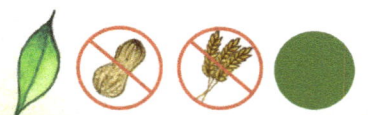

Herby Tomato Hummus

The flavours in this hummus are very Italian. This would be considered fusion food, where the flavours from one region are combined with those of another. Multi-cultural Australia is renowned for such recipes.

2 cups of cooked chickpeas (¾ cup of dried)
½ cup of chopped semi-dried tomatoes
2 tablespoons of tahini
1 clove of garlic
½ cup of basil leaves
¼ cup of pine nuts
¼ cup of olive oil
juice of 1 medium-sized lemon

1. If you are using dried chickpeas, cook according to directions on page 64.
2. Place all ingredients into a food processor and blend until smooth.
3. Serve with a selection of raw vegetable sticks, crackers or your favourite bread.
   May also be added to sandwiches or as a condiment in a meal.

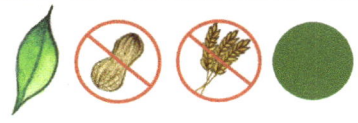

Almondy Hummus

In this recipe, raw almonds are used in place of the chickpeas. The flavour is completely different and very refreshing. Raw almonds are an excellent source of protein and calcium. They also help the body to reach its ideal pH.

1 cup of raw almonds (soaked in filtered water overnight)
¼ cup of tahini
1 clove of garlic
juice of ½ a medium-sized lemon
3 tablespoons of cold-pressed olive oil
⅓ cup of water
sea salt to taste

1. Drain the almonds and add with remaining ingredients to a food processor.
2. Blend until smooth.
3. Taste for seasoning. You may need to add more salt or lemon juice depending on your palate. If it is too thick, add more water a little at a time to produce a creamy consistency.

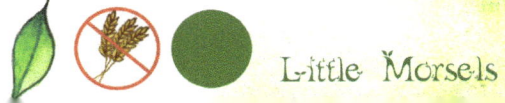

Cinderella Hummus

This version of hummus is a family favourite. The combination of pumpkin and lime is a match made in Heaven!

2 cups of cooked chickpeas (¾ cup of dried)
3 tablespoons of lime juice
¼ cup of tahini
1 clove of garlic
3 tablespoons of cold-pressed olive oil
1 cup of mashed pumpkin (275g of fresh peeled pumpkin will give you 1 cup of mashed).
½ teaspoon of sea salt
freshly ground black pepper

1. If you are using dried chickpeas, cook according to directions on page 64.
2. Place all ingredients into a food processor and blend until smooth. Season to taste.
3. Serve with a selection of raw vegetable sticks, crackers or your favourite bread. May also be added to sandwiches or as a condiment in a meal.

And still more Hummus ideas:

Try adding any of the following:

- Fresh herbs such as parsley, basil, oregano or mint
- Ground cumin or ground paprika
- Roasted capsicum
- Roasted or mashed sweet potato
- Cooked beetroot
- Roasted garlic (for a sweet garlic taste)

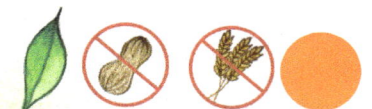

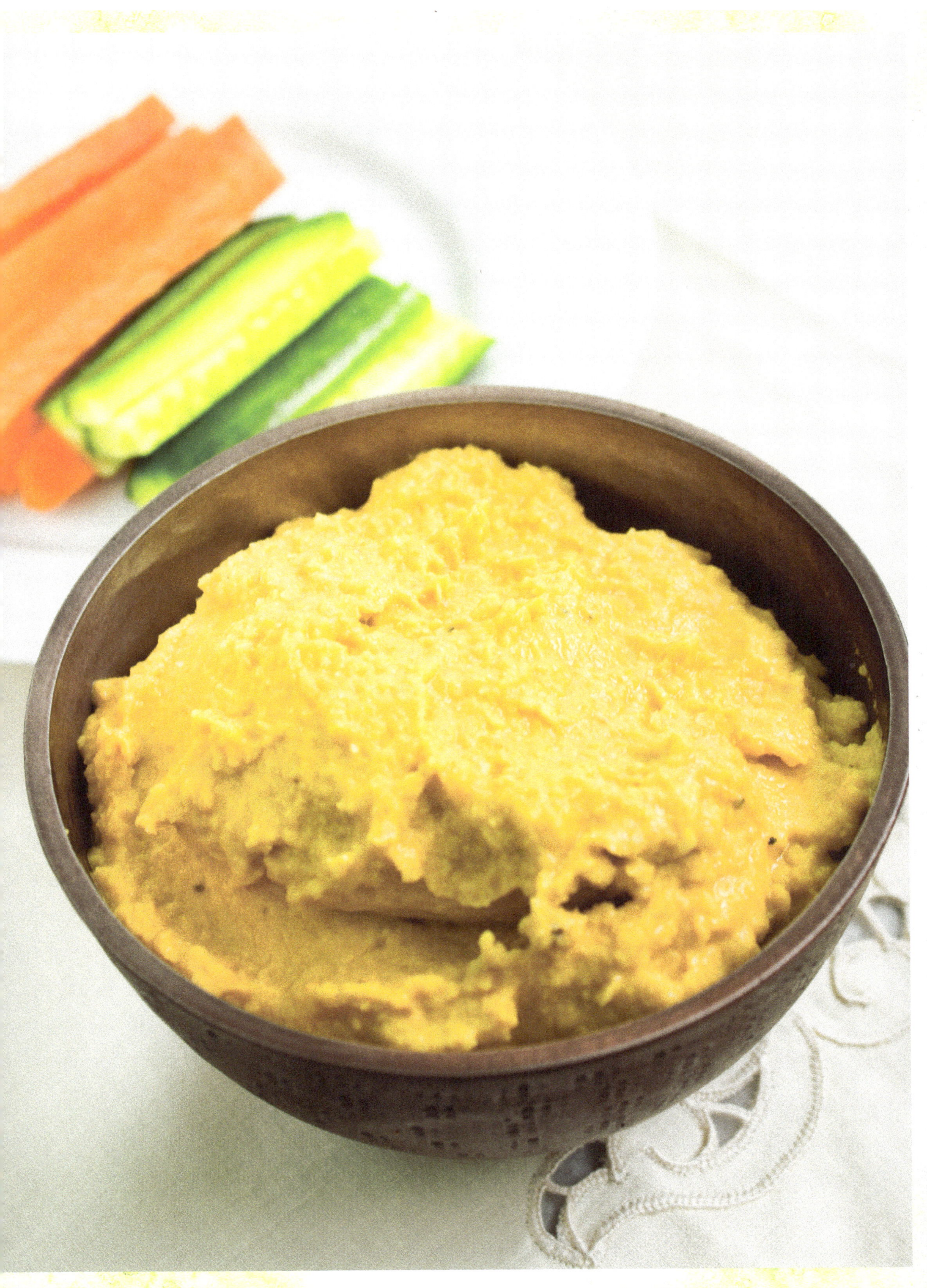

Making Your Own Crackers

Shop bought crackers are not only expensive for what they are, but they are often full of additives such as MSG, hydrogenated oils, sugar, artificial flavours and excessive table salt. Making your own is so quick and easy! Not only that, you get to decide on the flavour. You can make them plain or gourmet. You can mix things together that haven't been thought of before and you can make them any shape you like!

Following are a few recipes for some of our family's favourite flavours, and once you get used to making them you can start experimenting. There are a few tips I have learnt during my trial and error period of cracker making and they are listed below, as well as suggestions for presentation.

- The fan-forced setting on the oven seems to work better than the element setting. The crackers have less chance of burning.
- If you want your crackers to be crunchy, you need to watch them during the last 5-10 minutes of cooking. The ones on the outside edge will cook the fastest, so remove them after about 15 minutes of cooking time, and put the rest back to bake for longer.
- Crackers are ready when they are hard around the edges. They will harden up in the middle during the cooling time.
- Put them on a wire rack to cool so that no steam gets trapped underneath them.
- Wait until they are completely cool before you store them and always keep in an airtight container so that they stay crunchy.
- When being creative with the recipes, all you need is for the dough to be workable. It should be moist but not stick to your fingers when you handle it. Throw any vegetable, seed, nut, or herb/spice mix in.
- **To make the crackers look like the ones in a bought box**, roll your dough out on a piece of baking paper. Once the dough is thin (around 2mm), use a knife or pizza cutter to cut them into squares or rectangles. Then pierce each cracker a few times with a fork. Transfer the whole sheet with the ready cracker dough still on, over to the baking tray. Wait until after they are cooked to break them apart.
- **To make them into other shapes**, use your favourite cookie cutters. If you don't have any, use a glass or jar dipped in flour to make round crackers.

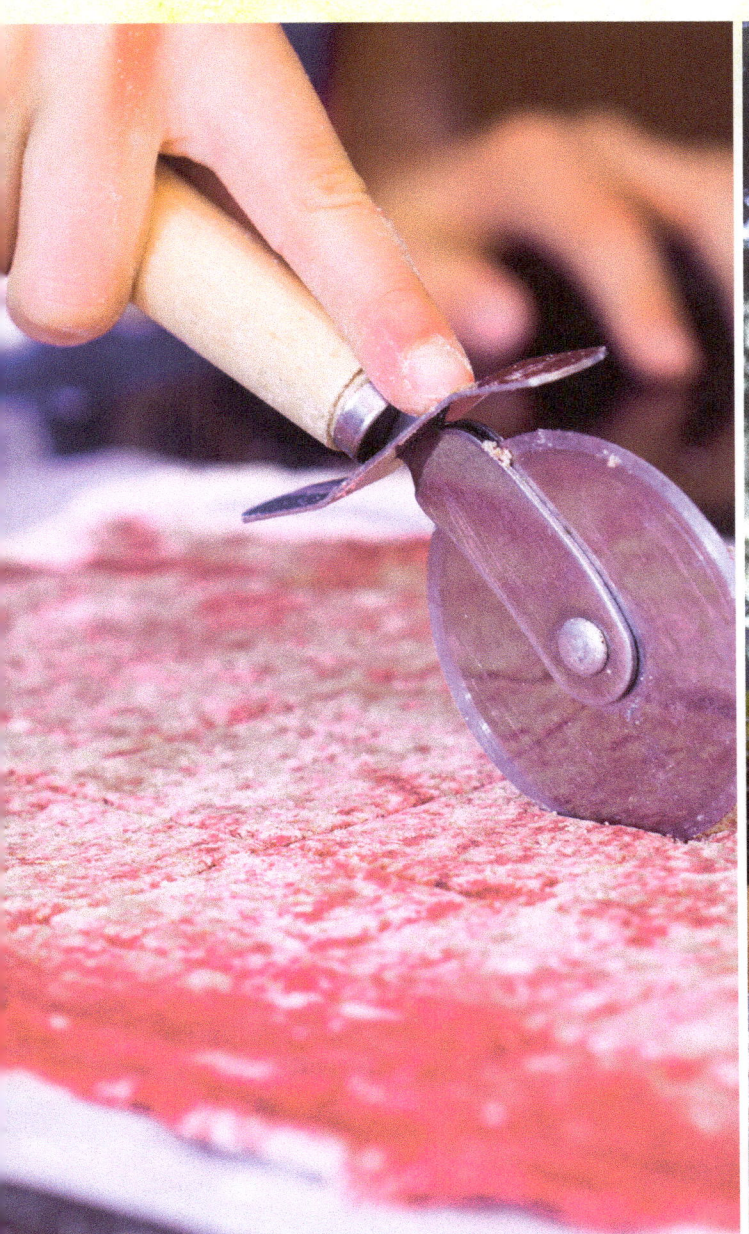
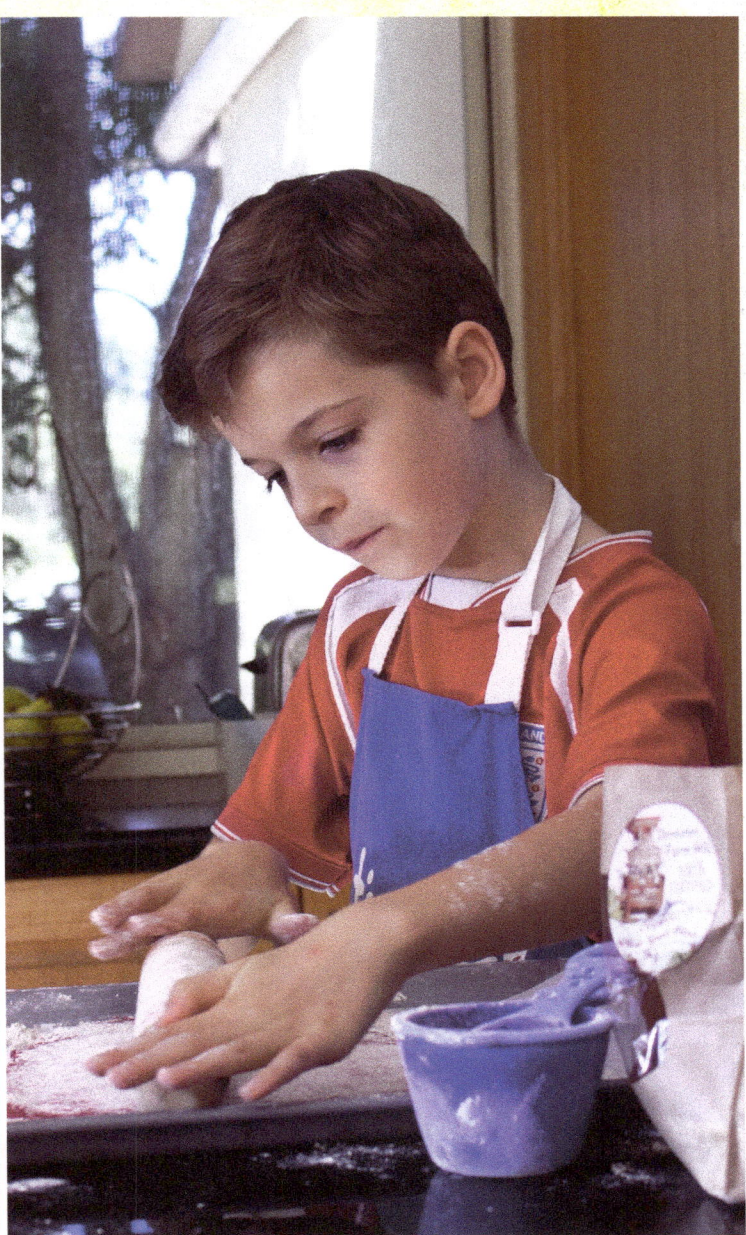
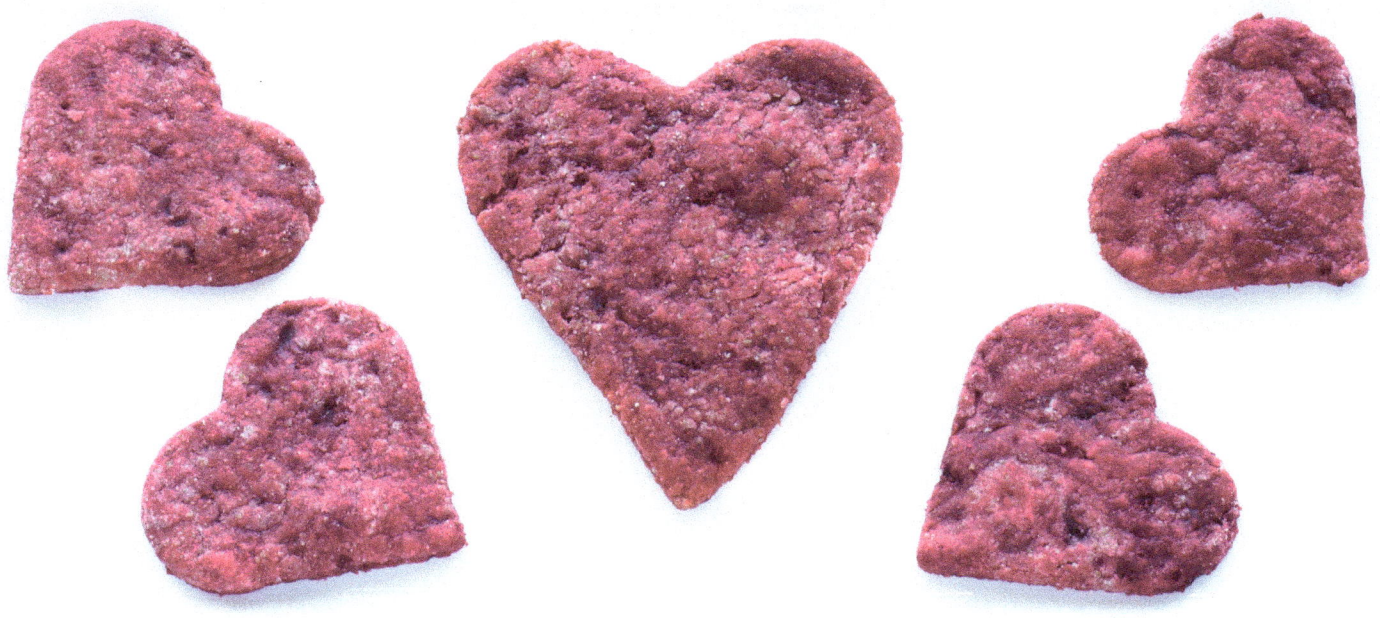

Heart's Desire Crackers

Little Morsels

Potato and Rosemary Crackers

Rosemary and potatoes are very good friends, especially with the addition of a little sea salt. These crackers complement most dips well and are tasty enough to be eaten on their own.

150g potatoes, peeled, steamed and mashed
1½ teaspoons of very finely chopped rosemary
¼ cup of oil
1 teaspoon of sea salt
1 cup of wholemeal wheat or spelt flour

1. Preheat the oven to 160 °C (fan-forced).
2. Puree the potato, rosemary, oil and salt in a food processor or mash with a potato masher.
3. Add the flour and mix into a workable dough.
4. Knead the dough and form it into a ball. It should be moist but not stick to your fingers. Add more flour if it is needed.
5. Roll the dough out on a well floured surface. It should be about 2mm thick.
6. Refer to the "Making Your Own Crackers" notes on page 104 for suggestions on shaping the crackers and for other helpful tips.
7. Bake for approximately 20 minutes. Thinner crackers and those on the edges will cook faster. Remove these and continue cooking the ones that are still soft. Crackers will crisp a bit more during cooling, but should be somewhat crisp when removed.
8. Leave on a cooling rack until they are cool.

Play Time!

- Use sweet potato instead of potato. You will need to add a little more flour as sweet potato contains a higher moisture content.
- Vary the herbs you use - choose from parsley, sage, basil, thyme, oregano, chives or even mixed herbs.

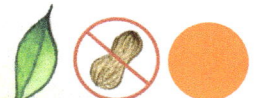

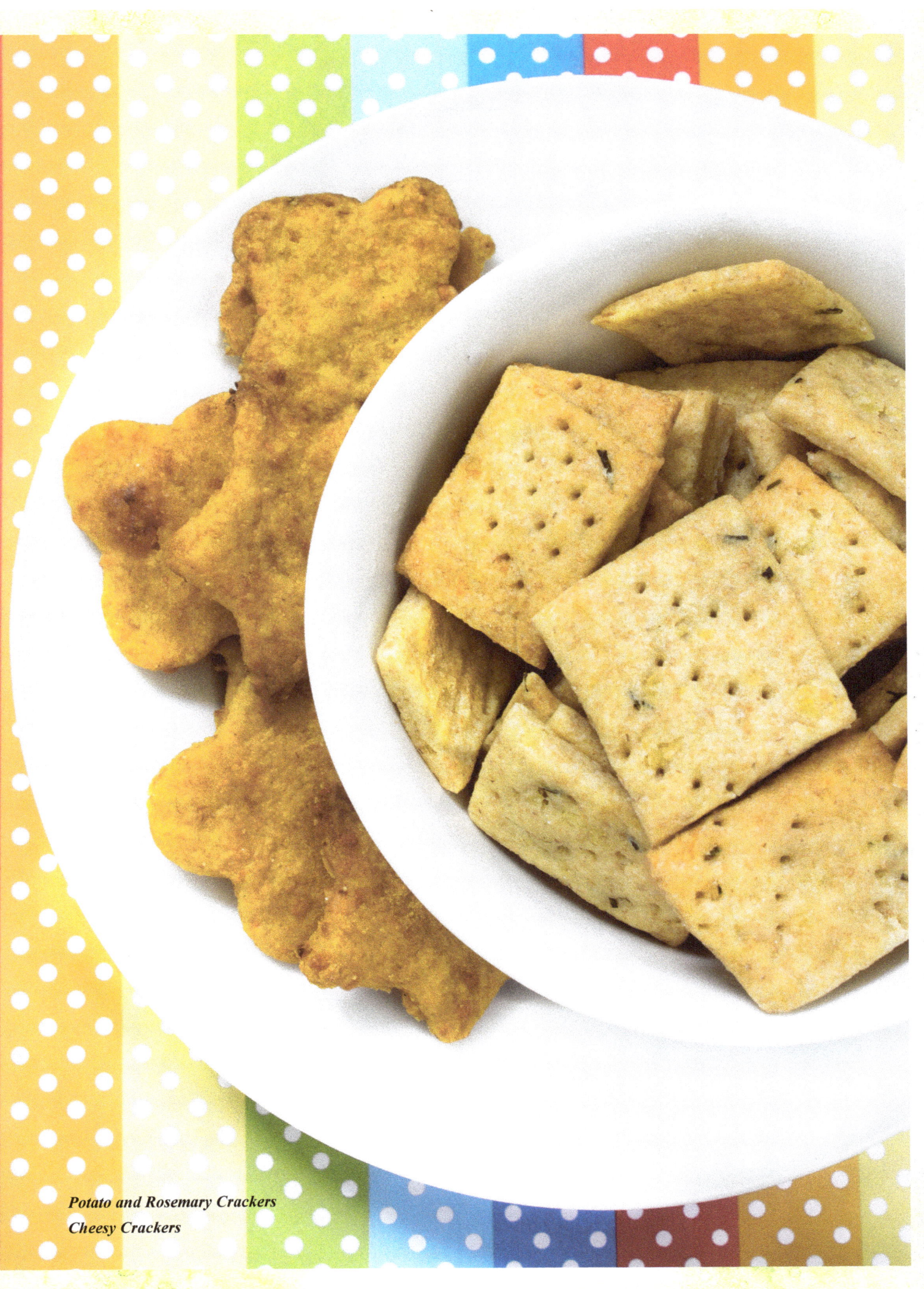

Potato and Rosemary Crackers
Cheesy Crackers

Popeye Crackers

These green crackers look so pretty with an orange or light coloured dip and they taste amazing with the combination of spinach, sesame seeds and salt.

120g fresh, trimmed spinach
¼ cup of oil
1 teaspoon of sea salt
1 ½ cups of wholemeal wheat or spelt flour
½ cup of sesame seeds

1. Preheat the oven to 160 °C (fan-forced).
2. Puree the spinach, oil and salt in a food processor or blender.
3. Add the flour and sesame seeds to the spinach mixture, either in the food processor or a mixing bowl.
4. Knead the dough and form it into a ball. The dough should be moist but not stick to your fingers. Add more flour if it is needed.
5. Roll the dough out on a well floured surface. It should be about 2mm thick.
6. Refer to the "Making Your Own Crackers" notes on page 104 for suggestions on shaping the crackers and for other helpful tips.
7. Bake for approximately 20 minutes. Thinner crackers and those on the edges will cook faster. Remove these and continue cooking the ones that are still soft. Crackers will crisp a bit more during cooling, but should be somewhat crisp when removed.
8. Leave on a cooling rack until they are cool.

Play Time!

- Try using other greens such as kale or sorrel.
- Instead of the sesame seeds, add some dill and or lemon zest: other friends of spinach. Always remember to add enough flour to make the dough workable.

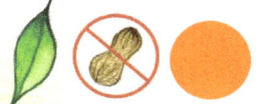

Cheesy Crackers

The addition of Parmesan in this cracker mix gives them a different texture. They are lighter and have a sharp taste which goes very well with refreshing dips such as Guacamole or Salsa.

120g trimmed carrot
¼ cup of finely grated Parmesan (those avoiding dairy, see playtime notes)
¼ cup of oil
½ teaspoon of sea salt
1 ½ cups of wholemeal wheat or spelt flour

1. Preheat the oven to 160 °C (fan-forced).
2. Chop the carrot into chunks and then pulverise in your food processor.
3. Mix the carrot, Parmesan, oil and salt in a food processor or blender.
4. Combine the flour and the carrot mixture until you have a soft dough. The dough should be moist but not stick to your fingers. Add more flour if it is needed.
5. Roll the dough out on a well floured surface. It should be about 2mm thick.
6. Refer to the "Making Your Own Crackers" notes on page 104 for suggestions on shaping the crackers and for other helpful tips.
7. Bake for approximately 20 minutes. Thinner crackers and those on the edges will cook faster. Remove these and continue cooking the ones that are still soft. Crackers will crisp a bit more during cooling, but should be somewhat crisp when removed.
8. Leave on a cooling rack until they are cool.

Play Time!

- Did you know that carrots come in more colours than just orange? Purple carrots are now becoming more common or if you grow your own you can produce pink, white and yellow varieties. These can make for some interesting crackers.
- Add some herbs such as parsley or thyme.
- Leave out the Parmesan for a dairy free version and add extra flavour with herbs or sesame seeds.

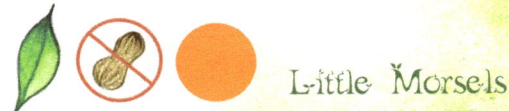

Heart's Desire Crackers

I love these crackers, not just because of the sweet and savoury taste but because they are so pretty!

120g fresh, trimmed and peeled beetroot
1 teaspoon of ground cumin
¼ cup of oil
1 teaspoon of sea salt
1 ½ cups of wholemeal wheat or spelt flour

1. Preheat the oven to 160 °C (fan-forced).
2. Roughly chop the beetroot and puree with the cumin, oil and salt in a food processor or blender.
3. Combine the flour and the beetroot mixture, either in the food processor, or a mixing bowl.
4. Knead the dough and form it into a ball. The dough should be moist but not stick to your fingers. Add more flour if it is needed.
5. Roll the dough out on a well floured surface. It should be about 2mm thick.
6. Refer to the "Making Your Own Crackers" notes on page 104 for suggestions on shaping the crackers and for other helpful tips.
7. Bake for approximately 20 minutes. Thinner crackers and those on the edges will cook faster. Remove these and continue cooking the ones that are still soft. Crackers will crisp a bit more during cooling, but should be somewhat crisp when removed.
8. Leave on a cooling rack until they are cool.

Play Time!

- If you don't like the flavour of cumin seeds, leave them out. You could try adding some mint instead, as mint and beetroot are very good friends.
- Caraway seeds are a nice substitute to cumin seeds, or even fennel seeds, which add an aniseed flavour.

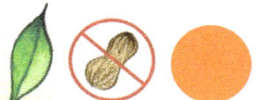

Platters and other Savoury Snacks

Below are ideas for platters as well as other savoury snacks. It is important to make sure that all snacks are not sweet. Although it is possible to sweeten foods with natural ingredients such as honey, maple syrup and dates, the high fructose contents of these foods is still not good for us in large quantities. The more sweet foods we have, the more we want. If a child grows up with a diet high in these sweet foods, this is what the palate will crave most, leading to possible problems later on.

Savoury Snacks
- Nuts (even better if they are soaked).
- Almonds, pepitas (pumpkin seeds) and sunflower seeds tossed with a small quantity of Tamari sauce in a frying pan.
- Air-popped popcorn.
- Home-made wedges served with guacamole and salsa (recipes included in this book).
- Guacamole and salsa served with plain salted corn chips.
- Salted, dried chickpeas (these are cooked and then dried in the oven with salt).
- Boiled eggs with a little home made chutney.

Platter ideas
- Dips on a platter with crackers, cherry tomatoes and vegetable sticks.
- Anti-pasta platters including olives, marinated vegetables such as semi-dried tomatoes, boiled eggs and artichokes with crackers or wholemeal breads.
- A platter of nuts, popcorn, cherry tomatoes, boiled eggs, cheese and vegetable spaghetti (made using a spiral vegetable slicer).

Rice Paper Spring Rolls

Rice paper rolls are as versatile as children's taste buds. Following is a list of suggested ingredients. There are no quantities, as making a rice paper roll is akin to making a sandwich. Choose your fillings and go for it! I don't suggest using all the ones I have listed, in fact doing this would make for too big a roll! Choose a tasty combination and try varying the ingredients which will in turn, train the taste buds. The only ingredient common to all rolls is the rice noodles. Also if you decide not to use the marinated tofu, I suggest a dash of Soy, Tamari or Teriyaki sauce to add flavour.

carrot, thinly julienned or peeled into strips
rice vermicelli or stick noodles (prepared according to directions on the packet and chopped)
cucumber, thinly sliced or peeled into strips
slices of marinated tofu cut into strips
avocado, thinly sliced
salad greens (snow pea sprouts, lettuce or rocket leaves)
fresh beetroot, grated
pickled ginger - finely sliced
snow peas - finely sliced
fresh mint leaves
fresh coriander leaves
capsicum, thinly sliced
rice spring roll sheets

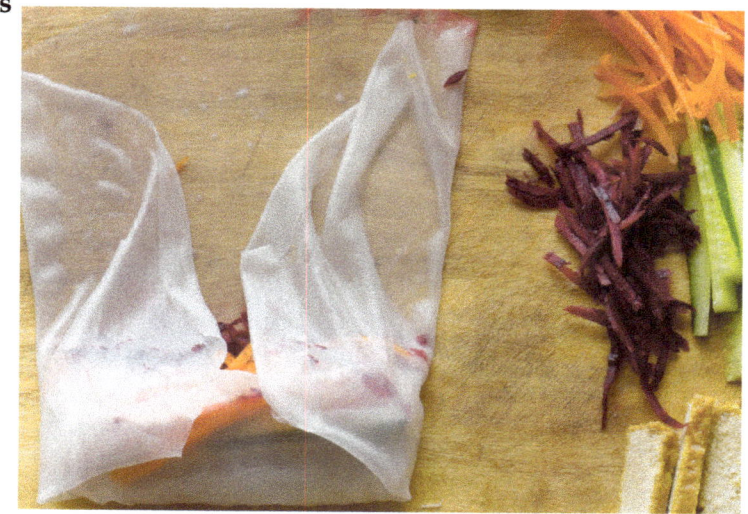

1. To prepare the roll, you first need to soften your dried rice sheet. Don't worry, it isn't hard. Put some water onto a dinner plate and submerge your sheet into it. Wait until it is soft and flexible like a big cooked noodle, then remove from the water and lay out on a plate or chopping board.
2. When filling your roll, be careful not to overdo it. Remember that it needs to be rolled and wrapped. Place a small amount of noodles to one side of the middle of the sheet and small amounts of other fillings on top.
3. Now roll the rice wrapper over the top and fold the sides over. Keep rolling until you have a neat little parcel. At first they will seem a bit delicate but after they have sat for a few minutes the wrappers will regain some of their toughness and be easy for little hands to hold. Of course these are yummy for big mouths too!

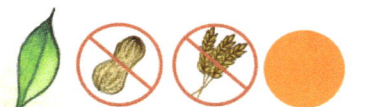

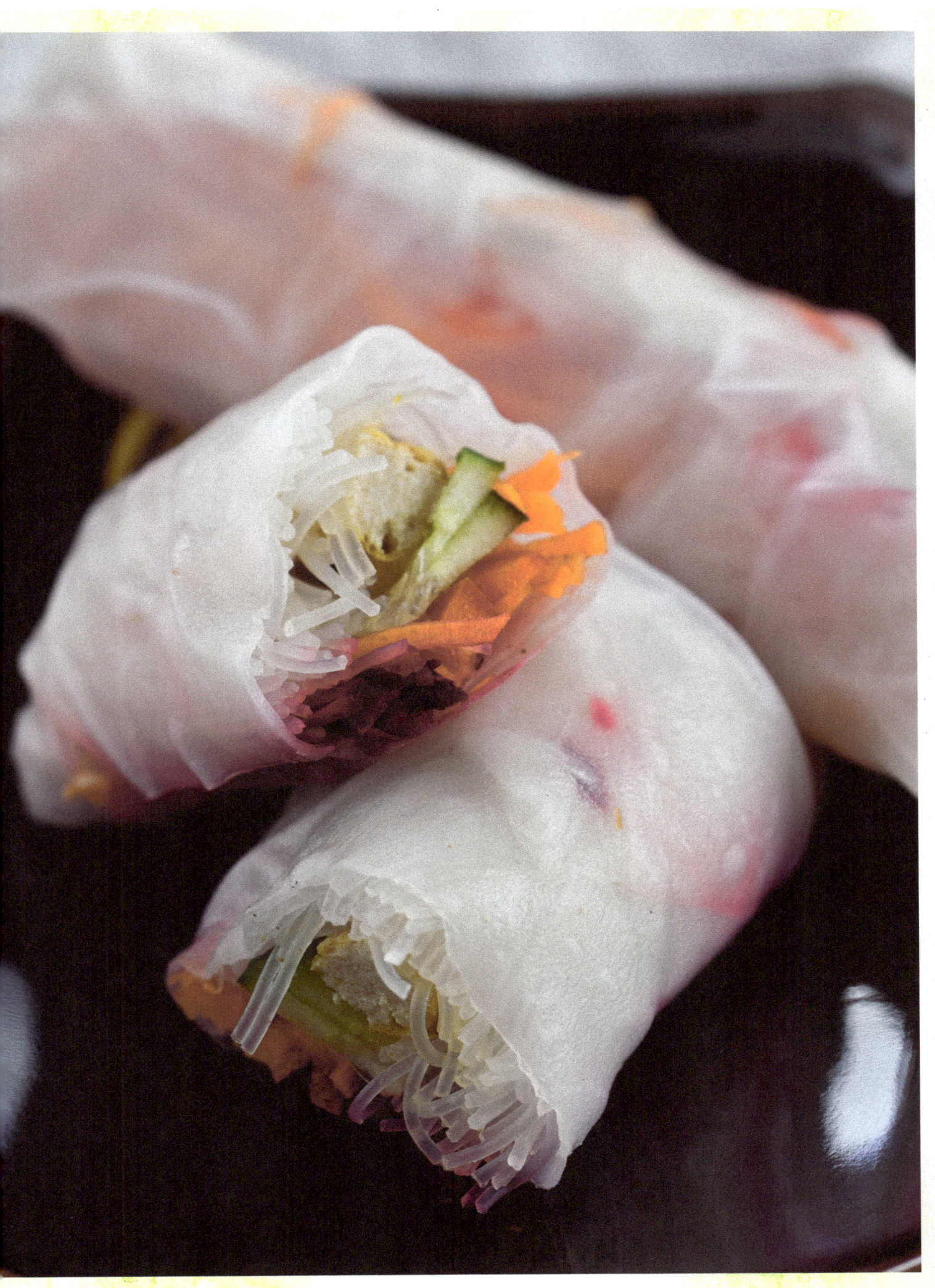

Never-lasting Nori Rolls

Like rice paper rolls, nori rolls are very versatile. You can vary your fillings just as you would a sandwich, providing a great variety of taste and nutrition. The task of rolling them may seem daunting at first, but once you get the hang of it, you will find it as easy as making a sandwich. In this recipe I have used brown rice, as it is more nutritious than white rice. Traditionally, white sushi rice is used.

quantity of brown rice (1 cup uncooked brown rice will make 6 rolls)
1 tablespoon of rice wine vinegar (Japanese seasoning) per 1 cup uncooked rice
sheets of nori

Choice of fillings. Pick from any of the following sliced ingredients

- **marinated tofu**
- **capsicum**
- **sprouts**
- **lettuce**
- **egg (boiled or slices of thin omelette)**
- **avocado**
- **cucumber**
- **pickled ginger**
- **beetroot (freshly grated or sliced, cooked)**
- **sun-dried or semi-dried tomatoes**

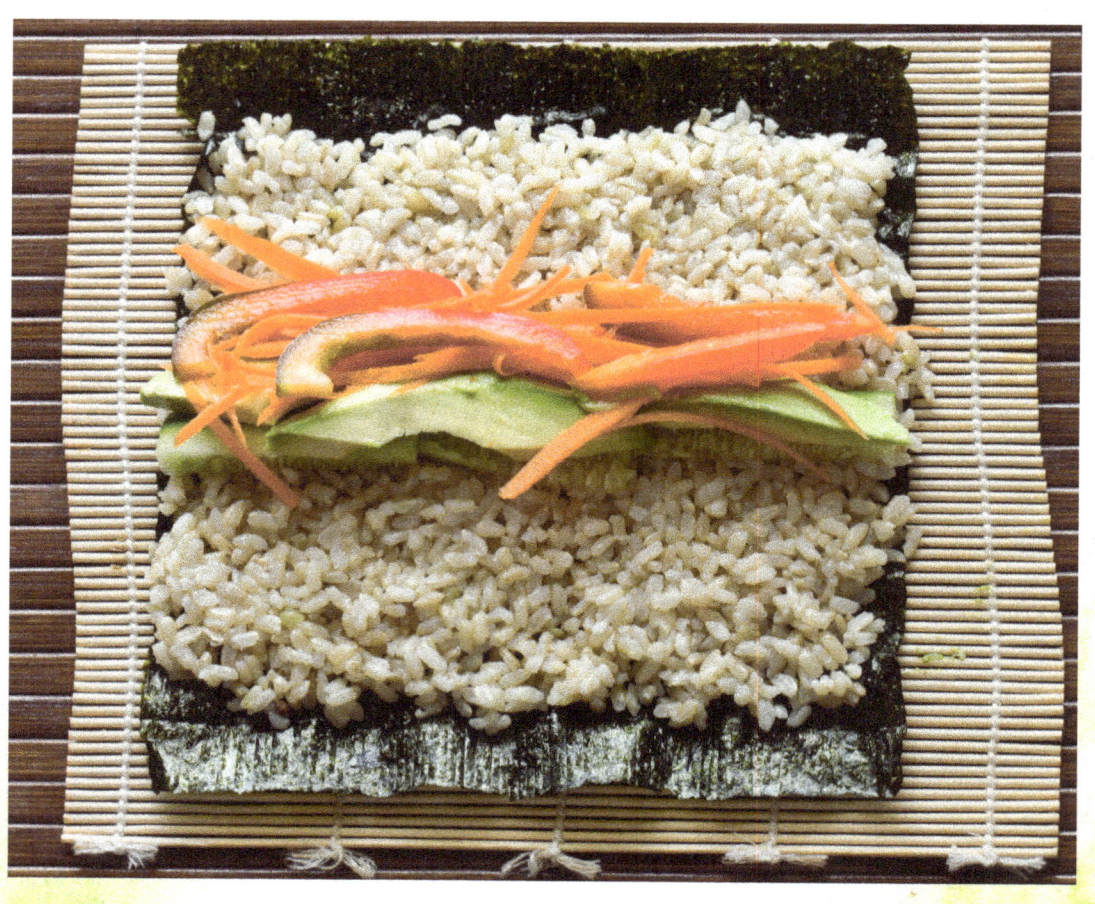

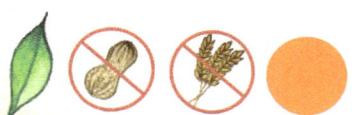

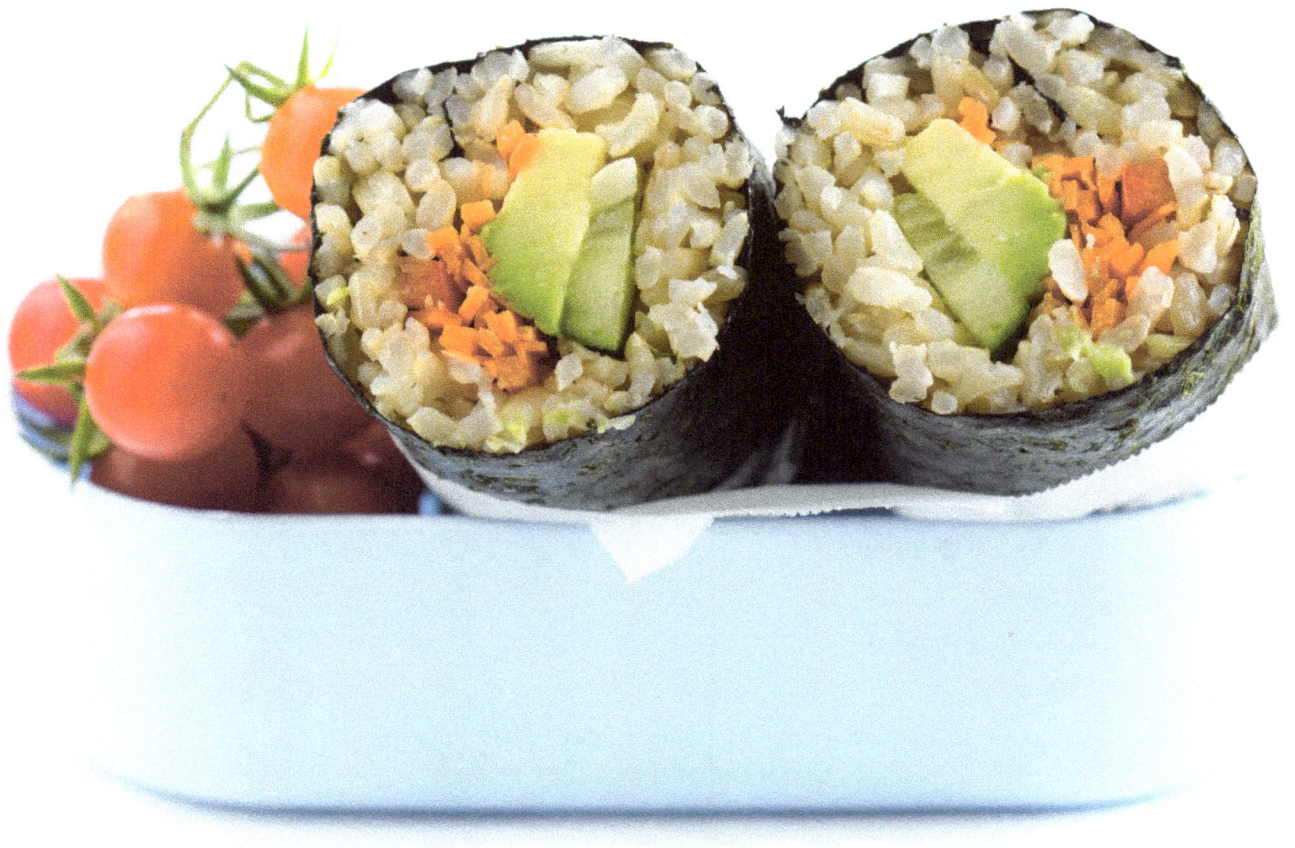

1. Cook brown rice according to instructions on page 68. However add just a little more water as you need the rice to be slightly sticky.
2. When the rice is cooked, stir the vinegar through and leave with lid on to cool.
3. Lay a nori sheet on either a sushi rolling mat or a flat surface. I don't use the mats as I find it easy enough to roll the nori without it. However I have provided a picture to the left of what it would look like using a mat.
4. Distribute a thin layer of rice as shown in the picture and lay your toppings across the centre.
5. Wet the edge furthest away from you and then roll the whole thing, supporting the middle as you go. It may be tricky at first, but keep practicing, as you will get the hang of it. It may be helpful to see the process demonstrated on Youtube.
6. Cut the long roll in half with a serrated knife and wrap one end in bakers paper or plastic to provide support while the rolls are being eaten.

These are a great school lunch. Just remember to put a little ice brick in with them to keep them fresh.

Not-Sausage Rolls with a Twist

In my first cookbook, Wild Vegan, I created a sausage roll recipe without meat.
This one is a gourmet version with the added flavours of herbs, Parmesan and lemon.
Makes 30 mini rolls

Filling

3 cups of hydrated TVP or a 300g bag of Quorn mince
⅓ cup of finely chopped parsley
1 tablespoon of fresh thyme leaves
¾ cup of peas, mashed
½ red onion, very finely chopped
2 garlic cloves, crushed
finely grated zest of one lemon
1 egg, lightly beaten
½ cup of grated Parmesan cheese (those avoiding dairy, see "Play Time" notes)

3 sheets frozen puff pastry
1 egg lightly beaten to glaze, or your choice of milk
sesame seeds to sprinkle on top

1. Preheat oven to 180°C convection or 160°C fan forced. Line a baking tray with baking paper.
2. Place all of the filling ingredients into a mixing bowl and mix well.
3. Cut pastry sheets in half and lay a generous amount of mixture down one side, leaving a 1-2cm edge. Press the mixture together into a sausage shape and roll the pastry over to encase it.
4. Lay out on trays and brush with beaten egg or milk and then sprinkle with sesame seeds.
5. Cut into mini rolls. It is easier to separate them after they are cooked.
6. Bake for 25-30 minutes until pastry is golden. Separate the rolls with a knife and serve warm with home made tomato sauce (the recipe for this is on the page opposite).

Play Time!

- Those avoiding dairy can leave out the Parmesan and add ½ teaspoon of sea salt.
- Try other seeds on top such as poppy, caraway or fennel.
- Vary the herbs you use: basil, sage, oregano, dill or marjoram.

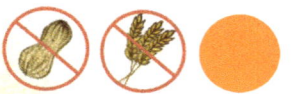

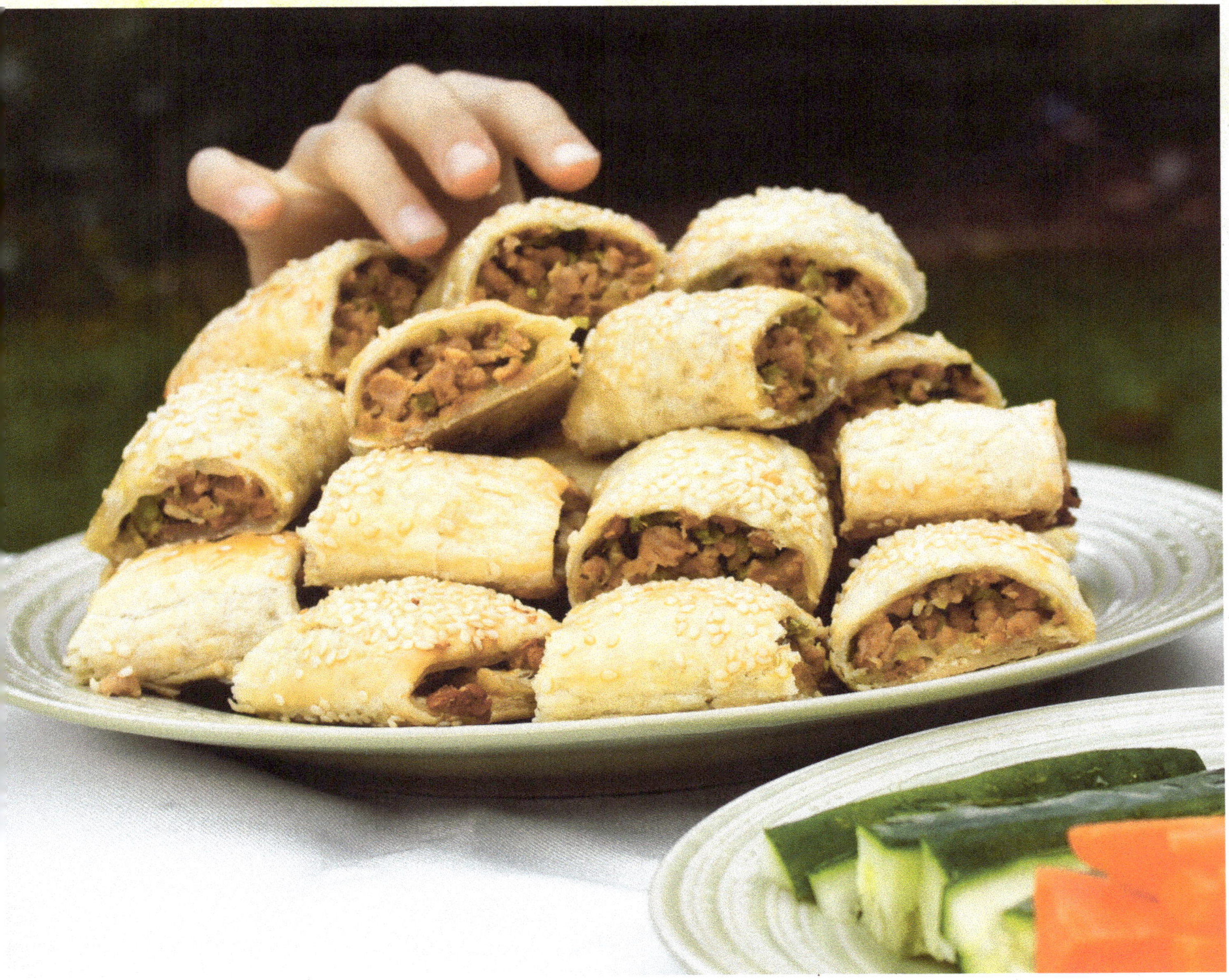

Better 'n' Bought Tomato Sauce

*Why buy tomato sauce when you can make your own?
Wait until tomatoes are in season and make up a big batch.*

1 large red onion, peeled and chopped
3 cloves garlic, roughly chopped
1 tablespoon of paprika (sweet or smoked)
1 teaspoon freshly ground peppercorns

2kg fresh tomatoes, roughly chopped
50g rapadura sugar
150ml apple cider vinegar
1 teaspoon of sea salt

1. Put all ingredients into a large saucepan, mix well and bring to the boil.
2. Reduce heat and simmer for half an hour, uncovered to reduce the sauce down. The longer you leave it, the thicker the sauce will be.
3. Leave to cool and then puree in a food processor.
4. Store in sterilised jars. If you don't want to deal with sterilising, this sauce will keep well in the freezer.

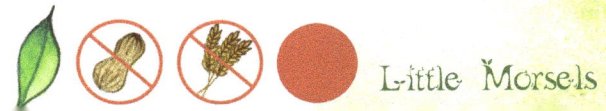

Golden Corn Cakes

The quinoa and besan flour in this recipe provide protein, making these little treasures a hearty meal. I serve them with a salad or Beautiful Brassicas (page 136).

Makes 17 cakes

500g pumpkin, peeled and chopped
2 cups of corn kernels (fresh or frozen)
½ cup of quinoa
1 cup of water (for cooking the quinoa)
2 teaspoons of mild curry powder
1 green chilli, seeded and chopped (optional)
1 cup of besan (chickpea) flour
½ teaspoon of sea salt
pepper to season
¼ cup of finely chopped coriander
oil for pan frying

1. Steam pumpkin and corn (if fresh) until both are soft. The pumpkin will need longer than the corn.
2. Meanwhile, place quinoa and water into a small saucepan and cover. Bring to the boil and then turn down to a simmer until the quinoa has absorbed most of the water. Leave to stand for 10 minutes to absorb remaining water.
3. Mash the pumpkin. It doesn't matter if the corn and pumpkin are together, the corn will withstand the masher.
4. Add the remaining ingredients to the pumpkin and mix well. The mixture will be quite wet. Don't worry it will firm up during the cooking.
5. With wet hands, shape mix into patties and pan fry until golden on both sides.
6. Serve with your choice of vegetables or salad. In this picture, they are also served with "Better 'n' Bought Tomato Sauce": recipe on the previous page.

Play Time!

- You can vary the flavour in this recipe by adding different herbs, a little curry paste (Thai or Indian) or by using sweet potato instead of pumpkin.
- Use half peas, half corn to add greens.

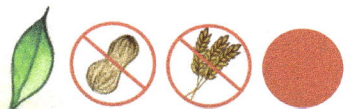

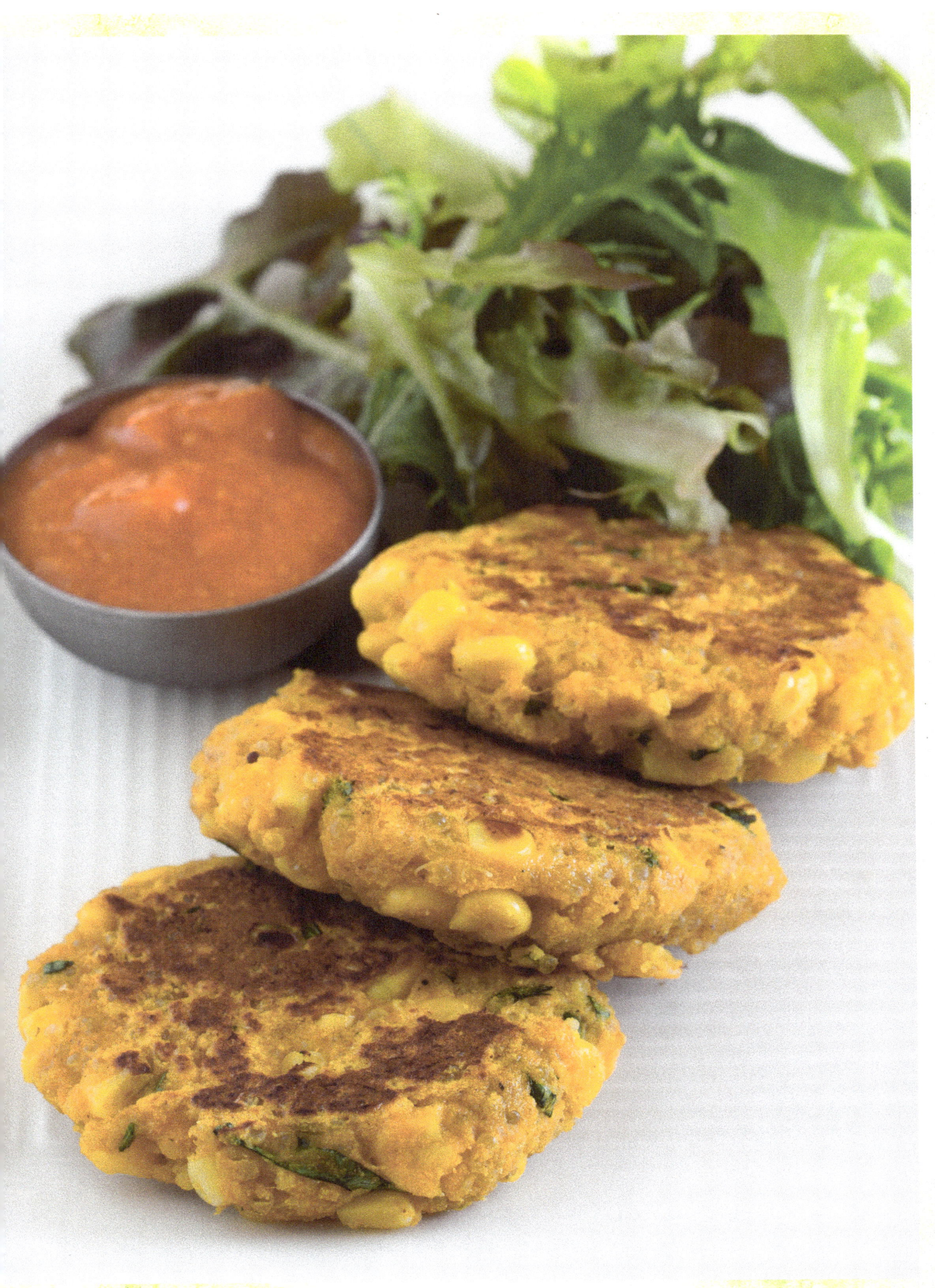

Greek Beanies

This is a very quick and flavoursome recipe. Beanies are great served with Slow Roasted Tomatoes (recipe on page 130), a green salad and Tzatziki (recipe below). Children may assist by mixing, shaping Beanies and flipping them in the frying pan.

Makes 17 Beanies

1 cup of dried cannelini beans, (soaked for at least 6 hours) or 2 ½ cups of cooked

150g feta cheese

an adult handful of each: chives, dill and mint

1 clove of garlic

1 small zucchini, grated

½ cup of besan (chickpea) flour

1 beaten egg

oil for pan frying

1. If using dried beans, drain and cook according to directions on page 64.
2. Put soft beans into a mixing bowl and mash lightly with a fork.
3. In a food processor, pulse feta cheese and add to the bowl.
4. Place herbs and garlic into the food processor and blend until finely chopped. Add to the bowl.
5. Add besan flour and egg and mix well.
6. Heat a large frying pan and coat the bottom in oil.
7. Form mix into patties and pan fry until golden on both sides.
8. Serve with Tzatziki and your choice of vegetables or salad.

Tzatziki

A very easy to make accompaniment. It is also great as a dip.

1 cup plain, pot set yoghurt

1 small clove crushed garlic

1 small Lebanese cucumber, peeled, seeded and grated

2 teaspoons of lemon juice

pepper and sea salt to season

1. Gently mix all ingredients in a bowl.
2. Set aside for half an hour before serving to allow flavours to develop.

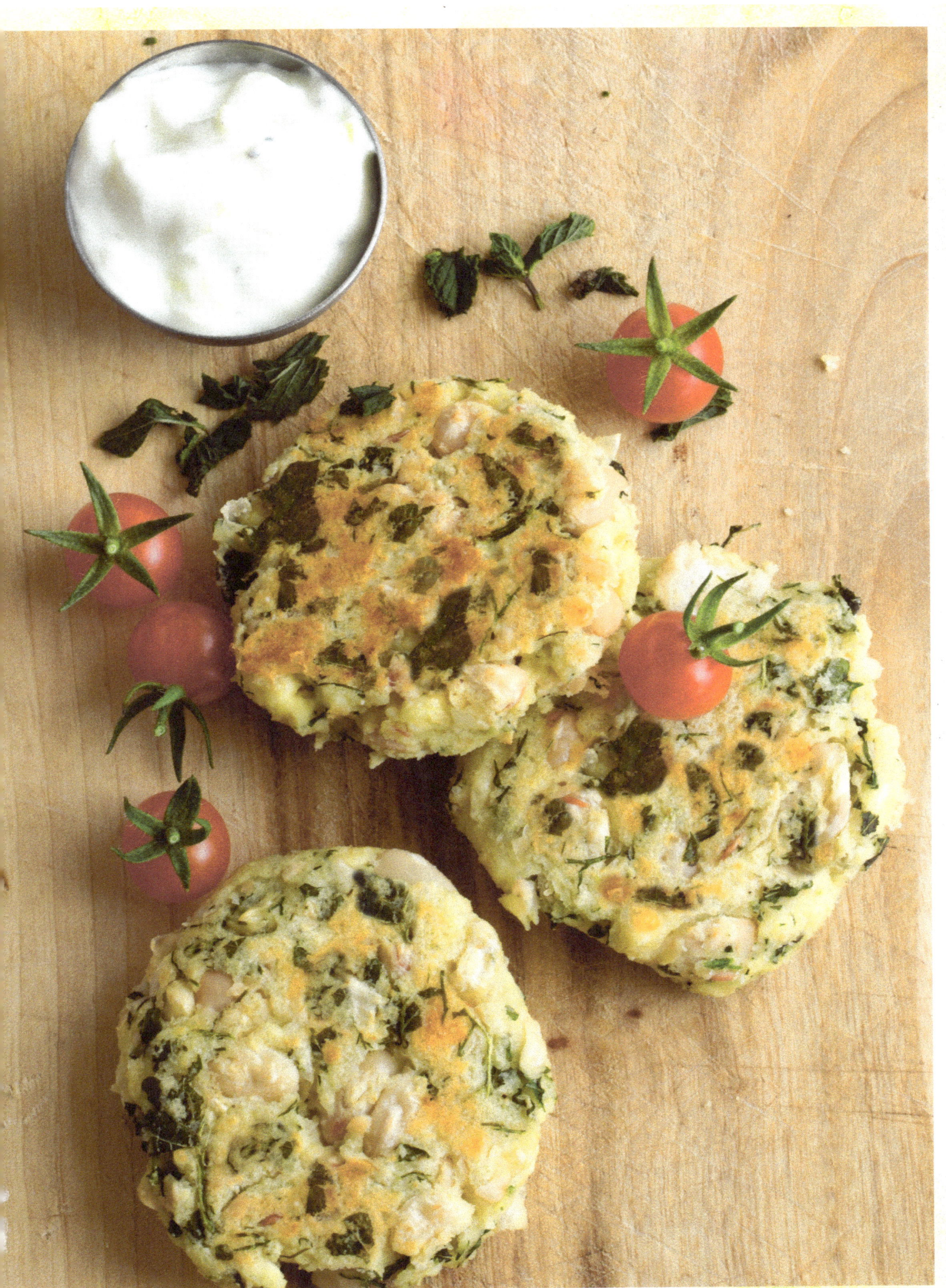

Nutty Chick-a-pea Burgers

These burgers are very quick to whip up if you do all of your chopping in a food processor. They are full of protein, vegetables and flavour. I either serve them on a bun with salad or with a rice and green salad for dinner. They are pictured here with flowering coriander and an edible nasturtium flower. Children can assist with the mixing, shaping and even flipping of the burgers in the pan.

1 ¼ cups dried chickpeas, (soaked for at least 10 hours) or 3 cups of cooked chickpeas
½ cup of natural peanut butter (at room temperature so it is a little runny)
2 cloves of crushed garlic
1 red onion, finely chopped
1 small bunch coriander
200g grated pumpkin
1 medium-sized zucchini, grated
3 tablespoons of Tamari or soy sauce
½ cup of besan (chickpea) flour
oil for pan frying

1. If you are using dried chickpeas, cook according to directions on page 64.
2. In a food processor, pulse the chickpeas and peanut butter. If you do not have one, mash them together with a potato masher. This will ensure that the peanut butter is spread evenly through the burger mix.
3. Add to large mixing bowl with remaining ingredients and mix well.
4. Form into patties and pan fry on both sides until golden brown.
5. Serve with your choice of vegetables or salad.

Play Time!

- Try using different vegetables in these. As long as they are grated or pulverised in a food processor, they will mix in well. The only vegetable I would specifically avoid is potato, as there is not enough cooking time and it would make the burger too starchy.
- Other herbs also work well. Try Thai basil, dill or parsley.

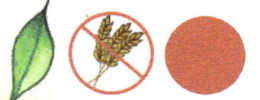

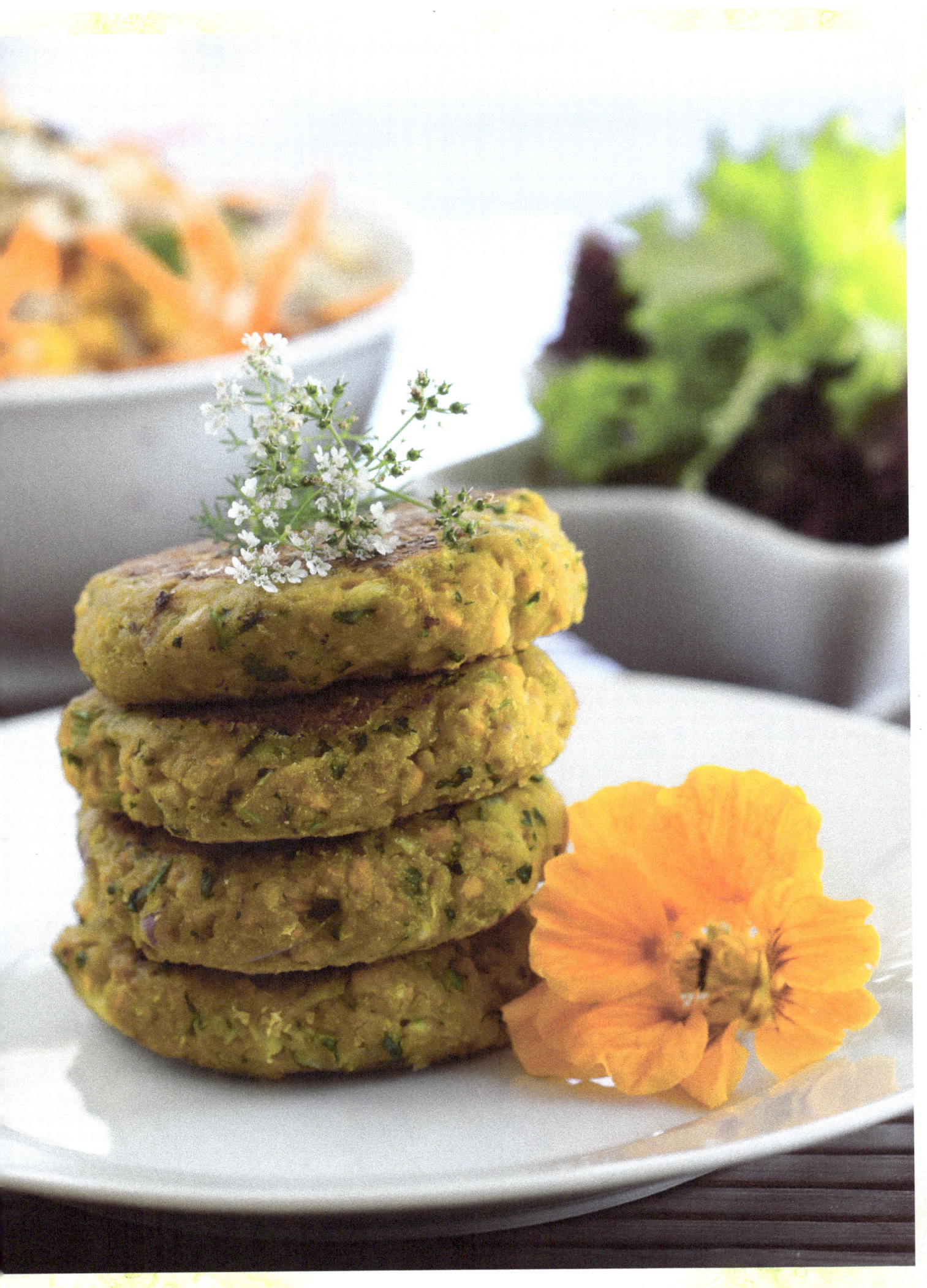

Little Morsels

Garden Burgers

These burgers take a bit longer to prepare than some of the others, but their flavour makes them worth it. Also if you make up a big batch, you can freeze them for another time. They will be a little soft in the frying pan, but leave them on a cooling rack for a few minutes and they will firm up. Children may assist by mixing and shaping the patties. Those who are more confident may enjoy flipping them in the pan as well.

Makes 15 burgers

750g mixed potatoes and sweet potatoes
1 cup of puy lentils, soaked for at least 6 hours
1 tablespoon of oil
1 red onion, finely chopped
1 large clove garlic, crushed
1 medium-sized carrot, grated
1 small zucchini, grated
1 teaspoon of sea salt
¼ cup of finely chopped dill leaves
½ cup of brown rice flour
oil for pan frying

1. Peel and chop the potatoes and steam until very soft.
2. Meanwhile, drain lentils and place into a saucepan with enough water to cover 2cm above them.
3. Bring lentils to boil, then turn down to simmer and cook for 20 minutes, or until they are tender, even mushy. Drain and cool.
4. Mash the potatoes with a potato masher in a large mixing bowl.
5. In a small saucepan, fry onion and garlic in the oil and stir over medium heat until tender.
6. Add the onion mix with all other ingredients, including cooled lentils to the potato mixture.
7. Form into balls and pan fry until brown and crispy on both sides.
8. Leave on a wire rack to firm up before serving. (This takes only a few minutes: you may wish to leave them in a warm oven so that you can serve them hot).

Play Time!

- Try besan flour in these burgers if you are out of rice flour.
- Use other herbs to flavour them such as coriander, parsley, sage or thyme.
- Add some curry paste/powder or spices such as paprika, cumin, garam masala.
- For a more European flavor add some chopped semi-dried tomatoes and basil.

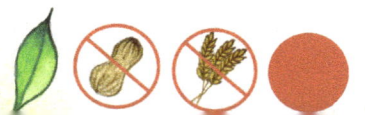

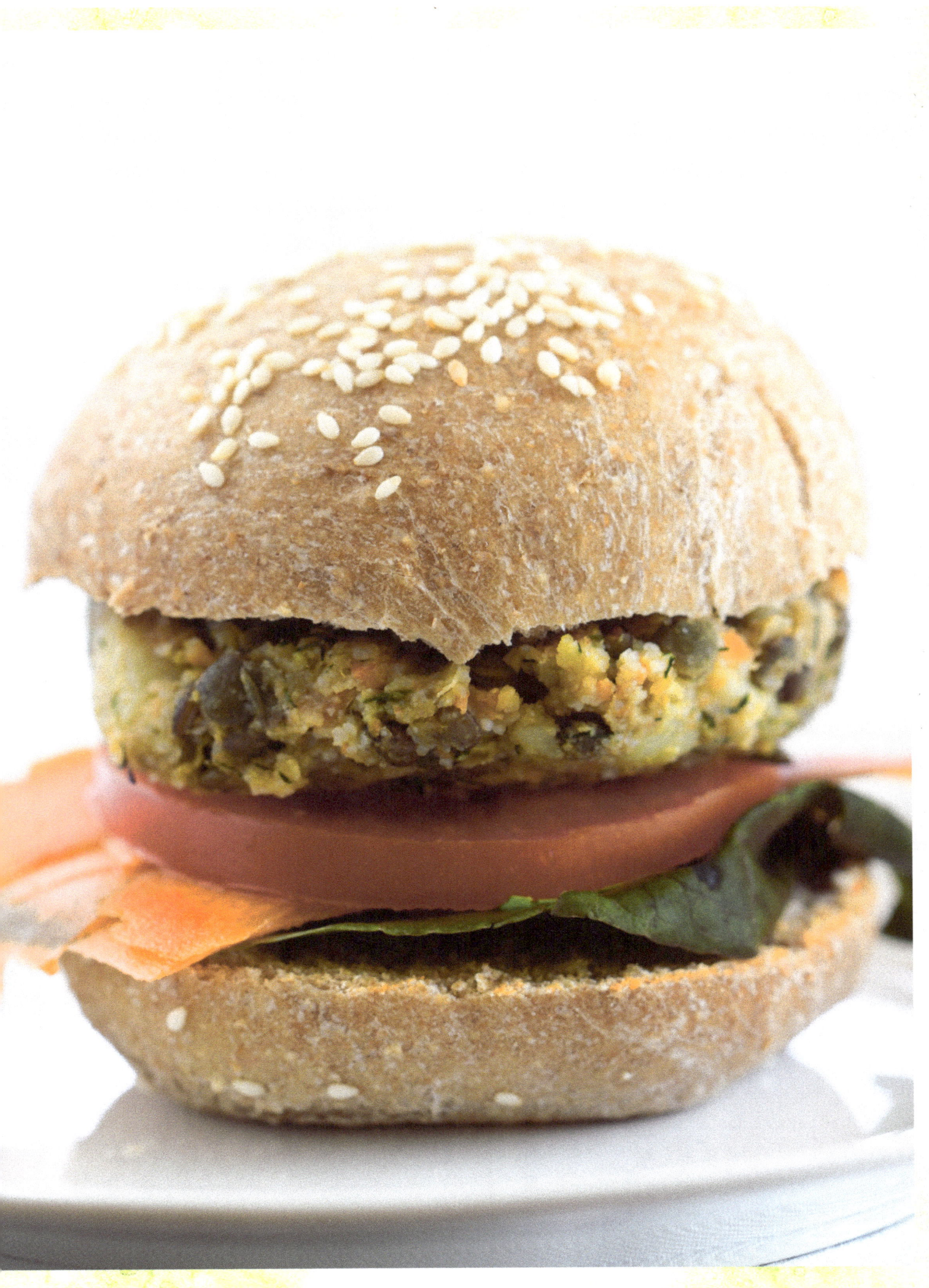

Mini Quiches

These make a delicious school lunch or even a snack for mum and dad (you may need two for a meal). I add a few sticks of salad vegetables to one of these for my kids' lunch boxes and they love them. They freeze really well too, so you can make a big batch and benefit for many days to come. I make my pastry from scratch, but there is no reason why you cannot use bought pastry for those times when you are not in the mood to make your own. On the other hand, children love to roll pastry and make the cases.

Makes 16 muffin-sized quiches

Wholemeal pastry
3 cups of wholemeal wheat or spelt flour
½ teaspoon of sea salt
125g cold, unsalted butter, cut into cubes
1 large egg
approximately 4 tablespoons of cold water (please read through the method to clarify)

Filling
5 eggs
100g semi-dried tomatoes, finely chopped
1 small or ½ large red capsicum, finely chopped
handful of basil leaves, finely chopped
½ cup of grated cheese (optional)
8 fresh cherry tomatoes, halved
sweet or smoked paprika (optional)

1. To make the pastry, pulse flour, salt and butter in a food processor until it resembles bread crumbs.
2. Add egg and pulse until it comes together. Different flours absorb more or less water depending on their coarseness and age. Different eggs will also contribute a different level of moisture to your mix. As pastry needs to be a particular consistency (i.e. not sticky but not dry) add cold water, 1 tablespoon at a time until the mixture comes together into a ball.
3. Form pastry into a thick disc shape and cover in plastic wrap. Refrigerate for 30 minutes. Careful not to leave it in for too much longer or you will end up with a rock that is almost impossible to roll out.
4. I use a standard sized muffin tin to make my quiches, but you could use individual tart cases as well. To prepare the muffin tin, I cut squares of baking paper and use these like a muffin case. I find that the quiches stick otherwise and it is a nice alternative to heavily greasing the compartments. Makes for easier washing up too!

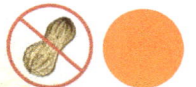

5. Preheat the oven to 180°C convection or 160°C fan-forced.
6. Roll the pastry out to about 3mm thick and cut a shape that resembles the area you will need. The great thing about this recipe is that the pastry is very easy to handle. You can fix tears and breaks easily by pressing the pastry together or adding small pieces.
7. Once your shells are ready, bake in the preheated oven for 15 minutes. While they are in the oven, prepare your filling.
8. In a medium-sized mixing bowl, beat the eggs until well combined.
9. Add the semi-dried tomatoes, capsicum, basil and cheese. Mix well.
10. Pour filling into each of the pastry cases and add a half cherry tomato to the top: seed side up. If you are using paprika, sprinkle lightly over the quiches.
11. Bake in the oven for 20-25 minutes or until the eggs are browned on top and firm to touch.

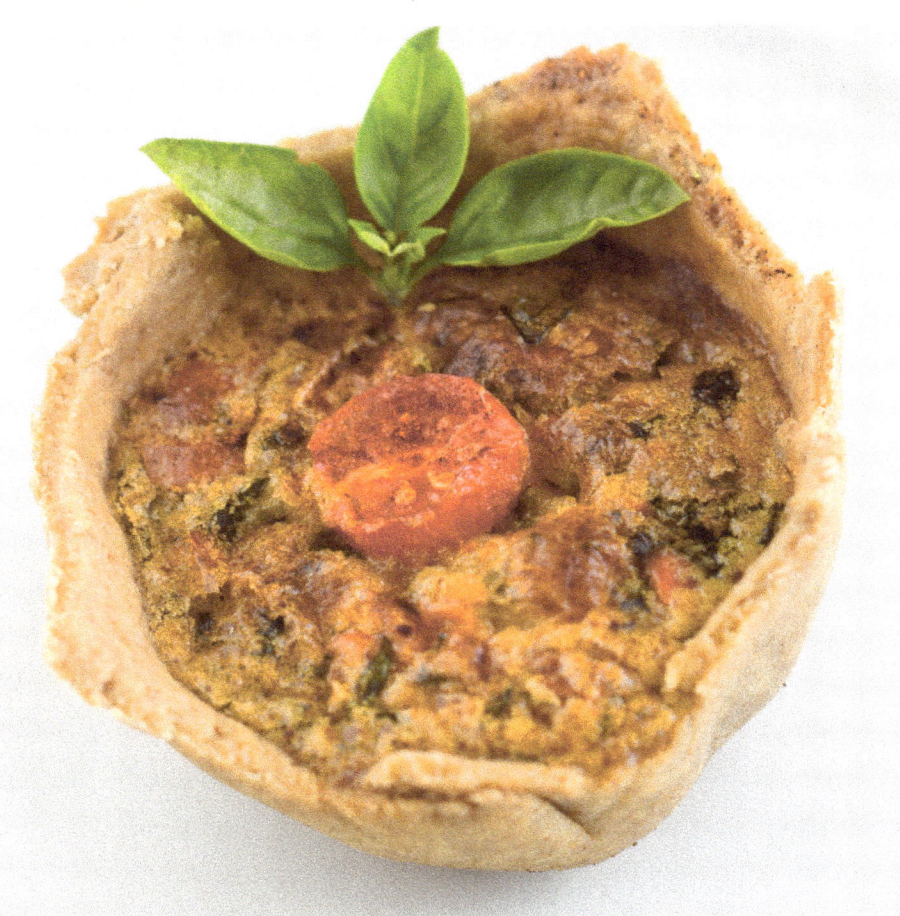

Play Time!

- Try adding other vegetables to the filling mix such as sliced, roasted pumpkin, sweet potato or chopped, steamed broccoli and cauliflower. Come up with your own favourite flavours!
- Try other herbs such as dill, parsley, sage or thyme.

Kids Eating Green!

- **Green Beginnings**: One of the easiest ways to have your child eat greens is to put them into their food right from the start and to continue as they grow. Of course many children go through phases where they decide they don't like certain foods or they are going to refuse anything healthy. Please see the information in the "Roots of Health" chapter on suggestions for getting through these periods (page 279).

- **Education**: It is important to educate your children about food from a very young age. Don't rely on school to do this for you: it is often a case of too little too late and many schools do not have a focus on nutrition. Just look at what has been available during recent years in the canteens! Education doesn't have to be boring either, it is a gradual process of letting a child know what is good fuel for their body and what is not. Which foods will give them strong muscles and make them grow taller, and which will make their bodies weak and more likely to get sick. If a child understands that the food they put into their bodies will make them feel good and grow up to be big strong adults, this will then have an impact on their choices. In terms of greens, there are so many varieties that provide many nutrients. Do some research and adapt what you find into a language your child will understand. We must sell the benefits to our children much the way a salesperson would sell a product to you in a shop. Make greens sound exciting and important as they are the "Super Heroes" of the vegetable kingdom.

- **Complementing Greens**: Make greens a part of another dish, chop into small pieces and include them in a saucy recipe such as a casserole or curry. This way the flavour of the sauce will complement the green and it gets a child used to the idea of eating greens.

- **Hide-and-Seek Greens**: For the really fussy child, you may at first need to puree the green and then add it to your dish. You may even need to disguise the colour by putting it into a darker sauce. This is not a long term solution however. The ultimate goal is for the child to eat greens without any protest.

- Taste Bud Training: Pick one particular green and give the child a small piece each night. It is only necessary that they eat that small piece. You may need to introduce a reward system for this (preferably not a sweet treat). After time, your child's palette will adapt to the new food. Explain to your child how the palette works (see Taste Bud Training on page 26).

- **Dressing Greens Up**: When it comes to raw leafy greens in a salad, I have found dressings to be the key. Make a dressing your child loves: get them to help you make it, maybe even allowing them to create their own concoction (scary I know). This dressing can only be eaten with a salad which includes leafy greens. I have found this encourages my children to eat foods such as rocket, English spinach and mesculin mix salads.

- **Grow your own greens**: They are so easy to grow and if your child is involved in the growing they are often more inclined to eat the food. My youngest son, Ryan was delighted to eat our first home grown harvest of lettuce when he was 3 years old after having flatly refused to put a raw leafy green near his mouth previously.

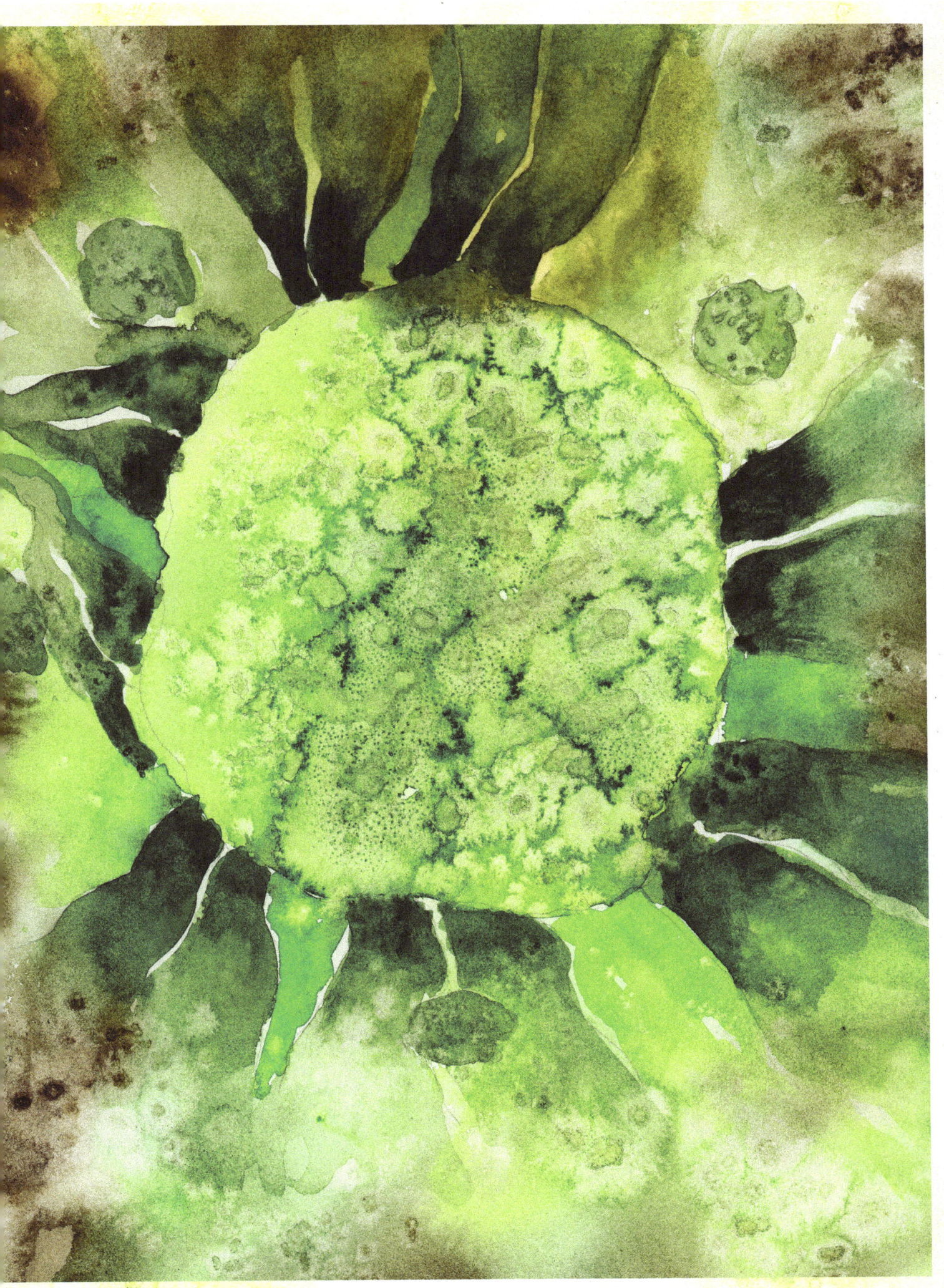

Little Morsels

Slow Roasted Tomatoes

These are heaven! There is nothing more I can say...
Serves 4-5 as a side

- 5 large, ripe tomatoes
- 1 clove garlic, finely sliced
- 1 tablespoon of rapadura sugar
- freshly ground, black pepper
- ¼ of a teaspoon of sea salt
- 1 tablespoon of balsamic vinegar
- few leaves of basil, torn

1. Preheat oven to 150°C convection which is the preferable setting. Otherwise, 140°C fan-forced.
2. Slice tomatoes in half and lay seeded side up on a lined baking tray.
3. Place a slice of garlic on each tomato.
4. Combine remaining ingredients, (except basil) in a small bowl and drizzle over each tomato.
5. Place in the oven and bake for 1-1.5 hours. Larger tomatoes will need longer.
6. Garnish with basil leaves and serve warm or at room temperature.

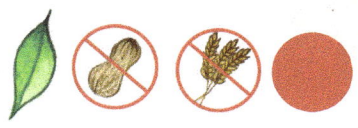

Garlicky Beans

This is a delicious side dish. I serve it with Greek Beanies (page 120) or rice and a salad. It tastes best when the beans are tender.
Serves 4-5 as a side

- 1 onion, finely chopped
- 1 tablespoon of oil
- 5 cloves garlic, crushed
- 450g trimmed, chopped green beans
- 450g tomatoes, diced
- ¼ teaspoon of cinnamon
- ¼ teaspoon of fresh pepper
- pinch of allspice
- 1 tablespoon of olive oil (to be added after cooking)
- 1 teaspoon of sea salt

1. In a medium-sized saucepan, cook the onion in the oil until tender.
2. Add the garlic and beans and stir over low heat. Place lid on the pan and leave them to sweat for 10 minutes, stirring occasionally.
3. Add tomatoes, cinnamon, pepper and allspice. Mix well and cook with the lid on for a further 10 minutes, until beans are tender.
4. Remove from heat and stir in the olive oil and salt.

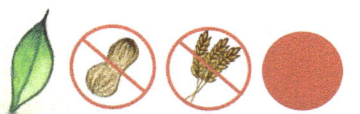

Little Morsels

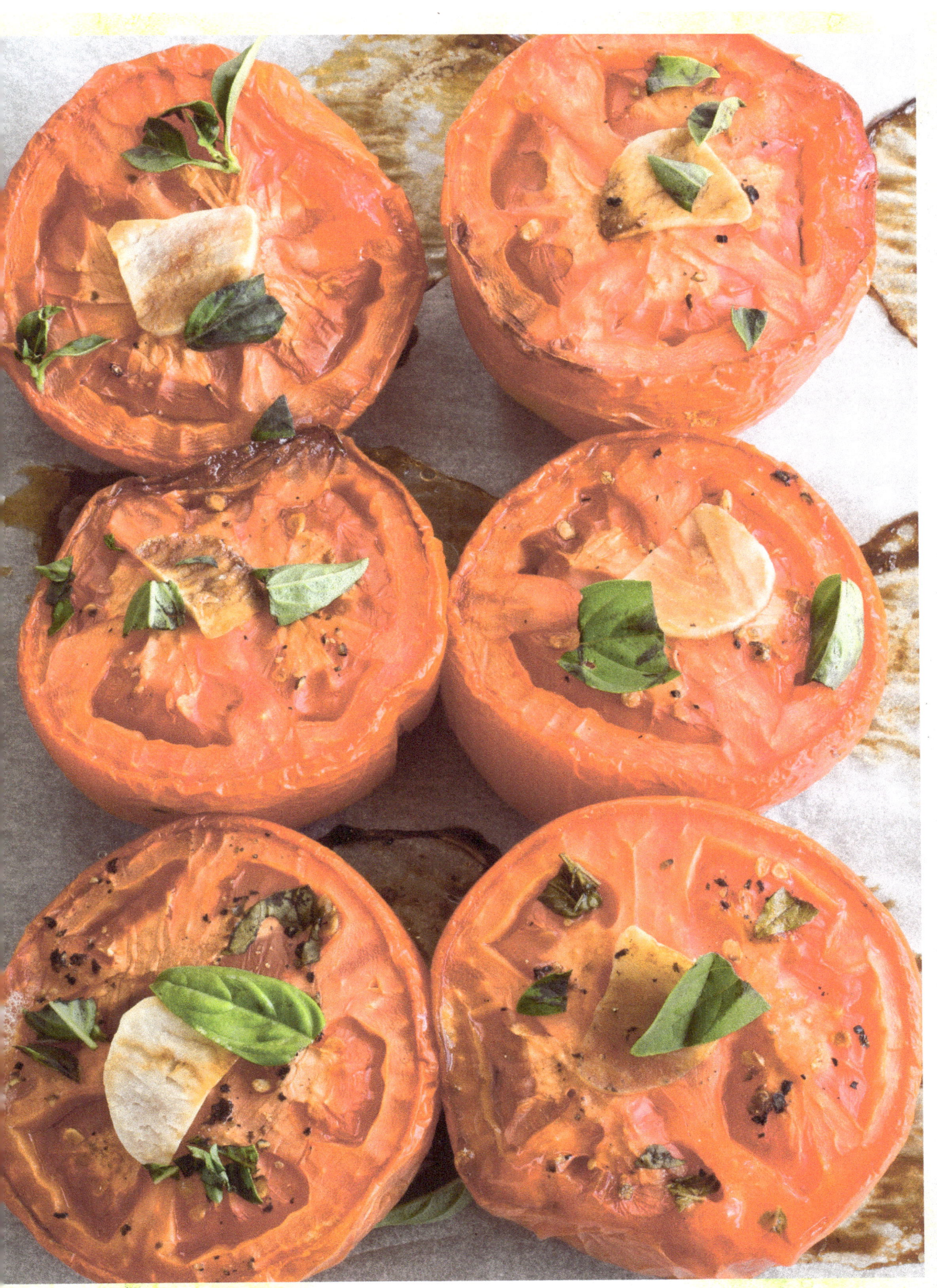

Maple glazed Treasures

You may use any root or hard vegetables for this dish such as swede, parsnip, beetroot etc. I have chosen the ones most readily available. Children may assist by whisking the flavours and tossing with the vegetables. Of course they may need to taste test as well.

Serves 4-5 as a side

1.2 kg cubed, peeled, potatoes, sweet potatoes and pumpkin
3 tablespoons of oil
⅓ cup of pure maple syrup
2 garlic cloves, crushed
1 ½ tablespoons chopped fresh rosemary
1 teaspoon sea salt
½ teaspoon freshly ground black pepper

1. Line a baking dish with grease proof paper.
2. Preheat the oven to 180°C convection or 160°C fan-forced.
3. Combine your vegetables in a large bowl.
4. Whisk remaining ingredients in a small bowl.
5. Add to vegetables and toss to coat.
6. Transfer mixture to prepared baking dish and bake for 40-45 minutes.

Play Time!

- If you don't have maple syrup, honey works well as a substitute.
- Grated ginger is a nice addition to this dish, especially if you are using the honey.
- If you don't mind a bit of spice, add a finely chopped chilli.

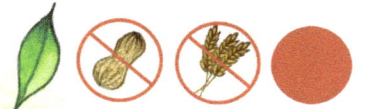

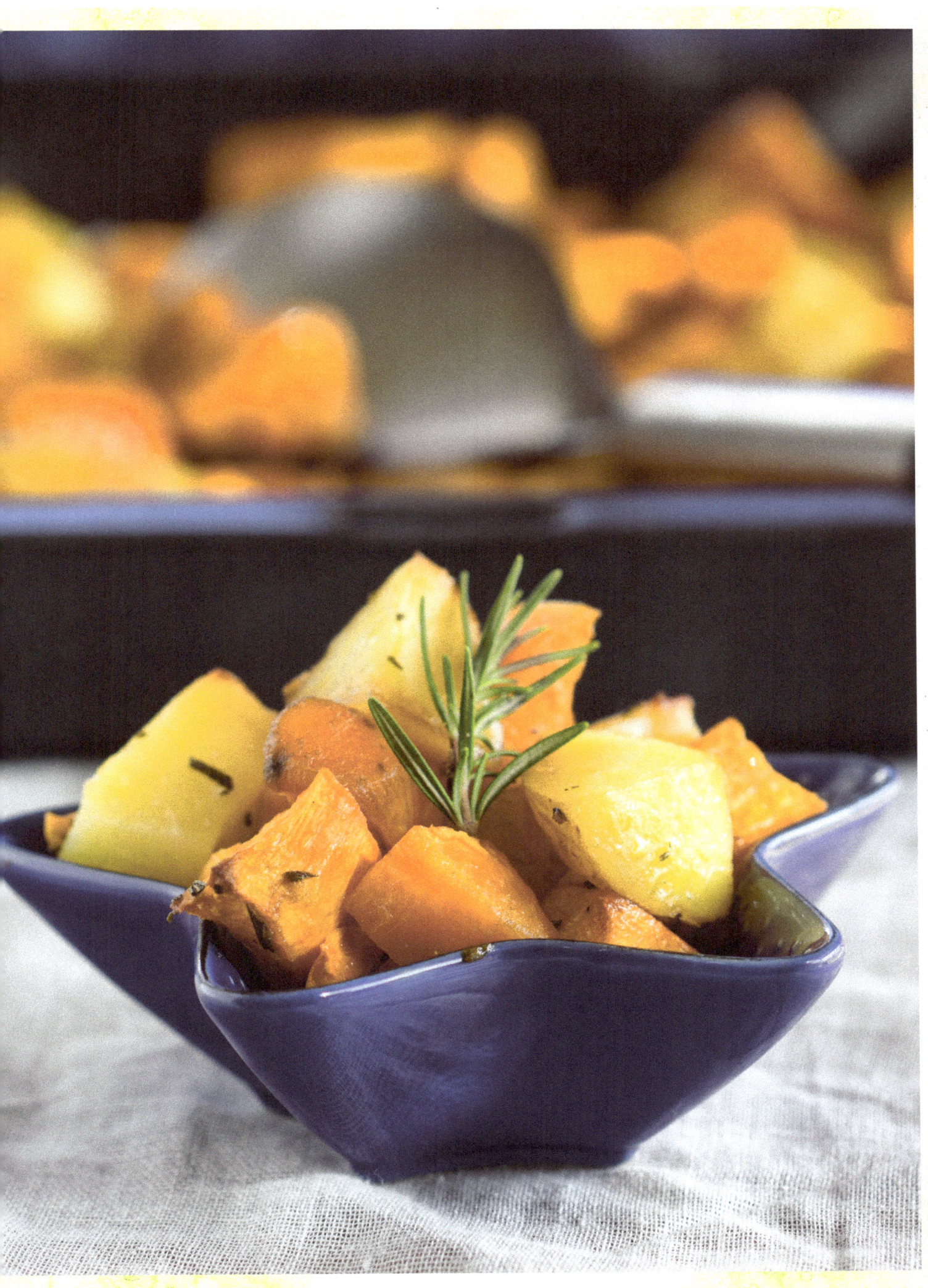

Honeyed Carrots

These are so yummy! Tarragon is one of those herbs that grows really easily, but which people often don't know what to do with. Here, it does a nice job of complementing the carrots and honey.

Serves 4-5 as a side

400g carrots, sliced
½ tablespoon of butter
2 tablespoons of honey
2 tablespoons of water
1 tablespoon of finely chopped tarragon

1. Place all ingredients into a small saucepan.
2. Cover and simmer over low heat for 10-15 minutes. The time will depend on how you like your carrots. Serve with a slotted spoon.

Play Time!

- Add other vegetables to this dish: greens such as broccoli and asparagus or cauliflower.
- Add some crushed garlic and grated ginger.
- Add a tablespoon of soy or Tamari sauce to introduce an Asian flavour.

Rose-Married Potatoes

Rosemary, garlic, salt and potato: what a great relationship these foods have and here they are in their shining glory!

Serves 4-5 as a side

1kg mixed potatoes and sweet potatoes
3 stems of fresh rosemary, leaves finely chopped
2 large cloves garlic, crushed
1 teaspoon of sea salt
2 tablespoons of oil
freshly ground pepper to season.

1. Preheat the oven to 180°C convection or 160°C fan-forced.
2. Peel and chop your vegetables into pieces. The size of your pieces does not matter, but it will affect cooking time. Longer for larger pieces and shorter for smaller ones.
3. Place remaining ingredients into a large mixing bowl and combine.
4. Add vegetables and toss to coat.
5. Place onto a large tray lined with baking paper and bake for approximately 40 minutes. Time will depend on the size of your vegetables, but as a rule, they should be browned and soft (test with a knife).

Play Time!

- Instead of cubing the vegetables, slice them thinly and they will be crispier.
- Use leftovers as a pizza topping.
- These potatoes can be pan-fried instead of done in the oven. They are also great done on the barbecue..

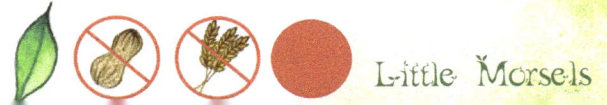

Beautiful Brassicas

Fresh and fast is the way to make this dish. With distinctly Asian flavours, it is a great accompaniment to burgers and patties, rice, noodles and other vegetable side dishes. As children become more confident in the kitchen, stir-frying is a great introduction to using the stove. They will learn how to tell when vegetables are cooked just enough and because it is a fast process, they will not have time to get bored with it. Also, experimenting with the creation of stir-fry sauces can be lots of fun.

Serves 4-5 as a side

500g chopped broccoli and cauliflower
1 tablespoon of sesame oil
1 clove of garlic, crushed
1 tablespoon of grated ginger
1 bunch of Asian greens (such as bok choi, pak choy or Chinese broccoli)

2 tablespoons of Teriyaki sauce
1 tablespoon of rice mirin
2 tablespoons of sesame seeds

1. Steam broccoli and cauliflower until just tender. Be careful not to overdo it, as you will be stir-frying them as well.
2. Heat sesame oil in your wok or frying pan and add the garlic and ginger. Add a little water to stop it sticking and burning.
3. Next add all of your vegetables. Toss them around for a minute or so, and then add your sauces and sesame seeds. Stir for another minute until greens are wilted and all vegetables are well coated. Serve immediately.

Play Time!

- If you double the sauce and add other sliced vegetables and tofu, this can be a complete meal, served with rice or noodles.
- If you like spicy food, add some finely chopped chilli.
- Herbs such as Thai basil, coriander and mint are a delicious addition.

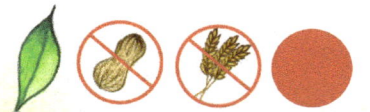

136 Little Morsels

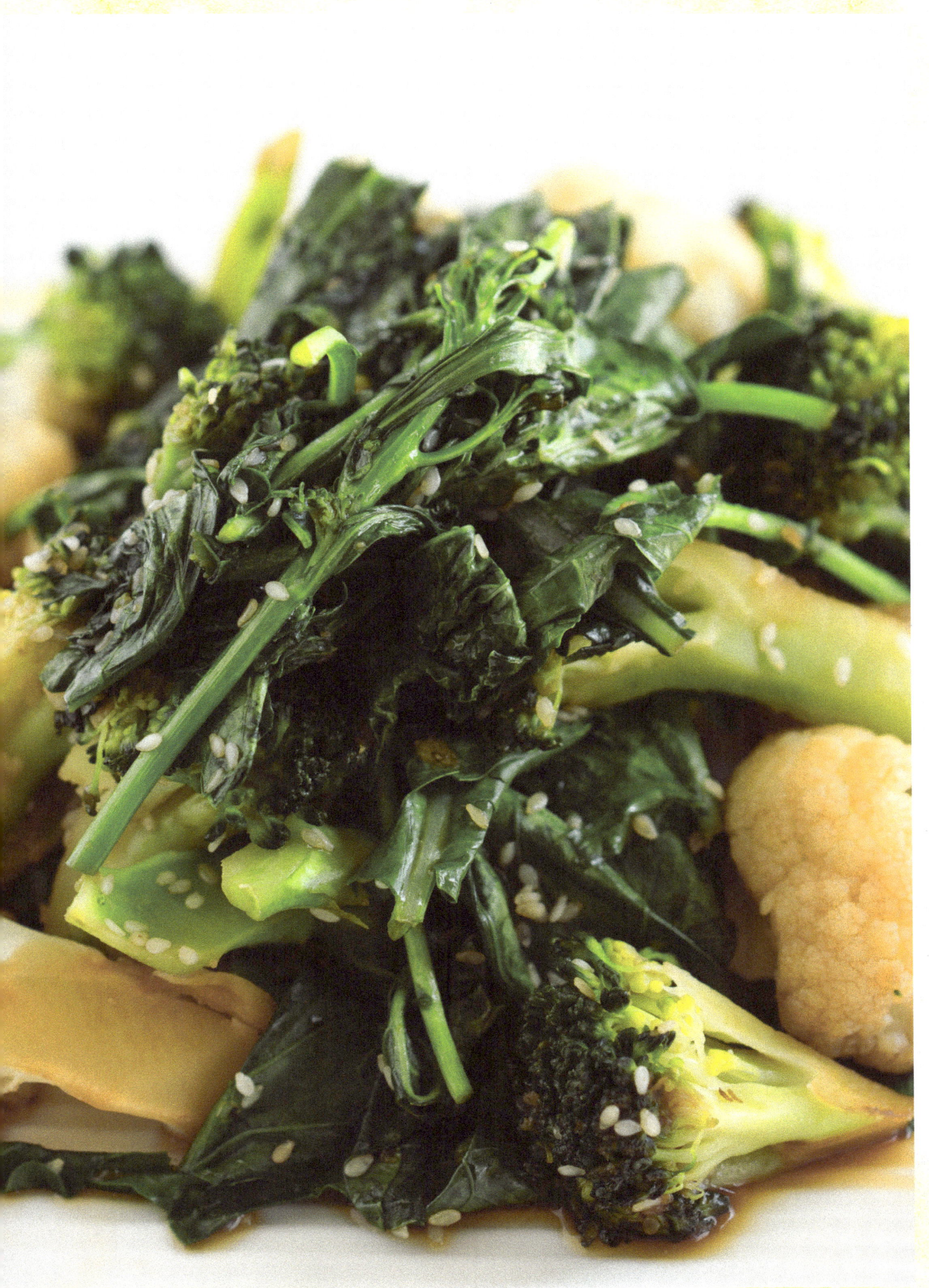

Lemony Peppered Greens

Lemon juice, salt and olive oil provide a great dressing to any steamed greens and it is such a simple dish to prepare. Adjust the various seasonings to your taste. Children may assist by creating the dressing and tossing the greens.

Serves 4-5 as a side

350g trimmed, chopped broccoli
100g of leafy greens (e.g. kale, spinach, collards, Chinese greens)
100g of snow peas
juice of 1 lemon
2 tablespoons of cold-pressed olive oil
pepper and sea salt to season

1. Steam greens until just tender. Harder ones such as broccoli will require longer than more delicate vegetables. Make sure that you don't overdo it or you will lose the goodness into the steaming water.
2. While the greens are steaming, combine the dressing ingredients in your serving bowl.
3. As soon as the vegetables are ready, add them to the bowl and toss to coat.
4. Serve immediately.

Shanta's Sesame Rice

This rice has so much flavour that it is sufficient as a meal with salad or some steamed vegetables. I like to have it as an accompaniment to a hearty salad and hummus. Children may enjoy grinding the sesame seeds and mixing the rice at the end.

Serves 4-5 as a side

1 ½ cups of brown rice
2 ½ cups of water
½ cup of sesame seeds
1 teaspoon of soy sauce
sea salt to season

1. In a medium-sized saucepan, place the rice and water.
2. Cover and bring to the boil, then reduce heat to low and simmer until most of the liquid has been absorbed.
3. Remove from heat and leave to steam for a further 10-15 minutes.

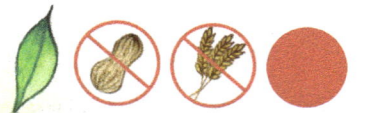

4. Meanwhile, toast the sesame seeds in an ungreased frying pan until brown.
5. In a mortar and pestle, grind the sesame seeds so that they split.
6. Add the sesame seeds to the rice with the soy sauce, then salt and mix well.
7. Taste for seasoning and adjust if necessary.

Crazy Coconut Rice

This dish is very simple to prepare and will provide a great lift to curries. I only serve it if the curry does not already have coconut milk/cream in it to avoid the meal being too rich. The whole spices are not a necessary addition to this recipe as it is still delicious without them.

Serves 4-5 as a side

1 ½ cups of basmati rice
1 tablespoon of ghee or oil
a tablespoon of whole, mixed Indian spices such as cardamom pods, curry leaves, cloves, cumin seeds.
1 x 400g can of coconut milk or the equivalent of powdered coconut milk and water
½ cup of water

1. Wash and drain your rice according to directions on page 68. Set aside.
2. In a medium-sized saucepan, heat the ghee or oil and add the whole spices.   Toss for a minute until they become fragrant.
3. Add the rice, coconut milk and water. Cover and bring to boil.
4. Reduce to a simmer over medium-low heat.
5. Once most of the liquid has been absorbed, remove from heat and leave to steam for another 10 minutes.
6. Fluff with a fork and serve.

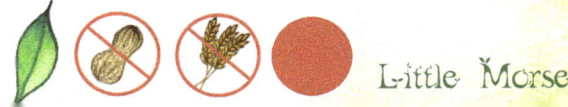

Queen Bee Wedges

These wedges have a great mixture of flavours and the edges become caramelised as the honey cooks. If you cut your potatoes ahead of time be sure to leave them in water so they don't go brown and do not mix with the sauce until you are ready to put them into the oven. If you do, the salt in the sauce will draw the moisture from the potatoes and you will have wedge soup!

1 kg roasting potatoes (e.g. King Edward or Desiree)
2 tablespoons of oil
1 loaded tablespoon of honey or rice syrup
½ tablespoon of dijon mustard
1 teaspoon of sea salt

1. Preheat the oven to 180°C convection or 160°C fan-forced.
2. Lay baking paper onto a large oven tray.
3. The potatoes may be roasted with the skin on or off. If you are going to have them peeled, do so, otherwise wash them well.
4. Cut your potatoes into wedges.
5. Make a sauce out of the remaining ingredients and toss with your potato pieces before laying them onto your tray.
6. Bake until soft inside and crispy outside. The time taken will depend on the size of your pieces but generally they should take between 30-45 minutes.

Play Time!

- Use a mix of sweet potatoes and potatoes.
- Add some crushed garlic and rosemary.
- Add herb salt instead of sea salt.
- Add some chilli powder.

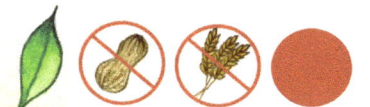

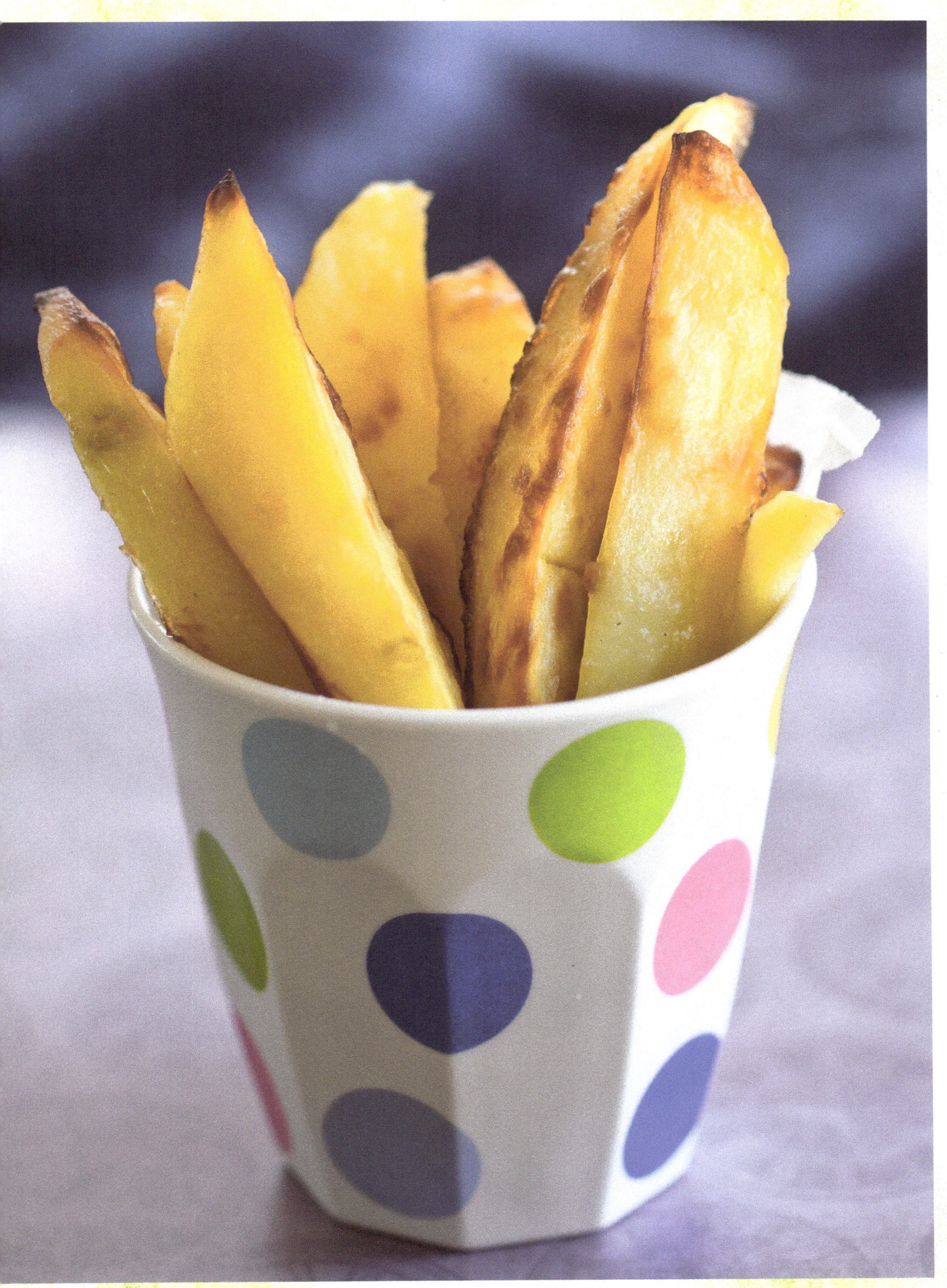

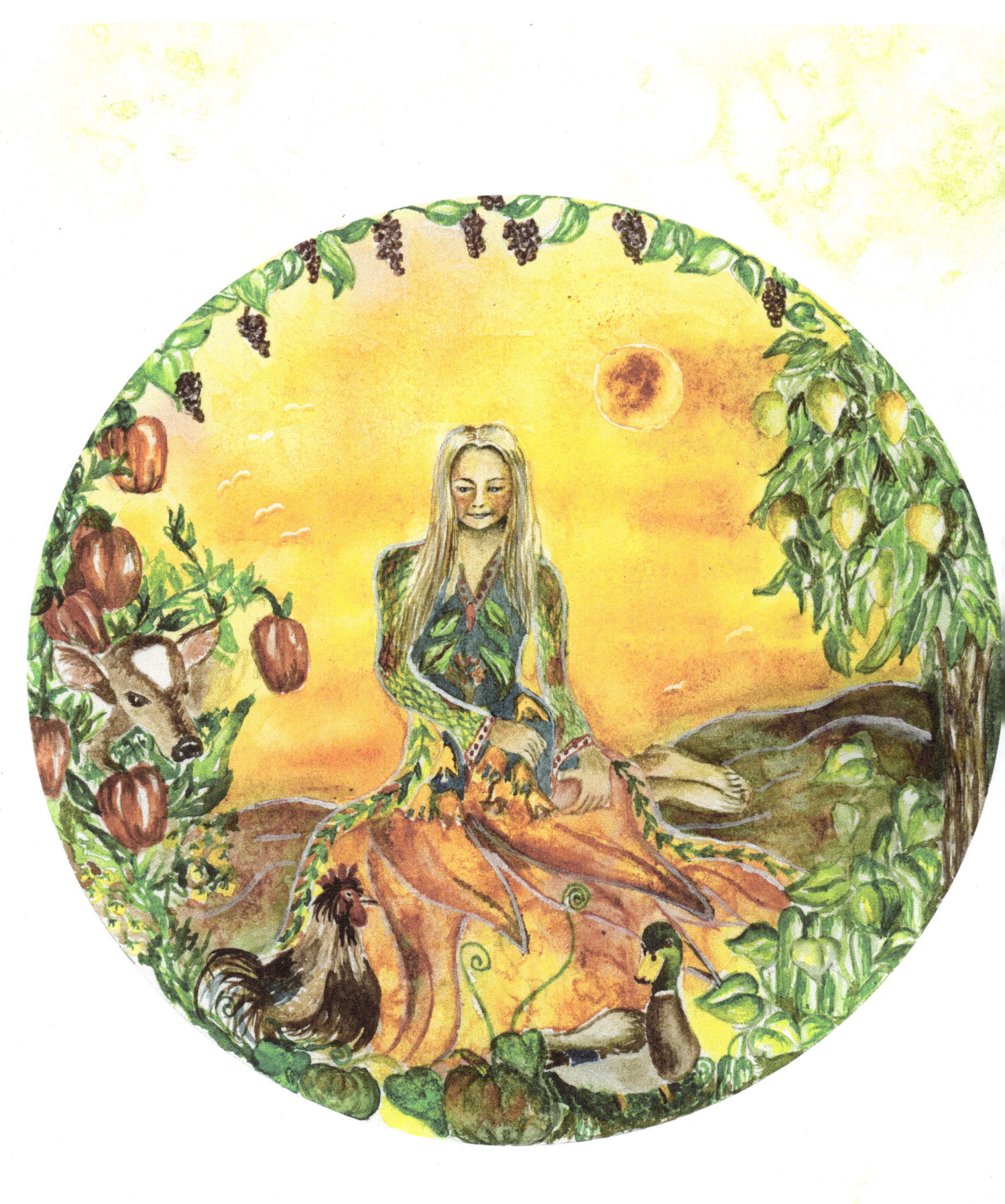

142 Gifts from the Garden

Gifts from the Garden

Salads are the key to feeling clean. With fresh, organic, raw ingredients, your body will become a place where disease finds it hard to live. Mix and match a variety of fruits and vegetables to make amazing combinations. Try these recipes and then experiment with your own.

Become a picture of health!

*"What is man without the beasts?
If all the beasts were gone, men
would die from a great loneliness of spirit.
For whatever happens to the beasts
happens to the man.
All things are connected."*

~Chief Seattle

Couscous Medley

One morning when I couldn't find anything to give the kids for their school lunch, I constructed this salad out of what I had. They loved it and so my frustration turned into a gift as now I make this salad often.

1 cup of couscous
1 cup of boiling water + 1 teaspoon of vegetable stock paste or 1 cup boiling vegetable stock
1 tablespoon of cold pressed olive oil
1 cup of cooked chickpeas or $\frac{1}{3}$ cup of dried (soaked for at least 10 hours)*
1 small capsicum, diced
1 small carrot, finely diced
1 small Lebanese cucumber, diced
1 cup of corn kernels
1 tablespoon of finely chopped parsley
1 tablespoon of finely chopped mint
juice of half a lemon
freshly ground pepper

If you do not already have some cooked chickpeas in the freezer and you want to use dried, I suggest you soak more than the $\frac{1}{3}$ cup required for this recipe. That way you will have stores for another time.

Optional extras/suggestions

sliced olives	diced avocado
finely chopped sun-dried tomatoes	sliced radish
chopped artichoke hearts	cherry tomatoes
sliced mushrooms	grated beetroot

1. If you are using dried chickpeas, cook according to directions on page 64.
2. In a saucepan or glass bowl, combine the couscous with your boiling vegetable stock, or water and stock paste. Stir quickly, then cover and leave for 5 minutes.
3. Drizzle olive oil over the couscous, fluff with a fork and allow to cool.
4. Add remaining salad ingredients and mix well.

Play Time!

- You can replace the couscous with rice or quinoa.
- Change the ingredients to suit your child's tastes. Sometimes if I have some leftover roast sweet potato or pumpkin, I add that in, other times I add more antipasto ingredients.

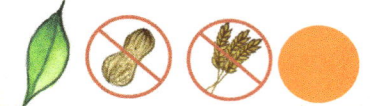

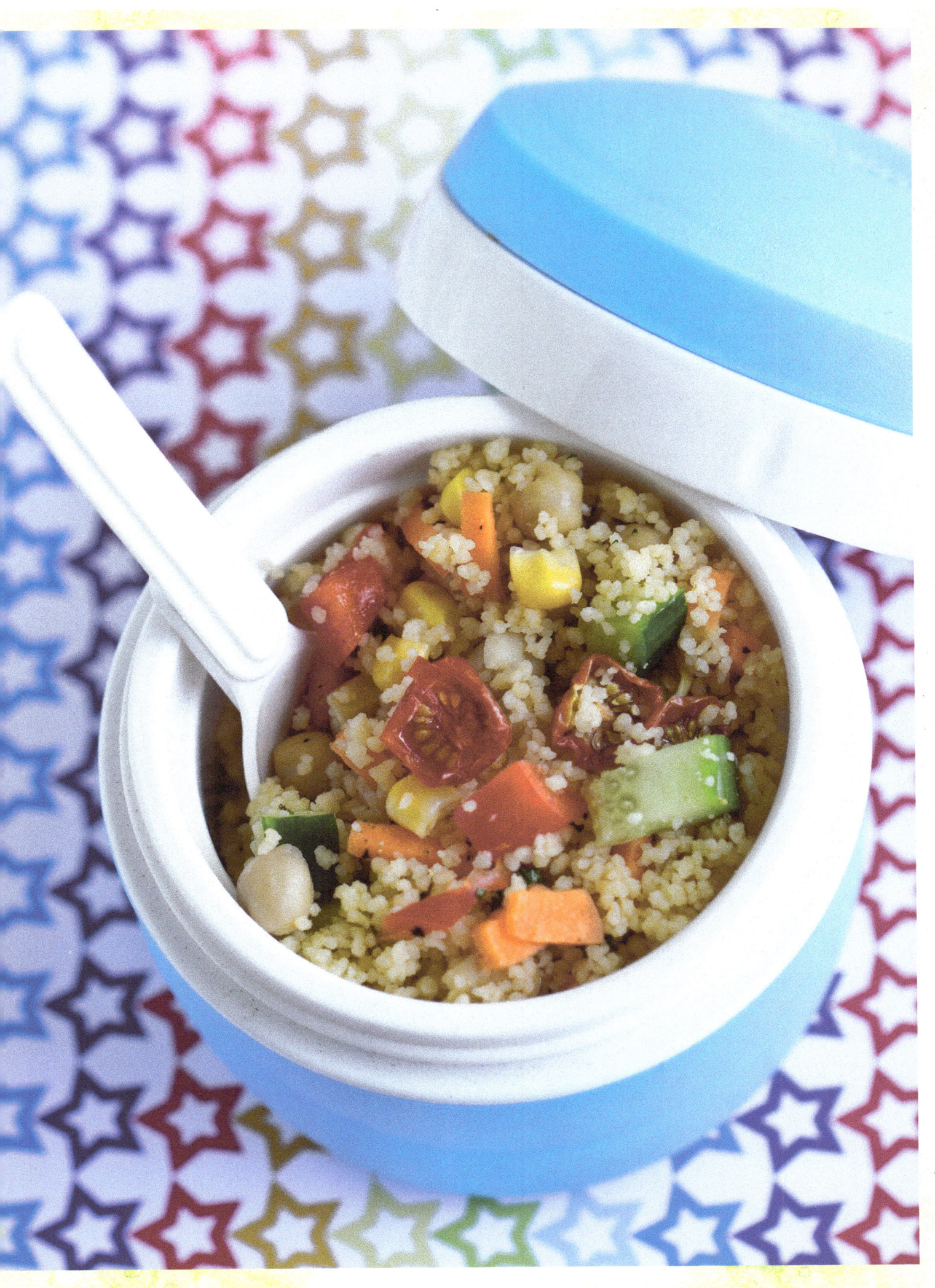

Lime, Pumpkin & Quinoa Salad

This is one of my favourite salads made with quinoa. I have always loved the combination of pumpkin and lime and it provides a fresh, sweet and sour flavour in this very substantial salad. Quinoa is very high in protein, making any salad it is in a potential meal in itself.

1 cup of quinoa
2 cups of water
½ teaspoon of sea salt
1 tablespoon of oil
1 medium-sized red onion, finely chopped
1 ½ tablespoons of white wine vinegar
200g grated pumpkin

Dressing
1 tablespoon of grated lime zest
1 tablespoon of grated ginger
juice of 1 small juicy lime
black pepper
handful of mint leaves, finely chopped.

1. In a small saucepan, combine, quinoa with water and sea salt. Bring to the boil, then reduce heat to low and simmer until most of the water has been absorbed. Set aside with the lid on until all water is absorbed and leave to cool.
2. Meanwhile, in a small frying pan, heat the oil and add the onion. Stir fry until tender and then add the vinegar. Cook for another couple of minutes, stirring often.
3. Add the pumpkin and cook for a couple of minutes. When pumpkin is soft but not mushy, remove from heat and leave to cool.
4. Combine dressing ingredients and when all hot ingredients have cooled, combine everything in a bowl and serve.

Play Time!

- Sweet potato works well if you want to substitute the pumpkin.
- Use lemon instead of lime when limes are out of season.
- Add other diced salad ingredients such as capsicum, cucumber, tomatoes, avocados and mung bean sprouts.
- Throw in some pumpkin seeds (pepitas).

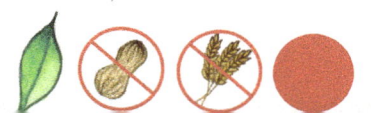

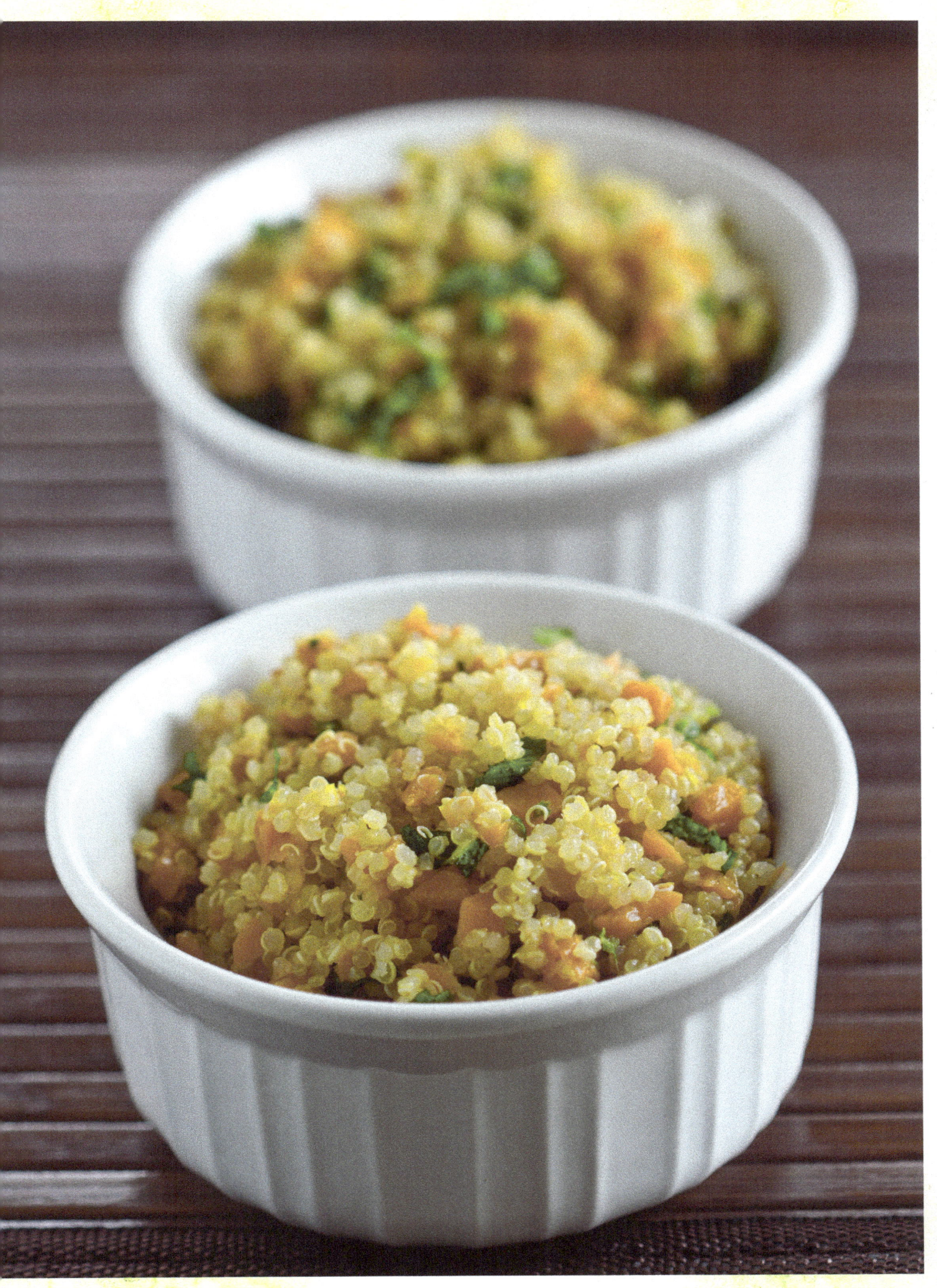

Aladdin's Salad

This salad combines flavours from the Middle East and tastes best when the salad vegetables are at room temperature.

1 red onion, finely chopped
1 clove of garlic, crushed
juice from ½ lemon
½ teaspoon of sea salt
freshly ground black pepper
¼ teaspoon of ground cinnamon
1 teaspoon of sumac
2 tablespoons of cold pressed olive oil
4 firm ripe tomatoes, diced
2 Lebanese cucumbers, diced
1 red capsicum, diced
handful each of parsley and mint, finely chopped

1. In a salad bowl, combine all of the ingredients down to and including the olive oil.
2. Leave to sit while you chop the other salad vegetables. This gives the onion time to soften and absorb the other flavours. Add remaining ingredients and mix well.

Play Time!

- The addition of avocado will add a creamy element.
- Play around with the herbs used. Dill or basil can be used in place of parsley.
- Throw in some semi-dried tomatoes for extra flavour.
- Use lime juice instead of lemon.

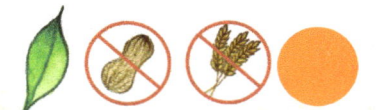

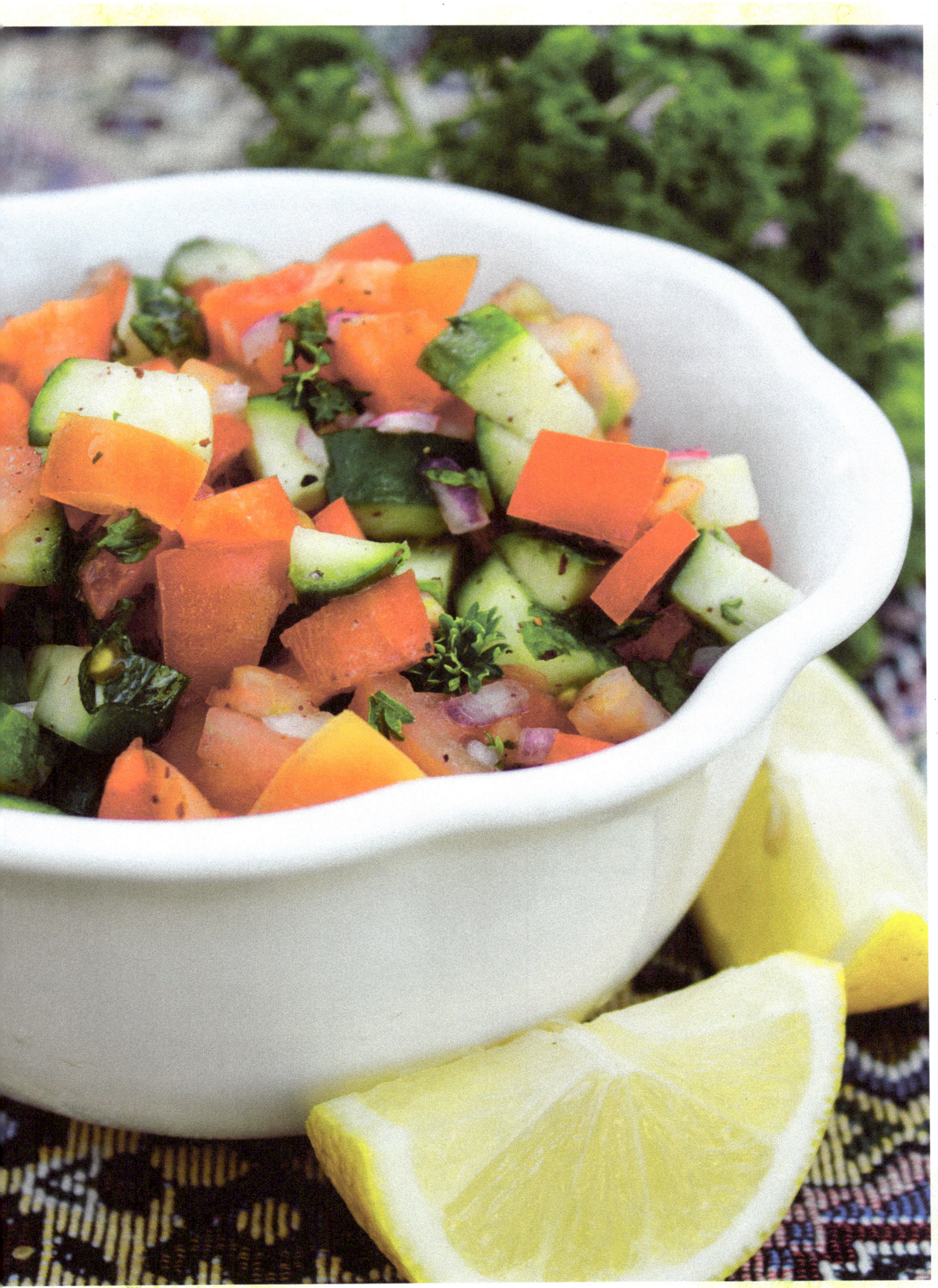

Rainbow Salad

This is one of the cleanest, most wholesome salads I make. It is bursting with flavour and nutrition, especially if the lentils are sprouted rather than cooked. (See page 64 for information on how to cook or sprout lentils).

Dressing

1 teaspoon of grated ginger
1 small clove of crushed garlic
1 tablespoon of olive oil
1 tablespoon of fresh lemon juice
1 tablespoon of fresh orange juice
1 tablespoon of Tamari or soy sauce
sea salt and pepper to season

¾ cup puy lentils, cooked until tender or sprouted
1 large cucumber, finely diced
1 large zucchini, grated or shredded
1 large carrot, grated, or shredded
1 large red capsicum, sliced thinly
½ small red onion, finely chopped
¼ cup of toasted sesame seeds (this can be done in a frying pan)
avocado slices to top

1. Combine dressing ingredients in a small bowl and set aside.
2. Place remaining ingredients (except avocado) into a salad bowl and toss with the dressing.
3. Top with avocado slices and serve.

Play Time!

- If you prefer your dressing sweeter, add a teaspoon of honey or agave syrup.
- Add some chopped herbs such as parsley, basil or mint for extra flavour.
- During the summer, throw in some mango or paw paw slices.
- Use lime juice instead of lemon.

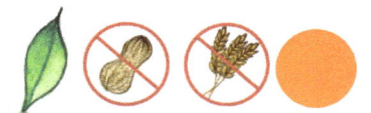

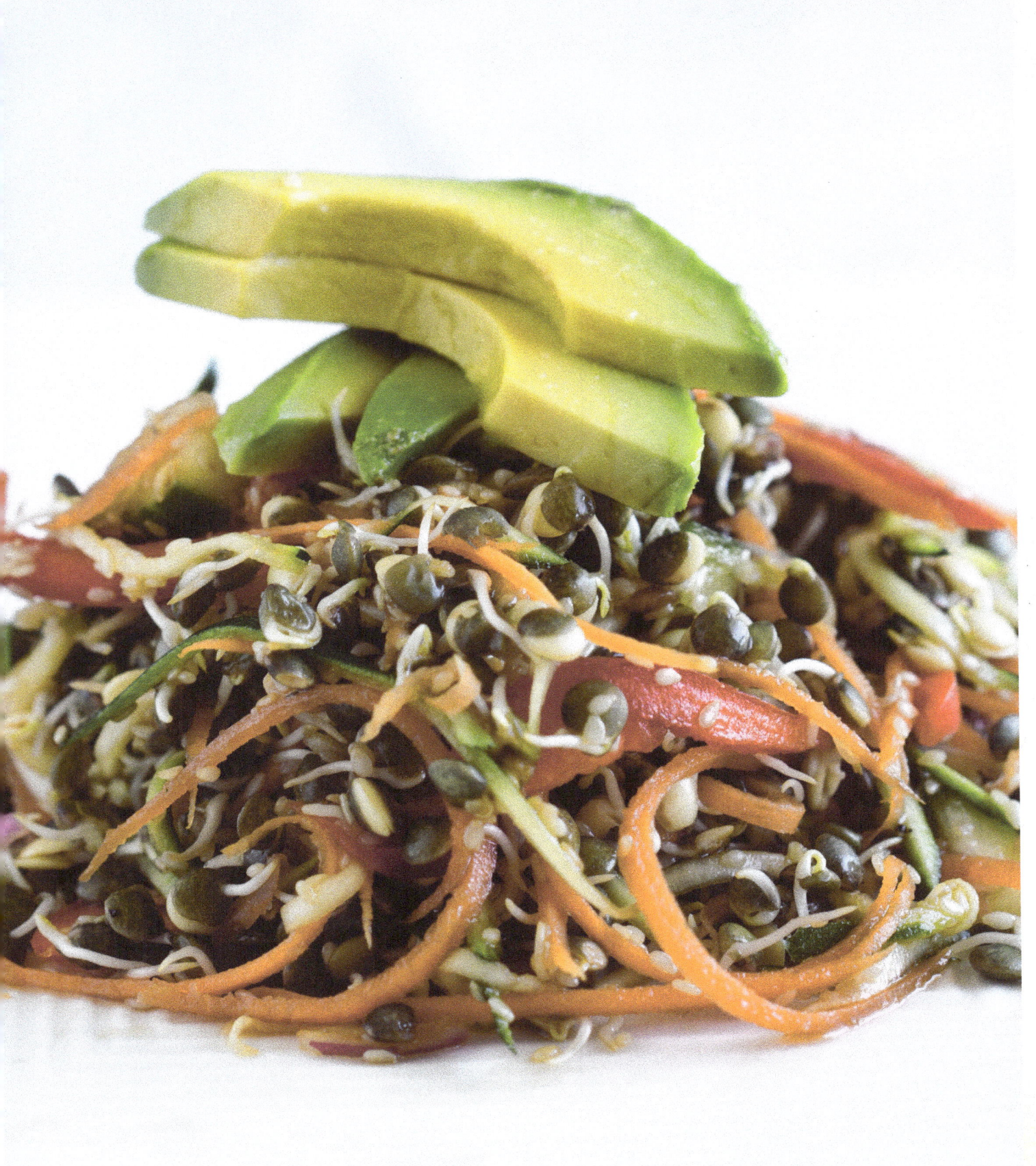

Tomato salad

This salad was inspired by bruschetta topping when my boys wanted to eat it with everything. Make sure you use good tomatoes for maximum taste. If you would like to use it as a topping for bruschetta, just cut the ingredients into smaller pieces.

- 750g varied tomatoes, diced (try to find different colours)
- 1 large avocado, diced
- 2 tablespoons of finely chopped basil
- 1 small red onion, finely chopped
- 1 small clove of garlic, crushed
- 1 tablespoon of balsamic vinegar
- 1 tablespoon of olive oil
- sea salt and pepper to season

Combine all ingredients in a large bowl. Serve at room temperature.

Posh Cucumber Salad

A refreshing little side dish that suits most meals.

- 450g Lebanese cucumbers
- 1 heaped tablespoon of finely chopped mint leaves
- 1 tablespoon of pomegranate molasses*
- ½ tablespoon of balsamic vinegar
- 1 tablespoon of olive oil
- sea salt and pepper to season

Pomegranate molasses is available at many delicatessens.

1. Prepare the cucumber either by dicing or peeling into strips.
2. In a salad bowl, mix the remaining ingredients together to form a dressing.
3. Add the cucumber and mint to the dressing and toss until well combined.

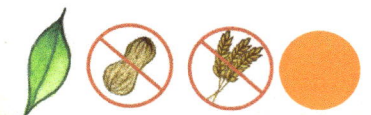

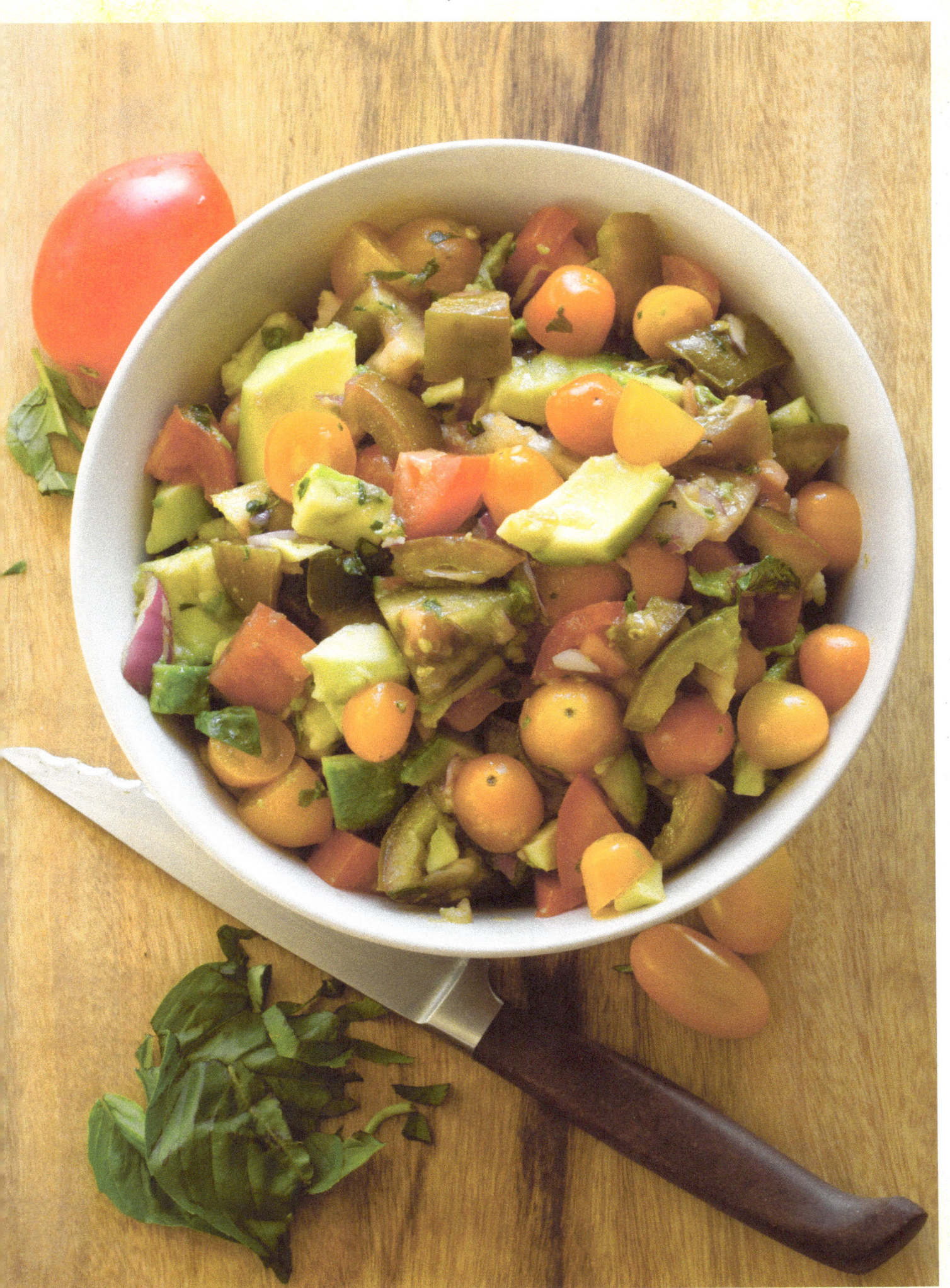

Balsamic Tomato Salad made with Roma, Kumato and Orange Cherry Tomatoes

Gifts from the Garden

Tabbouleh with a Spin

This slant on tabbouleh is rich in protein as it uses quinoa instead of the usual cracked wheat. It is also very flavoursome and is best made with sweet, juicy tomatoes. Don't skimp on the quality and you will be pleased with the result!

1 cup of quinoa

2 cups of water

½ teaspoon of sea salt

1 cup of cooked chickpeas or $\frac{1}{3}$ cup of dried (soaked for at least 10 hours)*

1 medium-sized Lebanese cucumber, diced

1 ½ cups of diced, fresh tomatoes

¼ cup of finely chopped parsley

¼ cup of finely chopped mint leaves

*If you do not already have some cooked chickpeas in the freezer and you want to use dried, I suggest you soak more than the $\frac{1}{3}$ cup required for this recipe. That way you will have stores for another time.

Dressing

3 tablespoons of olive oil

1 clove of crushed garlic

1 tablespoon of white wine vinegar

3 tablespoons of lemon juice

1 tablespoon of finely grated lemon zest

½ teaspoon of sea salt

freshly ground black pepper to taste

1. If you are using dried chickpeas, cook according to directions on page 64.
2. In a small saucepan, combine, quinoa with water and sea salt. Bring to the boil, then reduce heat to low and simmer until most of the water has been absorbed. Set aside with the lid on until all water is absorbed and leave to cool.
3. Meanwhile, in a small bowl, combine the dressing ingredients.
4. Once quinoa is cool fluff with a fork and add the remaining ingredients including the dressing. Give it all a gentle stir until well mixed.
5. Taste for seasoning, and if necessary, add more salt, pepper or lemon juice.

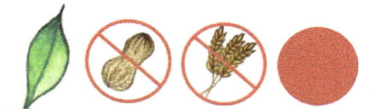

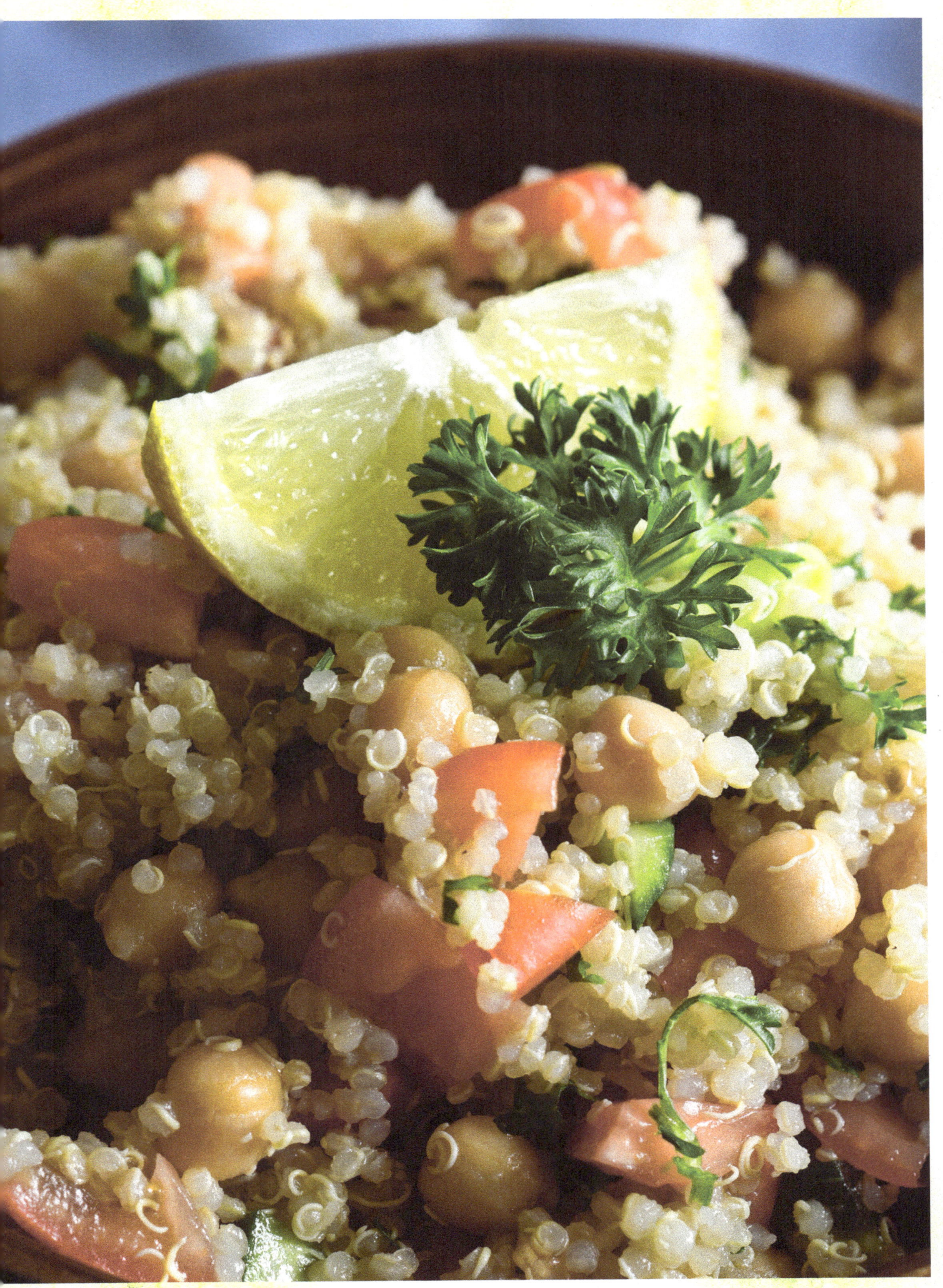

Sesame Rice Salad

*Because this salad is made with brown rice, it is filling enough to be a meal on its own.
It is also great as a side with vegetable fritters or other savoury h'orderves.*

1 ½ cups of brown rice
⅓ cup of sesame seeds, toasted
1 small carrot, shredded or grated
1 small red capsicum, diced
handful of snow peas, thinly sliced
¼ cup of finely chopped coriander
¼ cup of finely chopped chives

Dressing

¼ cup of fresh apple juice
1 tablespoon of balsamic vinegar
2 teaspoons of dijon mustard
1 clove of crushed garlic
1 tablespoon of soy or Tamari sauce
2 tablespoons of cold pressed olive oil

1. Using the instructions on page 68, cook the brown rice until tender. Leave to cool.
2. Combine dressing ingredients and set aside.
3. When the rice is ready, fluff with a fork and add to a salad bowl with the remaining ingredients, including dressing.
4. Mix well and serve.

Play Time!

- Try other salad vegetables such as tomatoes, grated beetroot, sliced mushrooms, sweet peas, corn kernels, grated zucchini, olives, avocado or grated squash.
- Add wild rice.
- Use different herbs such as dill, parsley or basil.

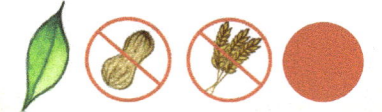

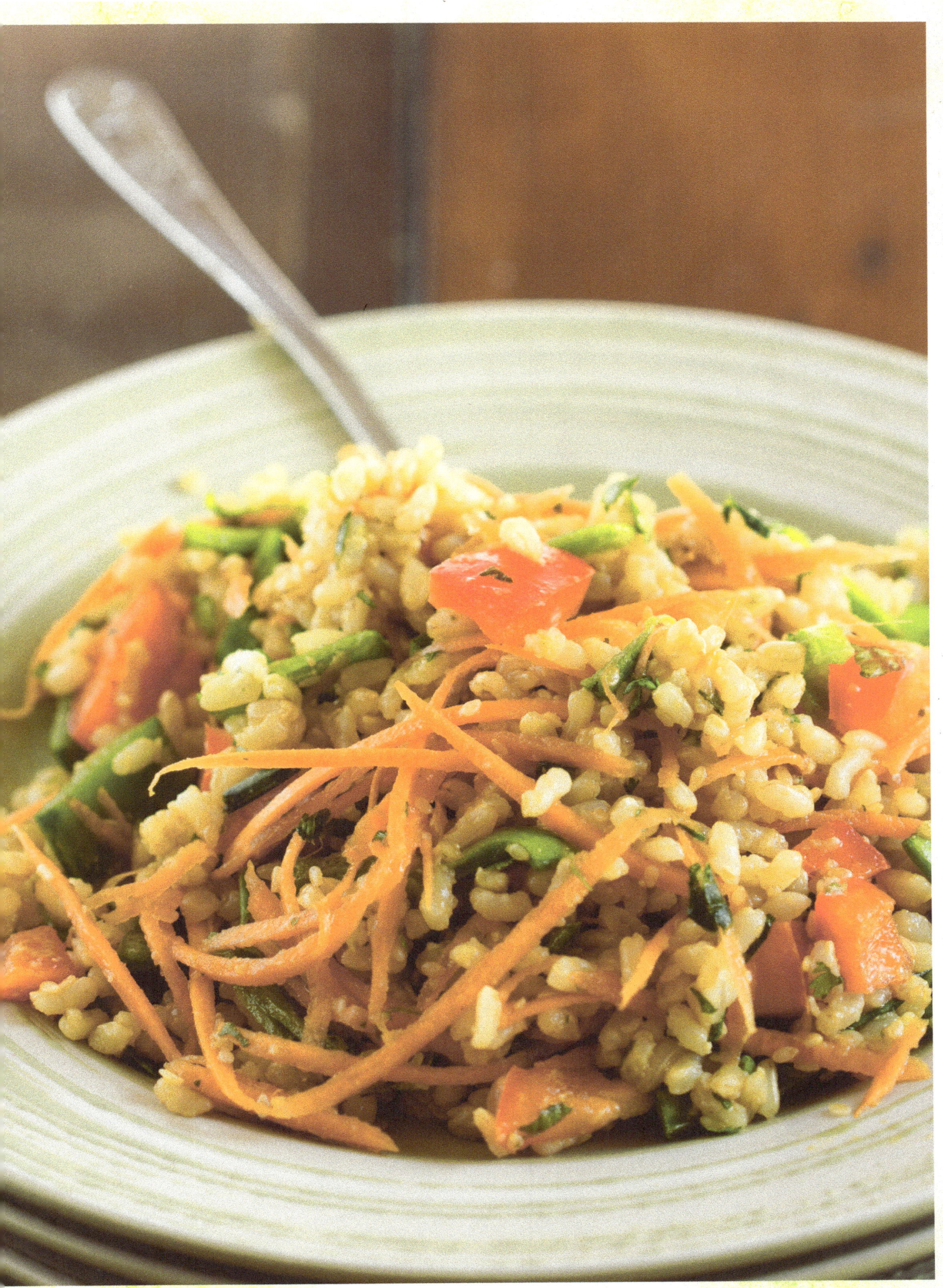

Gifts from the Garden

Wild Salad

Making a rice salad can be as easy as throwing what you have into some rice and making a dressing. Use this recipe as a base and try out different vegetables and herbs.

1 cup of basmati rice
⅓ cup of wild rice
1 cup of water
1 red capsicum, diced small
½ cup of corn kernels
1 medium-sized carrot, shredded
2 tablespoons of finely chopped chives
2 tablespoons of finely chopped parsley

Dressing

1 teaspoon of curry powder
2 tablespoons of white wine vinegar
1 teaspoon of honey or rice syrup
2 tablespoons of cold pressed salad oil (you can use olive, sunflower, safflower, etc.)

1. Cook basmati rice according to instructions on page 68.
2. Bring to boil the 1 cup of water and wild rice in a covered saucepan. Turn heat to low and leave to simmer until most of the water has been absorbed. This will take about 40 minutes. Remove from heat and leave to soak up remaining water.
3. Combine both rices and fluff with a fork.
4. Add remaining salad ingredients.
5. Whisk dressing ingredients and add to the rice mixture.
6. Combine and serve.

Play Time!

- Vary your vegetables or add extras such as olives, mushrooms or sun-dried tomatoes.
- Use other herbs such as coriander, basil or mint.
- Replace the basmati with brown rice to add bulk and nutrition.

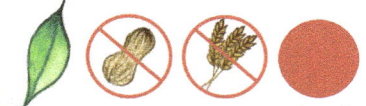

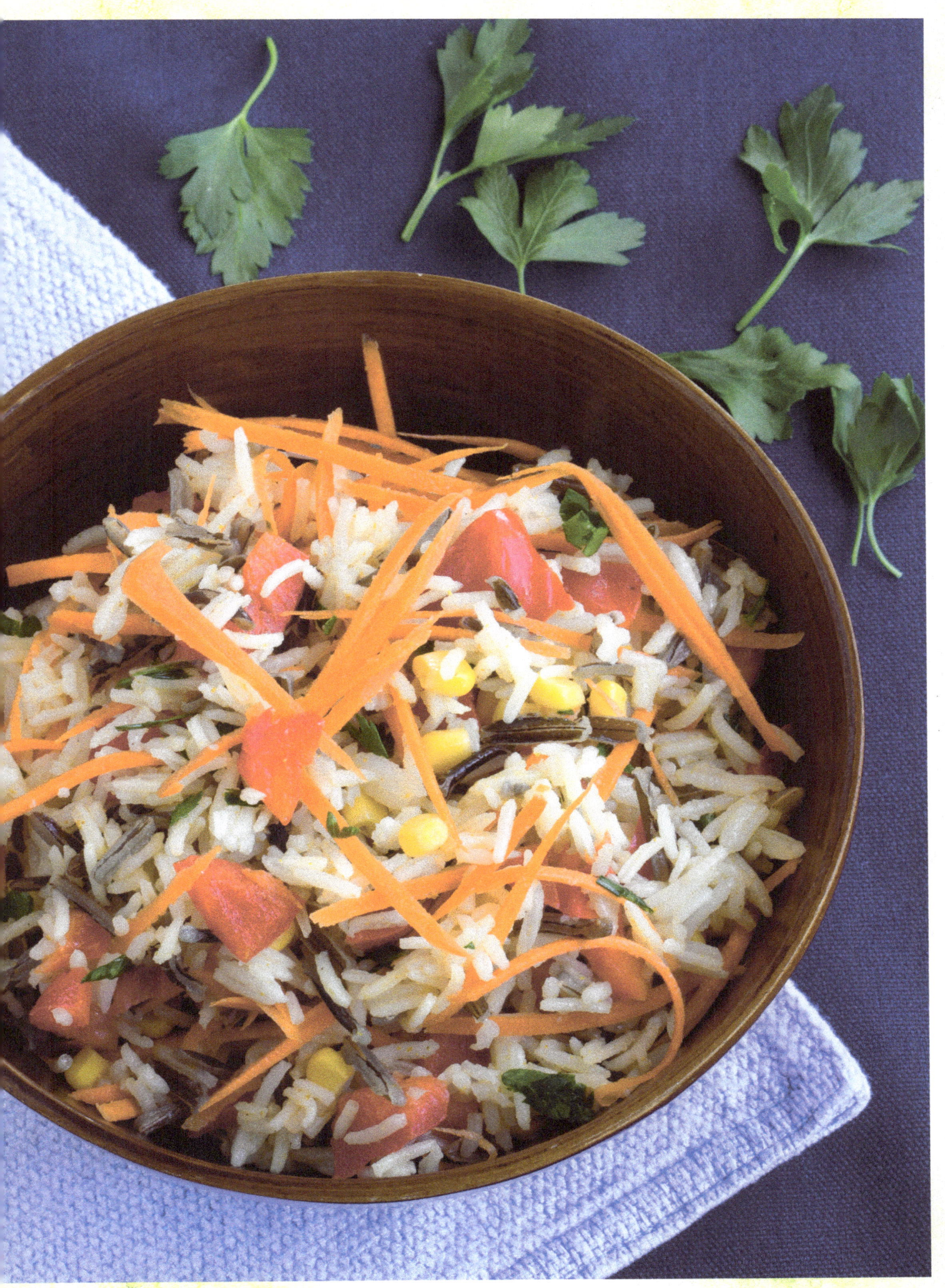

Gifts from the Garden 159

Asian Noodle Salad

*A refreshing dish that can be a meal in itself.
The combinations of salty with sweet and sour make it very special.*

150g glass or vermicelli noodles
1 small red capsicum, finely sliced
1 medium-sized carrot, shredded into strips
large handful of snow peas, finely sliced
½ cup of finely chopped, fresh coriander
½ cup of peanuts, pulsed into the food processor (or finely chopped)

Dressing
1 tablespoon of sesame oil
3 tablespoons of soy or Tamari sauce
2 tablespoons of agave or maple syrup
2 tablespoons of fresh lime juice
1 tablespoon of finely grated ginger
1 clove of crushed garlic

1. Soak noodles in boiling water until soft. Drain and rinse with cold water.
2. Put all salad ingredients, including the noodles into a large bowl and mix well.
3. Mix dressing ingredients and add to salad.
4. Stir until all ingredients are well coated.

Play Time!

- To make this salad nut free, substitute peanuts with toasted sunflower or pepitas.
- Vary the vegetables you use: add Asian greens, Chinese cabbage or cherry tomatoes.
- Add some marinated tofu for extra protein.

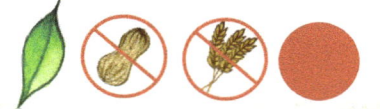

Gifts from the Garden

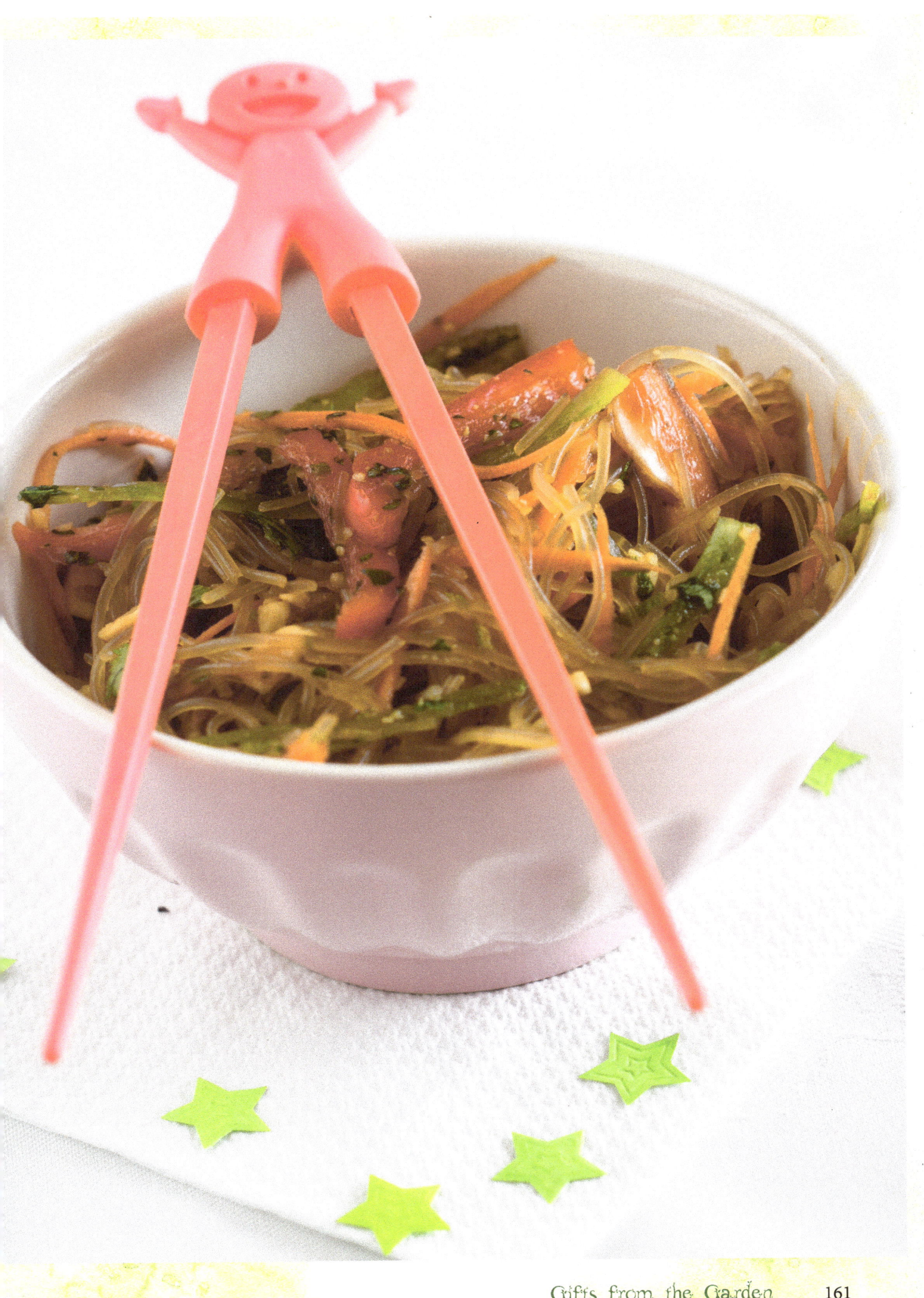

Rainbow Spaghetti Salad

This salad is made up of vegetables that have been prepared in a way that makes them look like spaghetti or noodles. You can buy a number of different appliances that do this from your kitchen shop. For vegetables that are awkwardly shaped, such as squash, radish and beetroot, I use a peeler that shreds. Presenting salads this way makes them a lot more interesting and appealing to children.

1 medium-sized zucchini
1 large yellow squash
1 medium-sized carrot
2 small radishes
½ cup of shredded beetroot

Dressing

1 tablespoon of sunflower oil
1 tablespoon of white wine vinegar
1 teaspoon of honey or rice syrup
½ teaspoon of dijon mustard
½ teaspoon of finely grated ginger
1 tablespoon of finely chopped mint
pepper and salt to season

1. Using your peeler or vegetable spaghetti maker, shred or peel all of your vegetables into spaghetti shapes. The radishes, I just thinly slice with a peeler.
2. Mix dressing ingredients and add to salad.
3. Stir until all ingredients are well coated and serve.

Play Time!

- Try any other dressing on this salad. When you gain confidence try creating your own dressing recipe!
- Add cooked or sprouted lentils or seeds to provide protein.
- Throw in other herbs such as coriander or dill.
- Add marinated tofu to make it a meal.

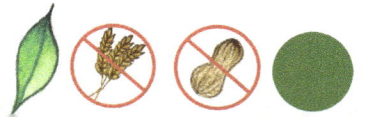

Gifts from the Garden

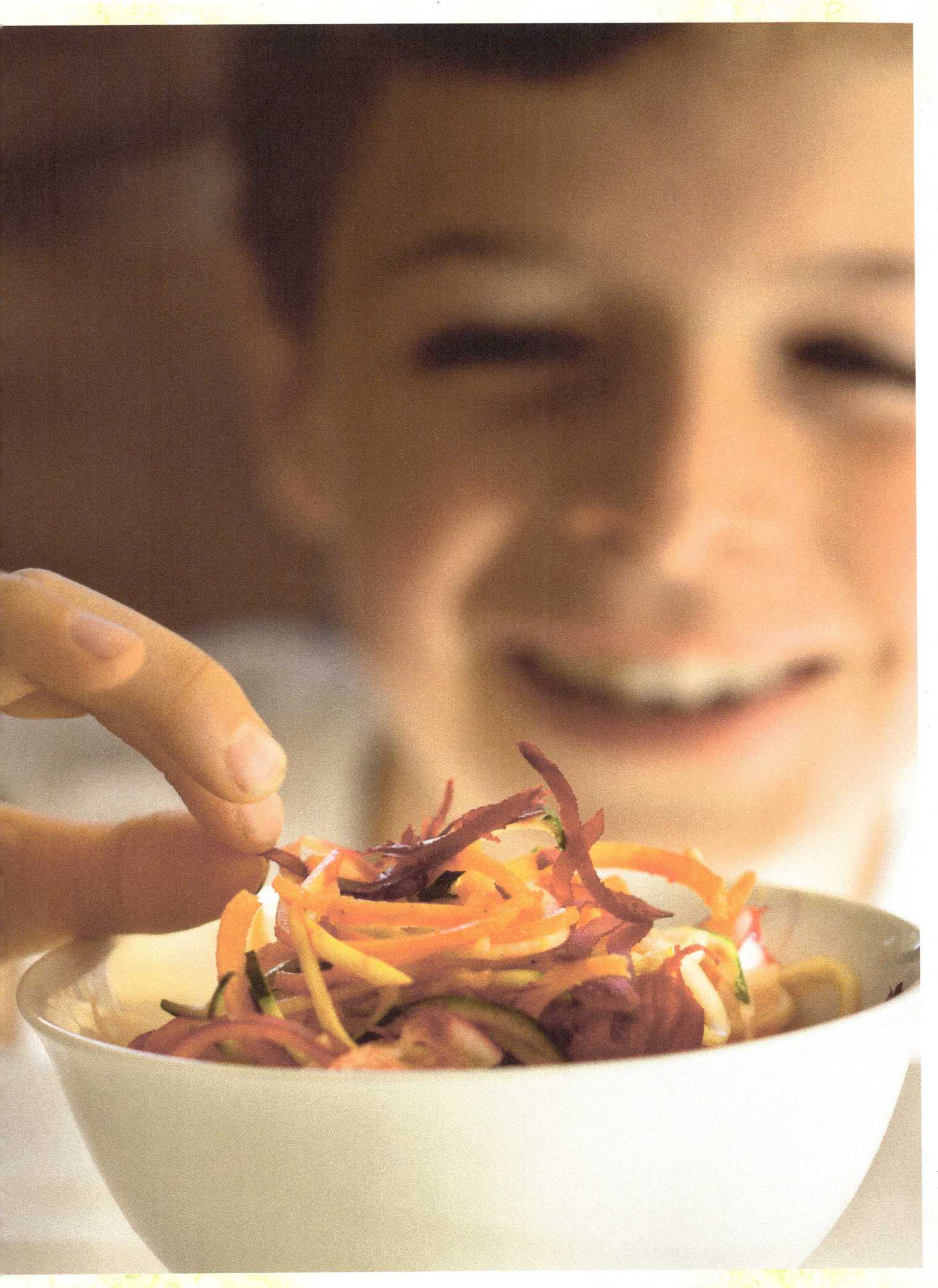

Gifts from the Garden

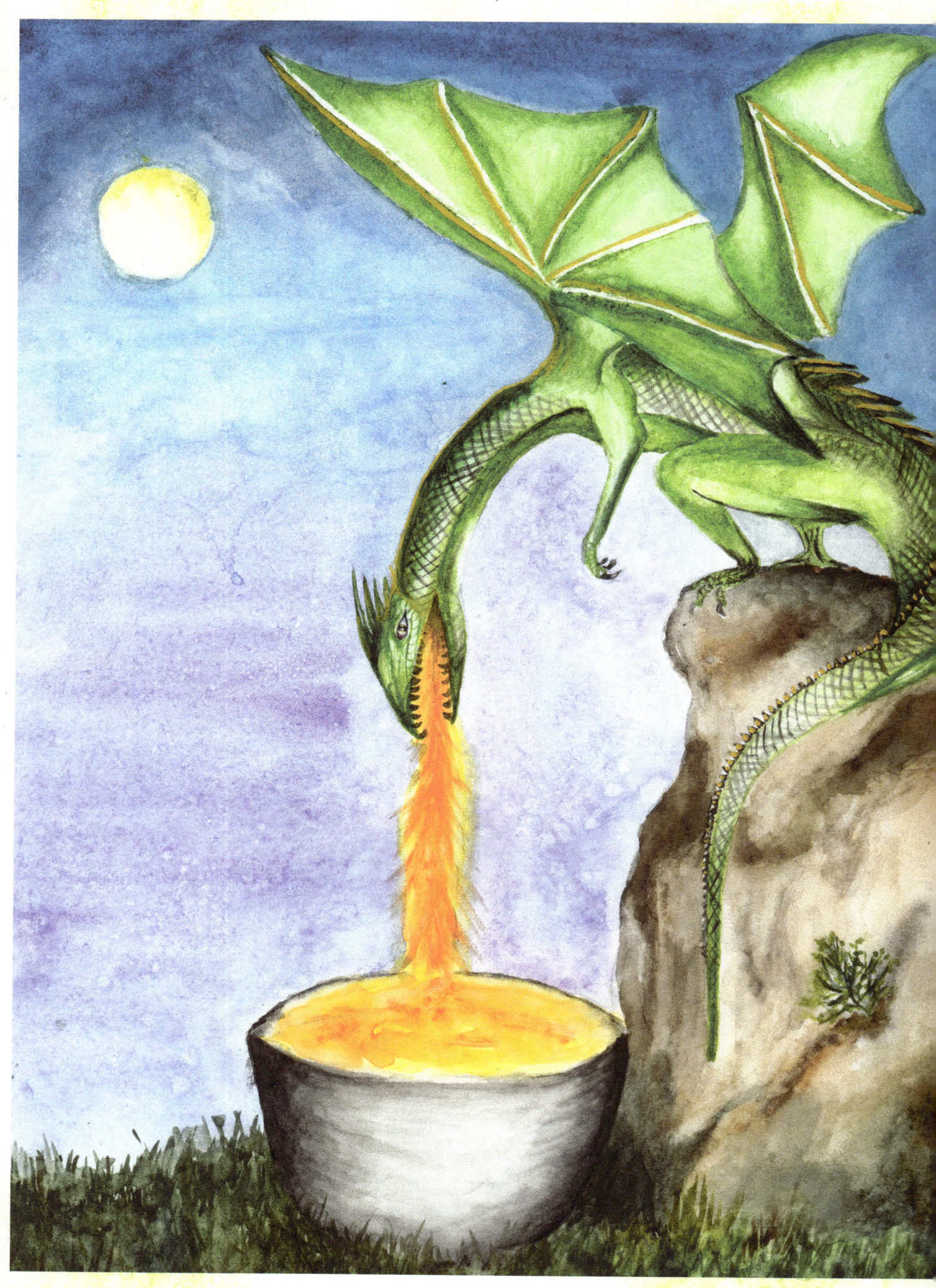

Beastly Brews

Beastly Brews

A soup can be a warm and comforting meal on a cold day or because they are so simple and quick to prepare, an alternative to take away. Making a soup can be a way of using up whatever produce you have left in the fridge or it can be an experimenting ground for new tastes and flavour combinations. Children can be a part of this process and as a result, learn how to mix different ingredients. Use the **Regional Flavours** guide on page 58 and the recipe for the **Soup of Endless Possibilities** on page 172 and you may come up with some new favourites on your own.

If your soup is too hot, add an ice cube and stir!

"To eat is a necessity, but to eat intelligently is an art."
~La Rochefoucauld

Vegetable Stock Concentrate

Making your own stock is easy and a great way to use up vegetables at the end of the week. If they are going a bit limp, they can be put to good use with this recipe. Most commercially made stocks are flavoured with MSG and contain other additives, best avoided. Even if they don't list MSG as an additive, chances are it has snuck in the back door through "flavours", "herbs and spices" or "yeast extract". When you make your own stock you will know exactly what is in it! This recipe is for a concentrate which may be added to water to make a liquid stock. Use 1 tablespoon of concentrate to 1 litre of water.

2 tablespoons of oil
1 large onion, roughly chopped
1 large clove of garlic, roughly chopped
400g of pulverised or grated raw vegetables (include different colours - e.g. zucchini, broccoli: including stalks, celery: including leaves, carrots, sweet potato, pumpkin, cauliflower, squash, cabbage)
1 large bunch of herbs, chopped: use a variety of two or three herbs (parsley, basil, dill, thyme, rosemary or sage)
2 bay leaves, torn
1 tomato or 1 tablespoon of tomato paste mixed with ¼ of a cup of water
150g sea salt

1. In a large, heavy-based saucepan, heat the oil and add onion and garlic. Stir-fry for a couple of minutes, until the onion softens.
2. Add remaining ingredients and mix well.
3. Put the lid on the saucepan and cook over low heat for 20 minutes, stirring often to avoid the vegetables sticking. If the mix becomes too dry, add a little water.
4. Once the mixture is very mushy, leave to cool.
5. Puree in a food processor and store in a sterilised jar in the fridge. This stock will keep for at least 2 months (if it lasts that long). If you use stock rarely, decanter into an ice cube tray. When the portions are frozen, remove from the tray and store in a container or bag in the freezer.

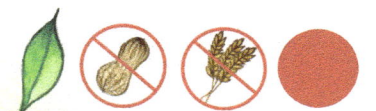

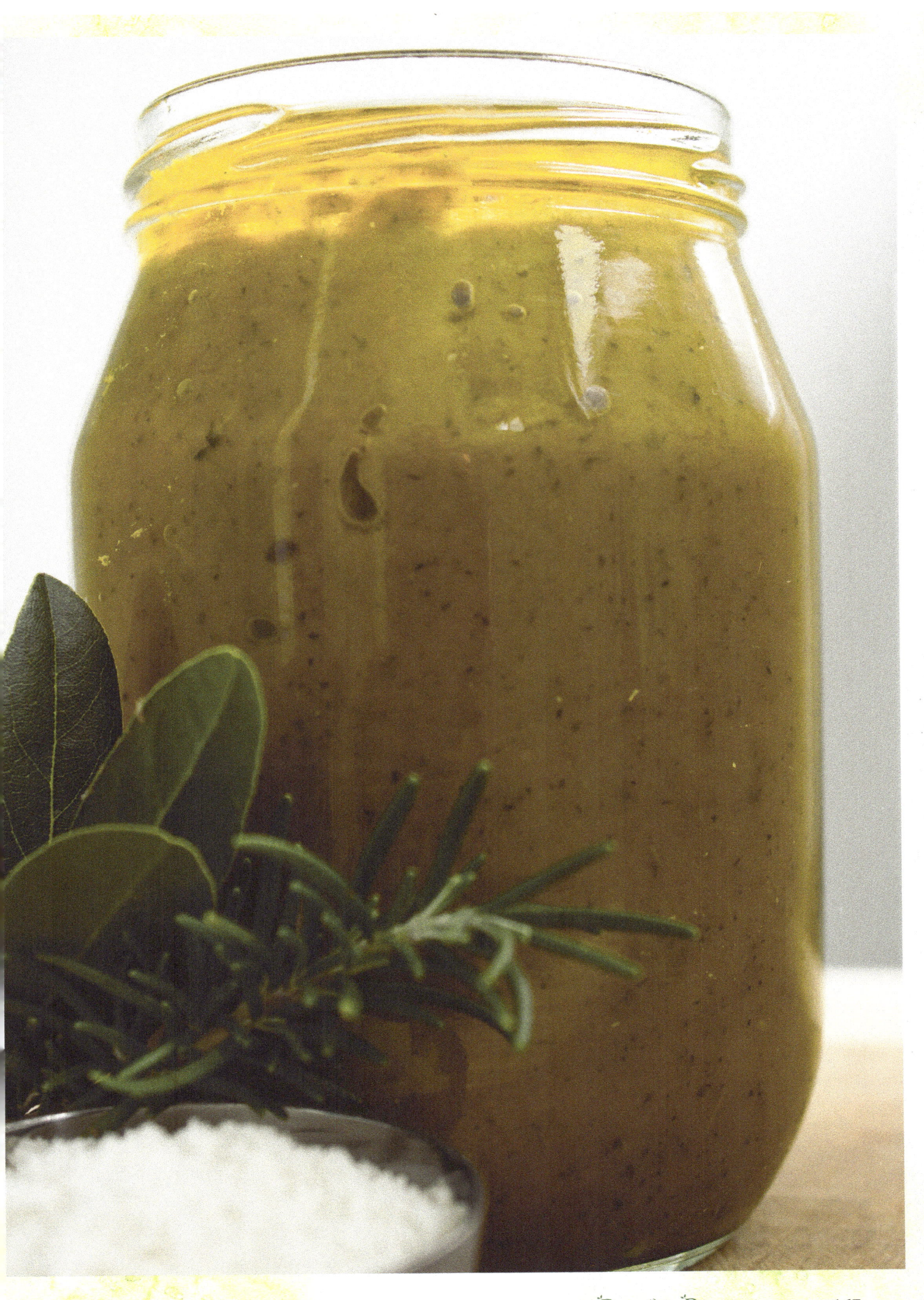

The Forest King's Soup

This soup is a favourite in our house and despite my son Ryan's suspicion of anything green, he wolfs it down. He loves the mintiness and the home-made garlic and herb pizza bread I serve with it. The rule is you don't get a second slice until your bowl is ¾ finished!

Serves 4-5

2 cups of green split peas, rinsed and soaked for at least 6 hours
1 tablespoon of oil
1 large onion, roughly chopped
3 cloves of chopped garlic
2 large sticks of celery, trimmed
5 cups of vegetable stock
500g of fresh or frozen peas
1 bunch of mint (approximately 30g), leaves only
pepper and salt to season

1. In a large saucepan, heat the oil and add the onion, garlic and celery.
2. Once the vegetables start to brown, add stock and drained split peas. Cover and simmer for 45-60 minutes. The longer you have soaked your split peas, the faster they will cook. Stir occasionally to make sure nothing sticks to the bottom of the pan.
3. Once the split peas have become more like a puree, add the peas and cook for a further 10 minutes. Turn the heat off and add the mint leaves. Puree your soup with a stick blender or leave to cool, then puree in a food processor.
4. Adjust seasoning to taste and add more water if you prefer a thinner soup.
5. You may also wish to add a little milk, cream or créme fraiche for a richer soup.

Play Time!

- Yellow split peas will work just as well in this soup. Of course it will not be as green.
- Other vegetables can be added: orange vegetables for a sweeter soup.
- Try other herbs for different flavours, e.g. dill, sage, parsley, lemon balm, coriander or basil.

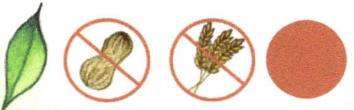

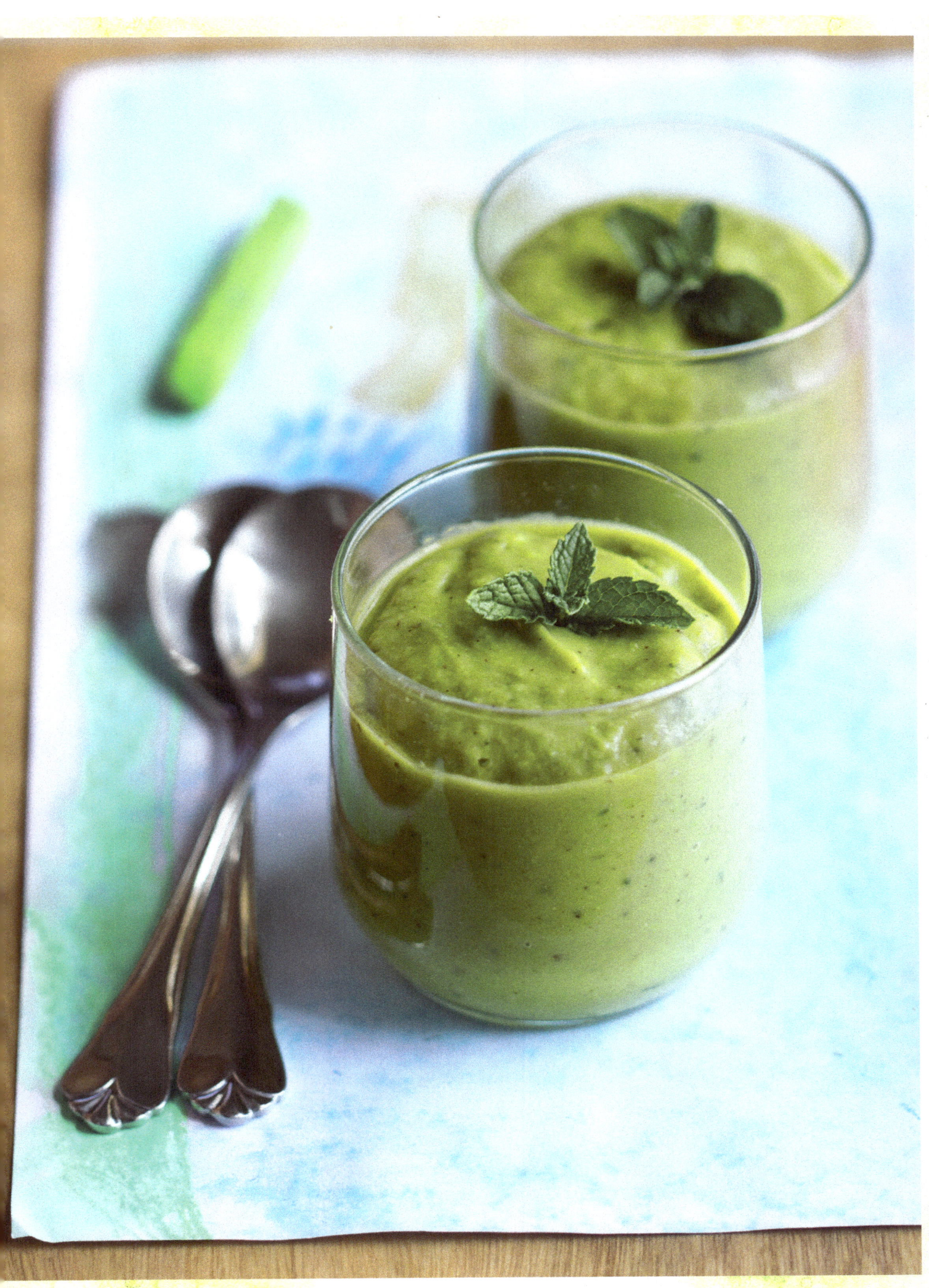

Fire Engine Soup

This is a very warming soup with spices and hearty lentils. It will make you feel great inside.

Serves 4-5

1 ¼ cups red lentils, soaked for at least 6 hours*

1 tablespoon of oil

1 onion, finely chopped

3 cloves of crushed garlic

1 tablespoon of grated fresh ginger

1 teaspoon of ground paprika (smoked is best, but not essential)

1 teaspoon of ground coriander

1 teaspoon of ground cumin

½ teaspoon of ground cinnamon

½ teaspoon of ground turmeric

½ teaspoon of ground nutmeg

1 litre of vegetable stock

350g of grated sweet potato (a food processor will do this job quickly)

700g bottle of passata

sea salt and pepper to season

¾ cup of chopped fresh coriander

* Red lentils do not require soaking in order to cook quickly. I soak them for health benefits (see page 64 for more information). If you do not have time, add more water to the mix as it cooks to maintain a soupy consistency.

1. Heat oil in a large saucepan over medium heat.
2. Add onion and stir-fry until tender. Add the garlic and ginger with the spices and stir for one minute.
3. Add the drained lentils and remaining ingredients, except seasonings and fresh coriander.
4. Stir to combine, then simmer covered for 25-30 minutes. Stir occasionally.
5. When the lentils are soft, season and stir in fresh coriander before serving.

Play Time!

- Pumpkin and carrot work just as well as the sweet potato in this soup. Try a mixture of all three.
- If you prefer smooth soups, Fire Engine Soup tastes just as good pureed.
- Add other mixtures of vegetables and herbs: parsley, basil and dill will also taste good.

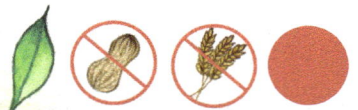

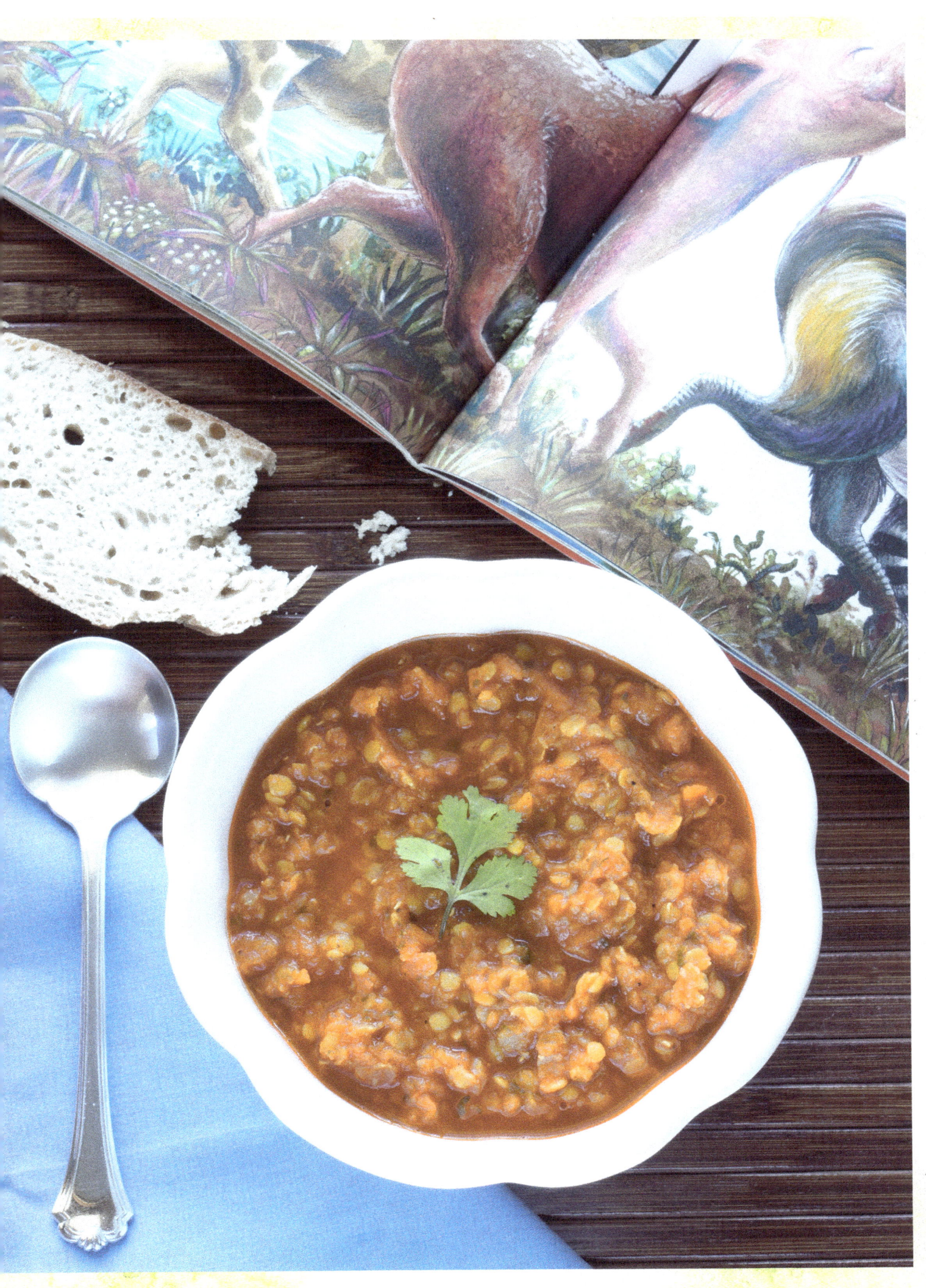

Beastly Brews 171

The Soup of Endless Possibilities

For a quick meal that could be dinner at night or a weekend lunch, make a soup with whatever you have in the fridge. I often do this the day before I go to the farmers markets so that I can use up the previous week's produce. Here is the basic recipe. Make sure you read it the whole way through before beginning, as this is written very differently to the other recipes in this book. It is non-specific and allows for ample creativity.

Serves 4-5

1 tablespoon of oil
1 onion, leek or bunch of spring onions, roughly chopped
2-3 cloves of roughly chopped garlic
1.3kg roughly chopped vegetables (whatever you have)*
1 litre of vegetable stock

*Beware of overdoing one particular vegetable if it has an overpowering taste. A lot of my soups have a base of the orange vegetables, such as carrot, pumpkin and sweet potato and then I add things like broccoli, celery, cauliflower, peas or cabbage.

List of other possibilities
1-2 tablespoons of sliced ginger
1 mild chilli, roughly chopped
1-2 tablespoons of curry paste
1 tablespoon of miso paste mixed with 1 litre of water (instead of vegetable stock)
1 cup coconut cream
1 cup of your favourite milk
fresh herbs such as thyme, rosemary, sage, parsley, dill, basil, mint, tarragon, fennel

1. In a large pot or pressure cooker, heat the oil and stir-fry the onion (or similar) and garlic. At this point you can also add fresh ginger and/or chilli. Add a little water to stop these ingredients sticking to the pan.
2. Next add the stock or miso and water.
   If you are using curry paste, stir-fry it before adding the stock.
3. Add the harder vegetables at this stage. If you are modifying quantities, as a general guide add enough stock to cover the vegetables. At this point also add any woody herbs such as rosemary, sage or thyme. Now cover the soup and let it all simmer until mushy. Pressure cookers will do the job a lot faster, but a large saucepan can be left to simmer on low for some time.
4. Once your harder vegetables are soft, add your fast cooking vegetables. Examples include broccoli, cabbage, zucchini, peas.

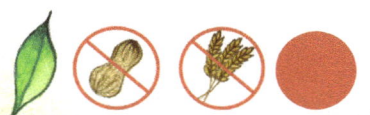

5. When the soft vegetables are cooked, it is time for seasoning and softer herbs. For a creamy soup, add coconut cream or a little of your favorite milk.
6. Puree the soup. You may wish to use a stick blender or food processor. Add more water if need be.

The variations to this kind of soup are endless and that is the positive thing about it. You can adjust according to your family's tastes and what you have available.

Hearty Lentil Soup

This soup is more chunky than the other lentil soups. It is very versatile as you can use whichever vegetables you have available and you can use other beans as well.

Serves 4-5

1 ½ cups cooked black eye or canellini beans or ½ cup dried, (soaked for at least 6 hours)
1 cup puy lentils, soaked for at least 6 hours
1 tablespoon of oil
1 large onion, finely chopped
2 cloves of crushed garlic
2 teaspoons of ground coriander
2 teaspoons of smoked paprika
2 tablespoons of tomato paste
3 cups of diced vegetables (separate harder longer cooking vegetables from the softer, fast cooking ones)
1.5 litres of vegetable stock
400g of chopped, fresh tomatoes or 400g of passata
⅓ cup finely chopped parsley

1. If you are using dried beans, cook according to directions on page 64.
2. Heat oil in a large saucepan and add the onion and garlic. Stir fry until tender.
3. Add the spices followed by the tomato paste and stir constantly, making sure that the mix doesn't burn.
4. Add the harder vegetables, stock, tomatoes and drained lentils. Mix well and leave to simmer with the lid on for 20-25 minutes. During this time give the soup a stir every 5-10 minutes.
5. When the harder vegetables have softened, add the soft/fast cooking vegetables and the beans. Leave to simmer for a further 5 minutes.
6. Before serving, stir in the parsley.

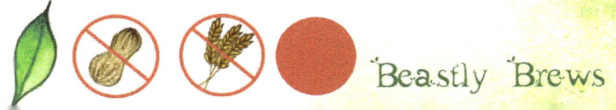

Mushroom Soup

This soup has a rich, deep flavour, owing to the variety of mushrooms included in the recipe. The lemon juice stirred in at the end is paramount to its delicious flavour.

Serves 4-5

1 tablespoon of oil
1 large red onion, roughly chopped
2 cloves of crushed garlic
200g mixed gourmet mushrooms* (e.g. shiitake, king oyster, porcini)
500g portabello mushrooms, roughly chopped
1.2 litres of vegetable stock
2 tablespoons of fresh thyme leaves
pepper to season
sea salt to season
juice of one lemon

*Fruit shops often have little trays of mixed gourmet mushrooms

1. Heat oil in a large saucepan, add the onion and stir-fry until tender.
2. Add the garlic and mushrooms. Cook until the mushrooms are soft.
3. Add the stock and thyme. Cover and simmer for 20 minutes.
4. Puree the soup with a stick blender or leave to cool and puree in a food processor.
5. Season with pepper and salt. Stir in the lemon juice before serving.

Play Time!

- There are many different types of mushrooms. Try different combinations as they have varying flavours.
- As your base you may wish to use button mushrooms instead of the portabello. They will give a lighter colour to the soup.
- For a more creamy mushroom soup, swap some of the water quantity for your favourite milk.
- If you like a bit of texture in your soup, puree only half and stir back into the pot.

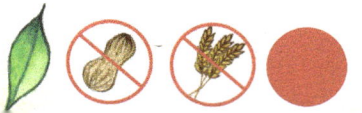

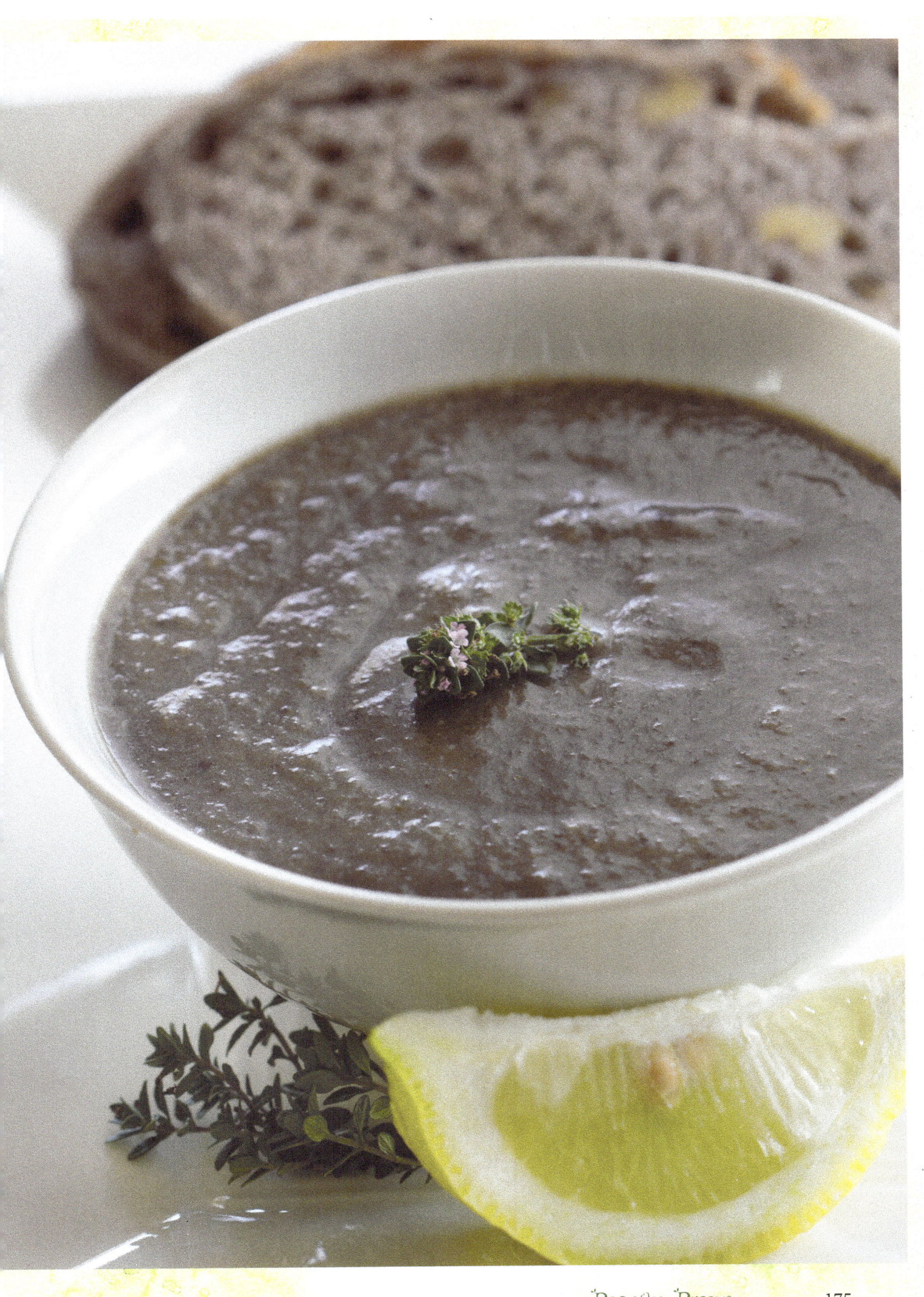

Tomato and Beetroot Soup

A soup rich in flavour and easy to make. The beetroot goes surprisingly well in a tomato soup and so provides a nice twist on the old favourite.
I like to do this soup in my pressure cooker, as it all happens a lot faster.

Serves 4-5

1 tablespoon of oil
1 large red onion, roughly chopped
3 cloves of crushed garlic
¼ cup of tomato paste
3 cups of vegetable stock
1kg tomatoes, roughly chopped
350g beetroot, trimmed, peeled and roughly chopped
2 large carrots, trimmed and roughly chopped
2 sticks celery, trimmed and roughly chopped
2 bay leaves
sea salt and pepper to taste

1. Heat oil in a large saucepan and add the onion and garlic. Stir-fry until soft.
2. Add remaining ingredients except salt and pepper and cover.
3. Bring to the boil and then turn down to a simmer until all vegetables are soft.
4. Puree with a stick blender or leave to cool and then puree in a food processor.
5. Season with salt and pepper to taste and serve.

Play Time!

- Instead of the carrot, try sweet potato or pumpkin.
- Add some basil leaves before pureeing as this herb always goes well with tomatoes.
- Try roasting your tomatoes before adding to the soup. If you do this, add them at the end. By leaving them in the oven until they are slightly charred, the flavour will taste "roasted".
- Add a little cream or yoghurt before serving for a richer soup.

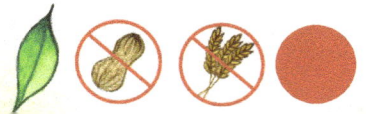

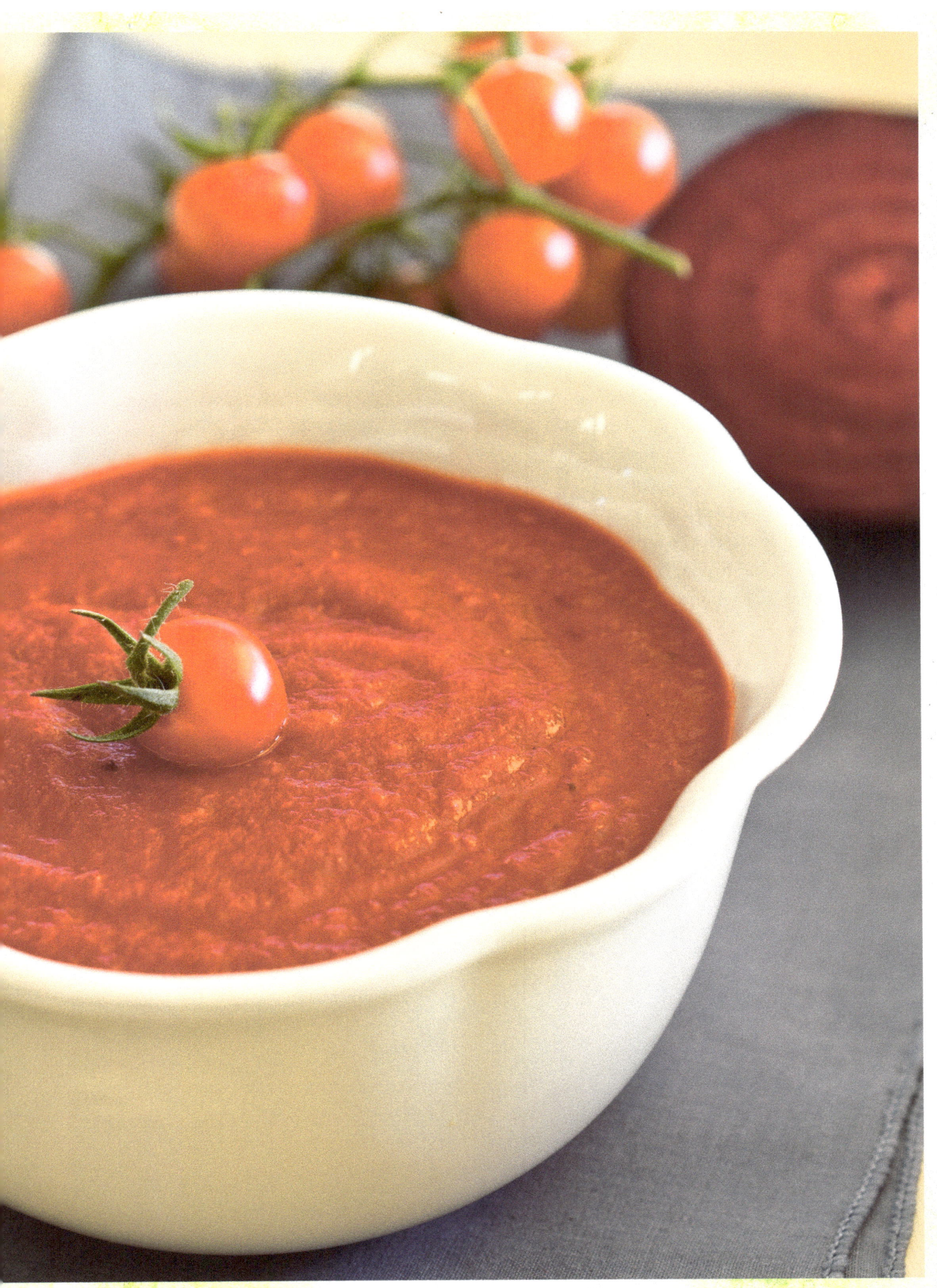

Pumpkin Soup

Pumpkin soup is one of those dishes that never needs to be the same. This is my basic recipe, but I like to vary it quite a lot. For beginners, especially children with plainer palates, this is a great start. Allow them to be involved in creating new flavours in this recipe. Check out the "Play Time"!

Serves 4-5

1 tablespoon of oil

1 large onion, roughly chopped

3 cloves of garlic, roughly chopped

800g peeled, diced pumpkin

550g peeled, diced potatoes

1 litre of vegetable stock

¼ cup of roughly chopped parsley leaves

sea salt and pepper to taste

dollop of yoghurt or cream or squeeze of lime juice - to serve

1. Heat the oil in a large saucepan and fry the onion until it is soft.
2. Add the remaining ingredients (except salt and pepper) and cover. Simmer on medium-low heat until the pumpkin goes soft. This should take about 20 minutes, depending on the size of your pieces.
3. Add the parsley, salt and pepper. Puree your soup using a stick blender or leave to cool and blend it in a food processor until smooth.
4. Serve with yoghurt, cream or lime juice.

Play Time!

- I often add sweet potato and/or carrots to my pumpkin soup for a varied flavour.
- As a base, I sometimes use a home-made Thai or Indian curry paste and then I add coconut cream before pureeing.
- Other herbs are a great addition too. Try coriander, dill, basil, sage or lemon balm.

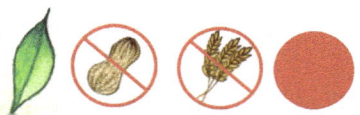

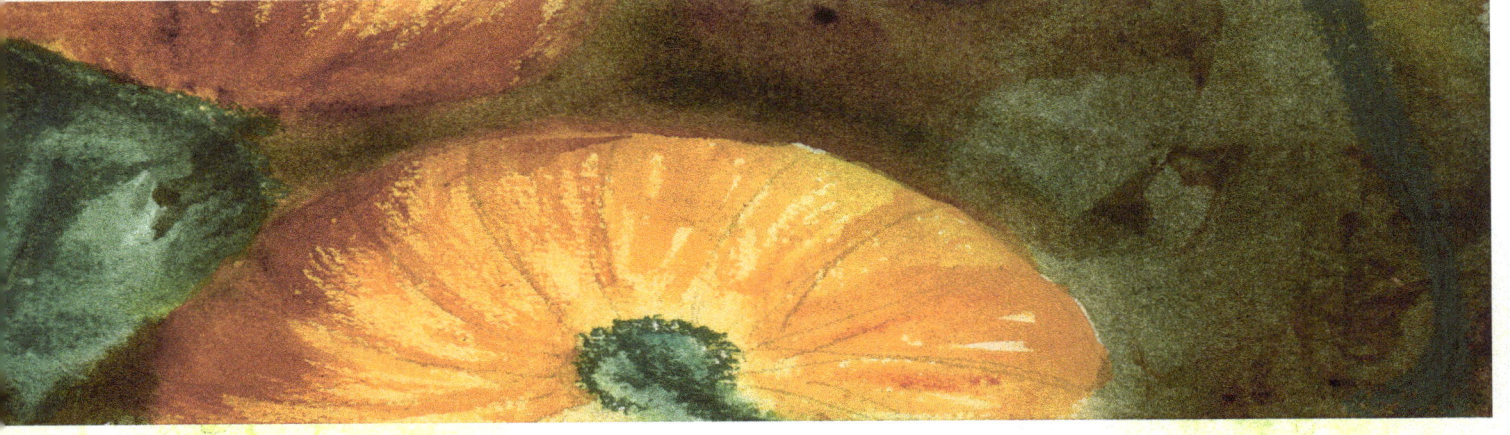

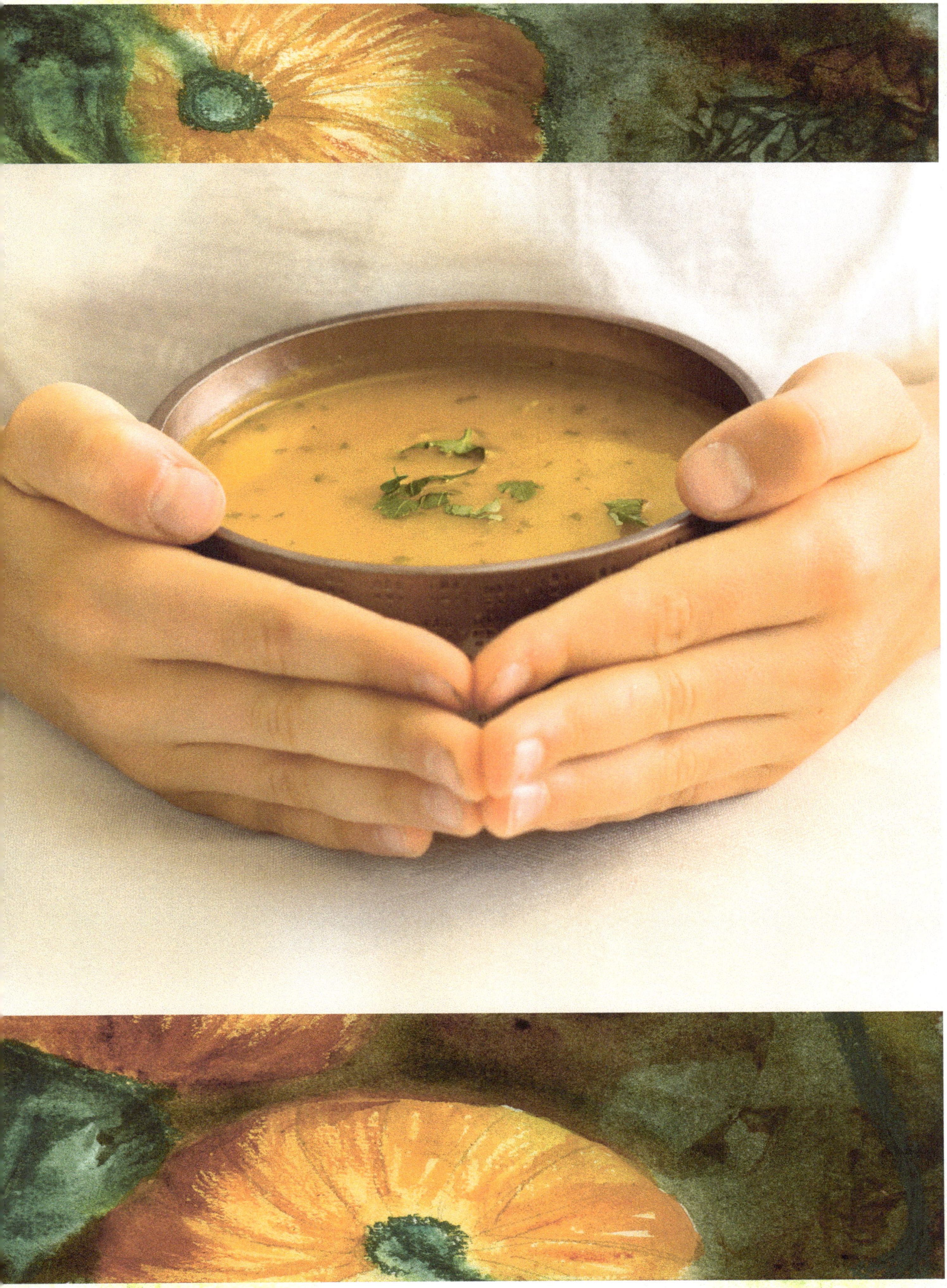

Beastly Brews

Turkish Red Lentil Soup

Whenever we go to a Turkish Restaurant, Ethan, Ryan and I like to order the Red Lentil Soup. This is my version which has the thumbs up from the family.

Serves 4-5

- **2 cups of red lentils, soaked for at least 6 hours***
- **1 tablespoon of oil**
- **1 large onion, roughly chopped**
- **3 cloves of crushed garlic**
- **1 small chilli, roughly chopped (optional)**
- **2 teaspoons of ground paprika**
- **2 teaspoons of ground cumin**
- **3 tablespoons of tomato paste**
- **1 ¼ litres of vegetable stock**
- **2 large carrots (approx. 250g), roughly chopped**
- **lemon juice to taste**

* Red lentils do not require soaking in order to cook quickly. I soak them for health benefits (see page 64 for more information). If you do not have time, add more water to the mix as it cooks to maintain a soupy consistency.

1. Heat the oil in a large saucepan and fry the onion until it is soft.
2. Add the garlic, chilli (if using) and the spices. Mix over low heat until the spices become aromatic.
3. Stir in the tomato paste and cook for a minute.
4. Add the stock, drained lentils and carrots then bring to the boil. Reduce heat and simmer until the carrots and lentils are soft. Stir occasionally. This should take about 30 minutes.
5. Puree your soup using a stick blender or leave to cool and blend it in a food processor until smooth.
6. Stir in the lemon juice before serving.

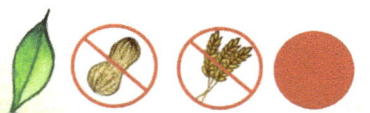

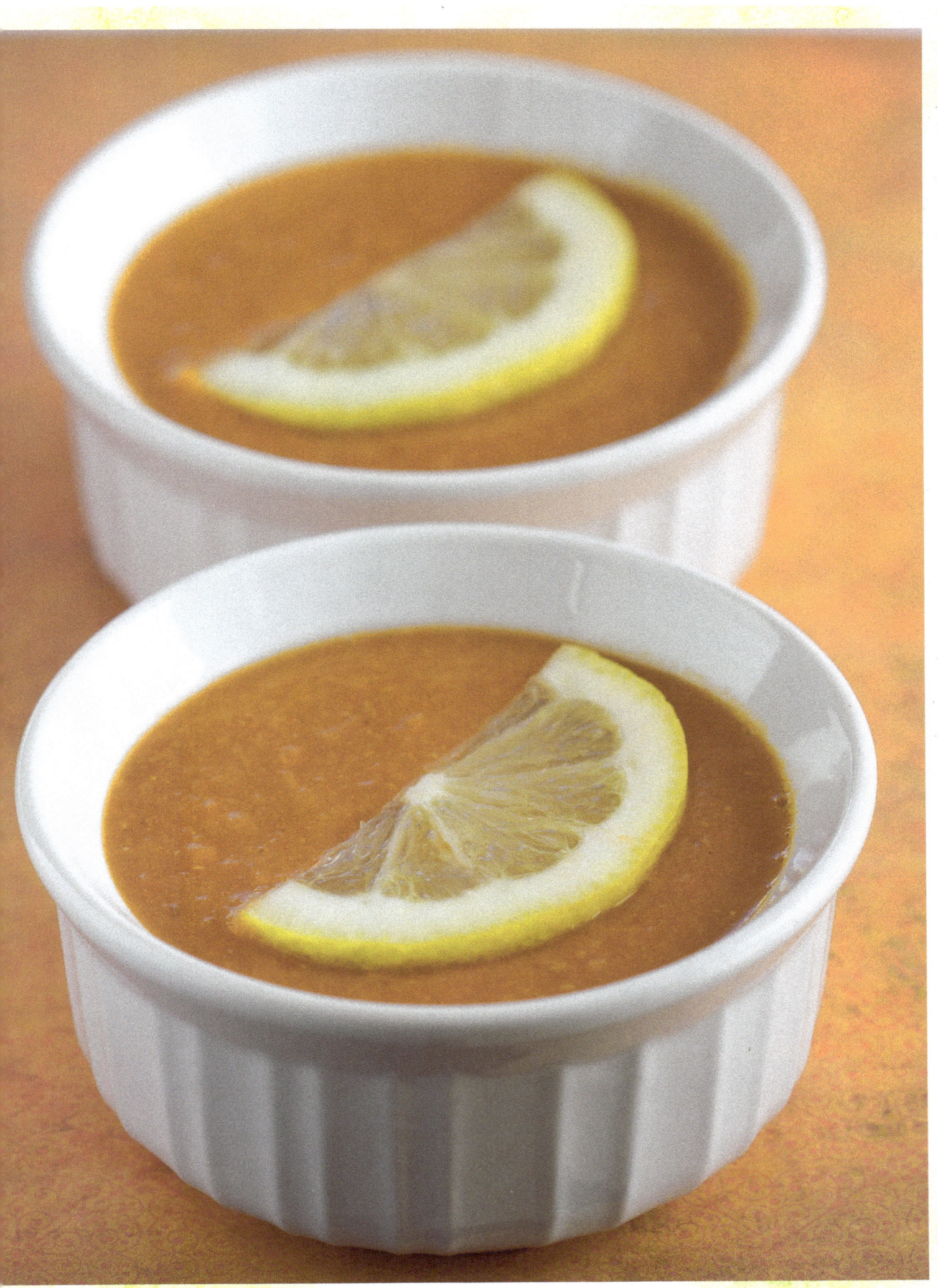

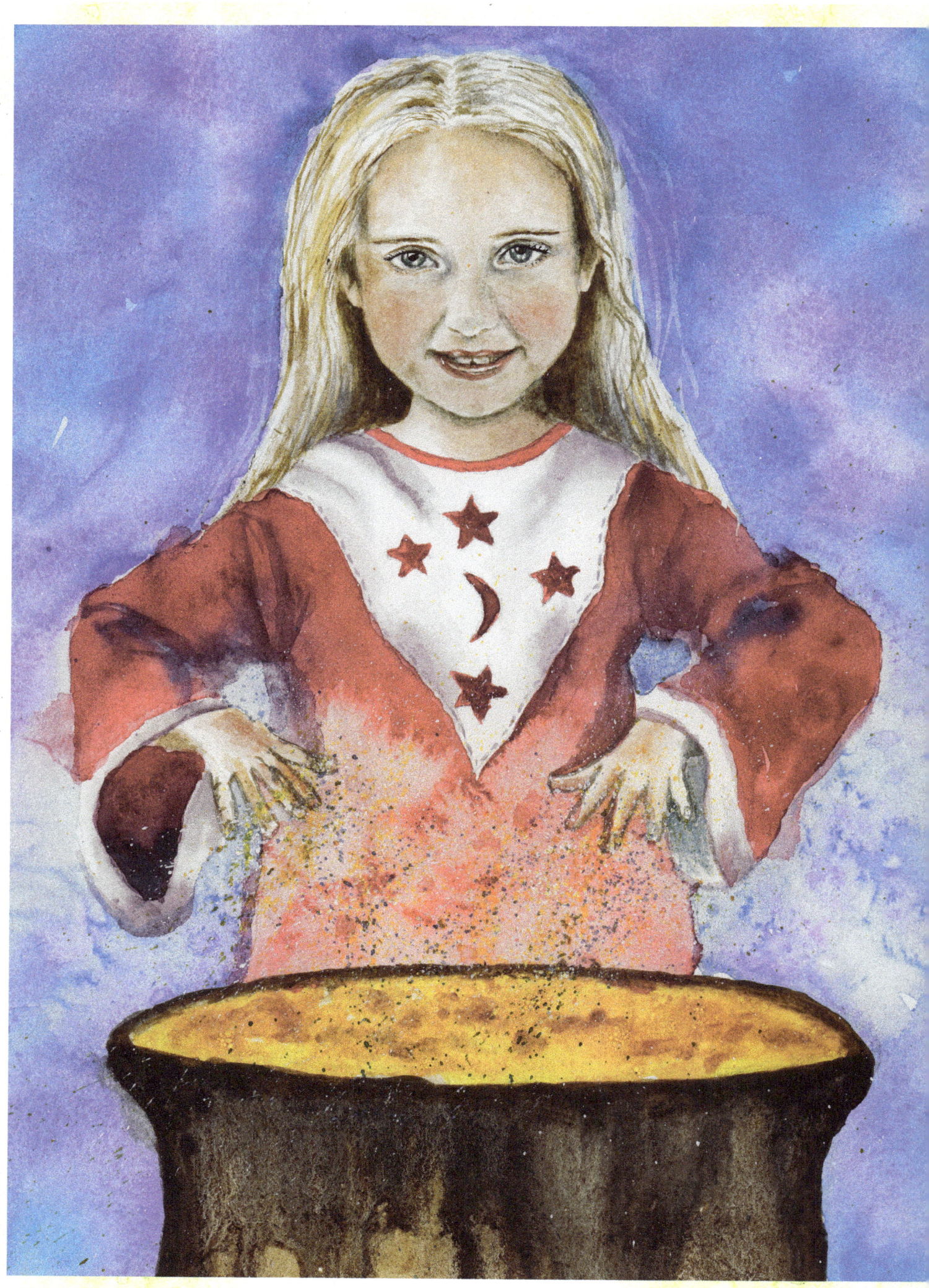

Magical Mains

Magical Mains

The evening meal is a time for sharing food and stories about your day. Use some of these tasty recipes to make a magical meal for your family. There is a wonderland of colour, texture and flavour, as well as plenty of "Play Time" hints for those feeling creative or adventurous.

We also make our main meals from a mixture of recipes in the "Gifts from the Garden" and "Little Morsels" sections where there is plenty of variety.
Your inspiration does not have to end here!

"Our bodies are our gardens, our wills are our gardeners."
~William Shakespeare

Pizzas

Making pizzas can be a quick meal or a long process of small steps, depending on whether you decide to make your own pizza dough, sauce etc. Regardless of that it does not need to resemble the high cholesterol fast food version. Should you decide not to make your bases at home, a great healthy alternative is Lebanese bread: preferably wholemeal. A sauce can be as simple as a thick passata, seasoned with a little pepper and salt, and of course when making your own pizzas you can choose from a wide range of healthy toppings. See the topping list below for suggestions.

Serves 4-5

I like to make our own bases because the kids love to knead the dough and roll it into unusual shapes (anything but round!). Of course assembling toppings is a job most kids enjoy too, as it allows them a high level of control: we all know how they love that.

Pizza dough - If you don't feel like making the dough, try wholemeal Lebanese bread as a base

7g sachet of dried yeast
250ml warm water
1 tablespoon of honey or rice syrup
1 ½ cups of unbleached spelt or wheat flour
1 ½ cups of wholemeal spelt or wheat flour
1 teaspoon of sea salt
1 tablespoon of oil

1. In a small bowl, combine the yeast and warm water. Leave to sit for 10 minutes and then stir in the honey.
2. In a large bowl, combine the flours and salt.
3. Add the flour and salt to the liquid and mix to form a dough.
4. Knead the dough for at least 5 minutes. This will develop the gluten in the flour.
5. Grease a bowl with the oil and place the dough inside. Cover with a wet cloth and leave to proof for an hour, during which time it will double in size.
6. Divide the dough into portions and using a flour dusted rolling pin, roll out on a floured surface into bases.

Pizza sauce

1 small onion, roughly chopped
2 cloves garlic, crushed
2 cups of really ripe chopped tomatoes or 400g of passata
¼ cup tomato paste
2 tablespoons of fresh chopped herbs, e.g. basil, marjoram, oregano, thyme or parsley. If you need to buy your herbs, rather than buying multiple bunches, basil is a good all rounder.
1 teaspoon of balsamic vinegar
sea salt and pepper to season

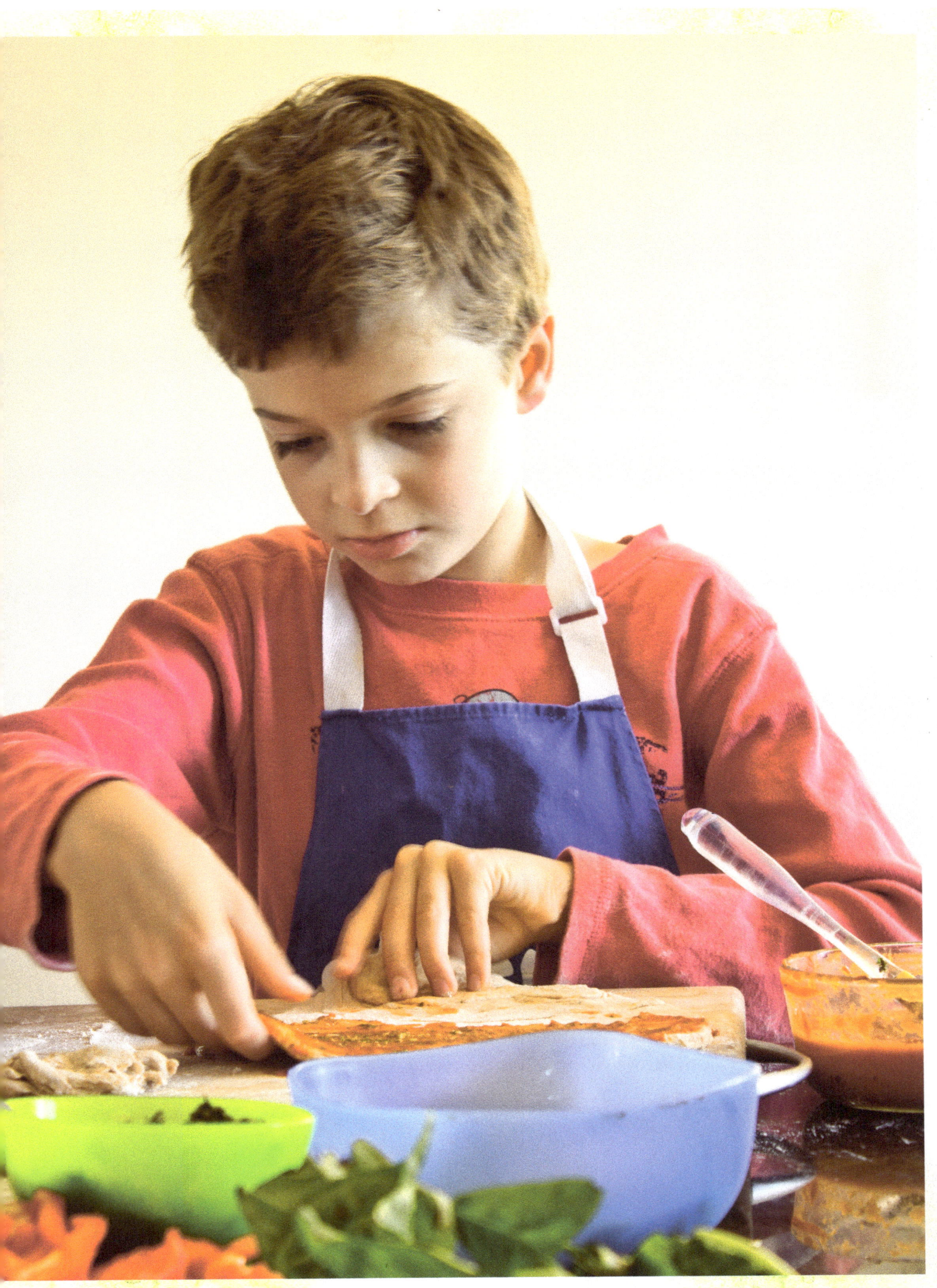

1. Heat the oil in a small saucepan and add the onion and garlic. Stir-fry until tender.
2. Add remaining ingredients and simmer with the lid on for 10 minutes.
3. Taste for seasoning and then puree with a stick blender or in a food processor.

Pesto (*Dollop on before you add the cheese so that it melts together or add after it is cooked.*)

leaves from one bunch of basil (a bunch being approximately 60g including stems).
¼ cup of pine nuts
30g Parmesan cheese (optional)
1 small clove of garlic
½ cup of oil (if you are cooking the pesto, use oil, otherwise, olive oil is best)
sea salt to taste

Place all ingredients into a food processor and blend until smooth. Adjust seasoning to taste.

Suggestions for Topping Ingredients

diced onions   **sliced capsicum**
diced pineapple   **chopped sun-dried tomatoes**
sliced mushrooms   **olives**
chopped artichoke hearts   **grilled eggplant slices**
grilled zucchini slices

roasted vegetables e.g. pumpkin, sweet potato, potato (when you next make a roast dinner, make extra vegetables to chop up for your pizzas the following night).
gourmet cheeses such as bocconcini, mozzarella and haloumi
egg: crack a raw egg over the pizza before baking and it will cook into the other toppings

Cooking your Pizza

There are three different ways to cook a pizza at home (provided you don't have your own wood-fired pizza oven).

- The first is to lay the pizza on a tray and bake it in a moderate oven (moderate meaning 180°C).
- The second is to use a pizza stone. The stone should be preheated in a moderate oven and then the assembled pizza placed on top and put straight back into the oven. This will create a nice crispy base. To transfer the pizza, either use a large pizza spatula or assemble it on a piece of baking paper that may then be lifted onto the stone.
- The third way is to pan-fry the pizza base, assemble the pizza while it is in the frying pan and then grill the top in the oven once the bottom is browned.
- Try them all and see which works best for you.

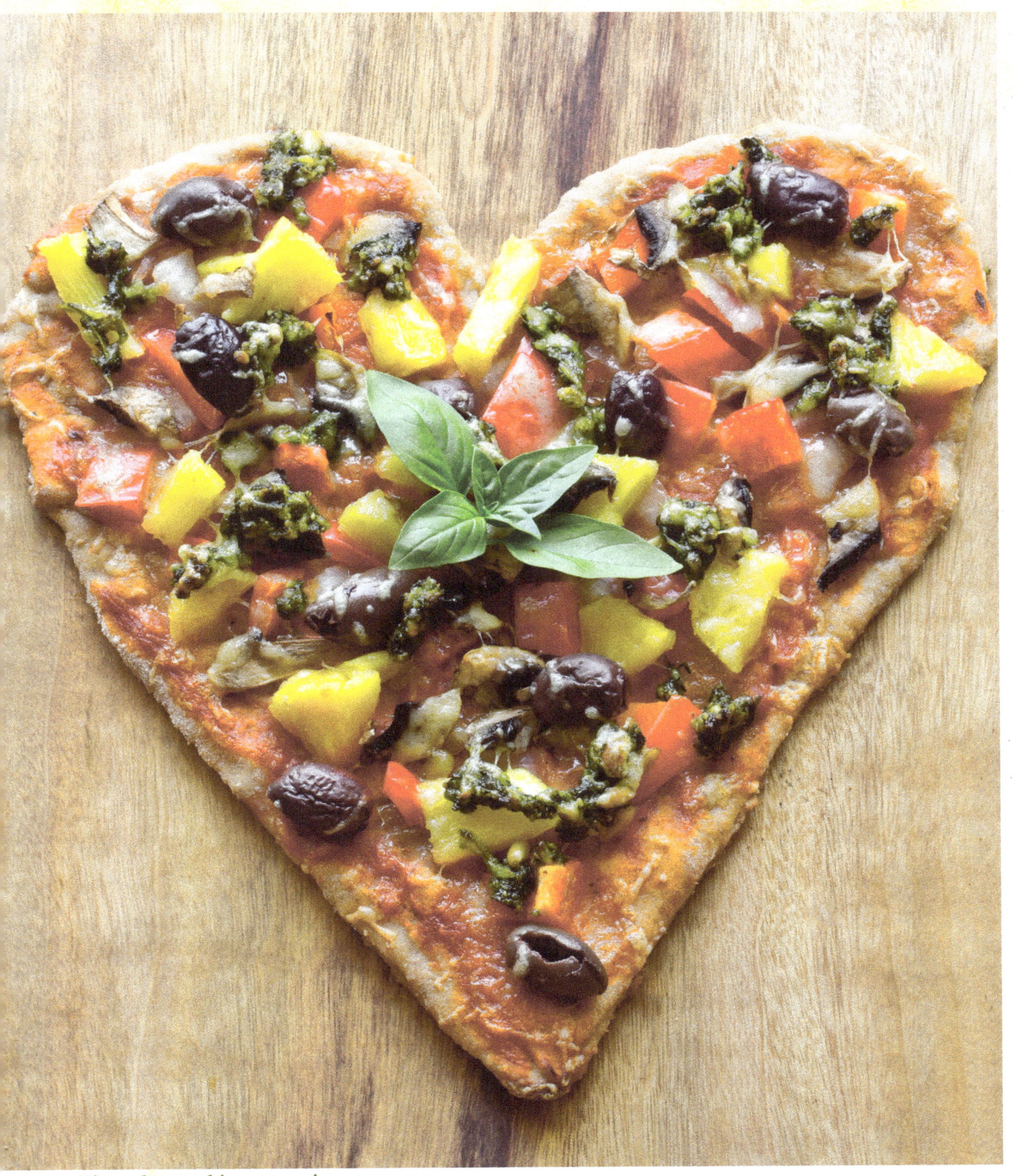

Tips when making your pizza

- Adjust your topping quantity to the thickness of your base - a very thin base will not support a lot of heavy toppings
- Beware of adding a large quantity of very wet toppings such as juicy tomatoes and pineapple as the base will become soggy.
- If adding a raw egg before cooking, crack it over the fully made pizza just before putting into the oven. The cheese and barrier of other toppings will stop it from soaking your base.

Nachos

We love Mexican food, so this is a favourite at our house. I don't always serve the combination of beans and toppings as nachos, sometimes they are burritos, or just served with rice on a plate. You can also do tacos. Mix and match, make it as simple or as intricate as you like.

Serves 4-5

2 cups of dried pinto or borlotti beans (soaked 8-10 hrs) or 5 cups of cooked
1 tablespoon of oil
1 large onion, finely chopped
3 cloves crushed garlic
2 teaspoons of Mexican Seasoning*
2 tablespoons of tomato paste
400g of diced fresh tomatoes
½ cup of water
1 x 200g bag of plain corn chips
grated cheese for topping

Extra Toppings
Either 1 quantity of guacamole (page 98) or diced avocado
Either 1 quantity of salsa (page 98) or diced tomatoes

*Mexican Seasoning Recipe
2 teaspoons of sea salt
1 teaspoon of pepper
2 teaspoons of paprika
1 tablespoon of ground cumin
1 teaspoon of onion powder
1 teaspoon of garlic powder
1 teaspoon of chilli powder
1 teaspoon of dried oregano

Combine all ingredients and store in a jar.

1. If you are using dried beans, cook according to directions on page 64.
2. In a large saucepan, fry the onion and garlic in the oil until tender.
3. Add the seasoning and tomato paste. Stir to mix and add a little water if it starts to stick.
4. Add the cooked beans, tomatoes and water. Simmer over low heat for 15 minutes.
5. Meanwhile, preheat your oven to 180°C convection or turn on your grill.
6. In a large baking dish or small individual dishes, lay out your corn chips.
7. Grate cheese over the corn chips and then spoon your bean mix over the top. Top with more grated cheese and bake in the oven until the chips start to brown and the cheese melts (usually about 10-15 minutes). If you are cooking under a grill, make sure you watch it closely to avoid burning the top.
8. Serve with toppings.

Play Time!

- To make a dairy free version of this, omit the cheese and do not bake. Assemble the corn chips followed by the warm bean mix, salsa and guacamole.
- As a dip: In a large dish, layer the beans, then salsa and guacamole. Serve with corn chips.

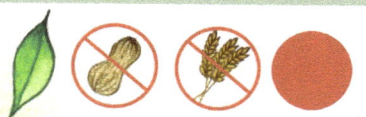

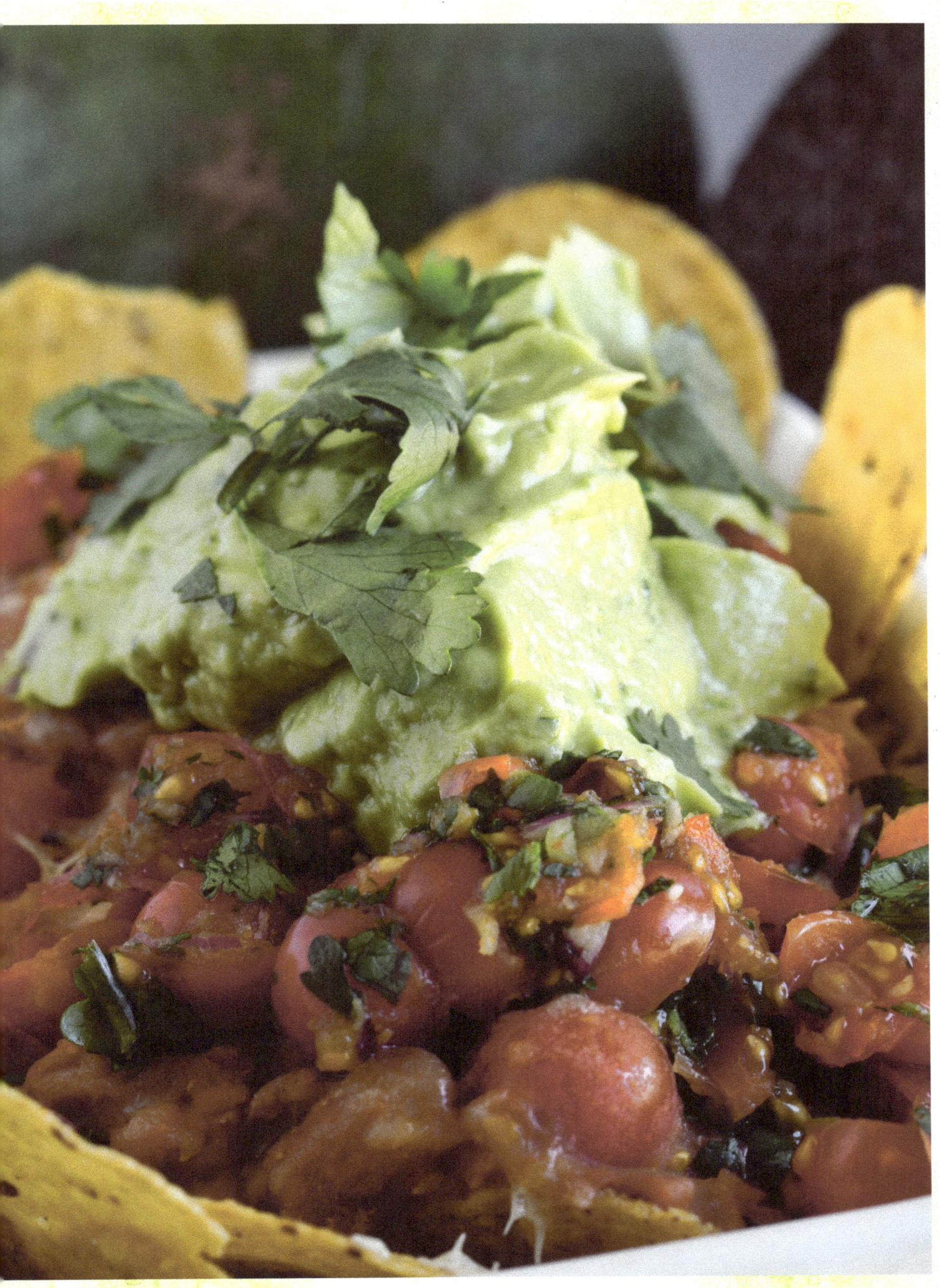

Shepherd's Pie

This is a hearty meal, perfect for winter. It has plenty of protein and nourishing vegetables, as well as the comfort of mashed potatoes. You can make this in one large baking dish or two smaller ones. I like to do the latter so that I can freeze one for another night. As children get older and become more confident in the kitchen, meals such as this may be created with a little help from an adult.

Serves 8-10 (freeze one for later)

1 ½ cups either puy or brown lentils, soaked for at least 6hrs
1 tablespoon of oil
1 large onion, finely chopped
3 cloves garlic, crushed
2 sticks celery, finely chopped
2 carrots, sliced or pulverised in a food processor
¼ cup tomato paste
1 x 700g bottle of passata
½ cup of water
1 tablespoon of vegetable stock concentrate
1 bay leaf
600g finely chopped or pulverised vegetables. (For harder vegetables such as pumpkin, sweet potato or swede, allow longer cooking time. Add faster cooking after removing the mix from the heat).
½ cup finely chopped parsley
sea salt and pepper to season.

Topping

1.5kg potatoes, peeled and chopped
½ cup of milk
30g butter or 2 tablespoons of oil
¼ teaspoon of ground nutmeg (freshly grated is even better)
1 teaspoon of sea salt
freshly ground pepper to season
finely chopped parsley to garnish

1. Drain and rinse the lentils and set aside.
2. In a large saucepan, fry the onion and garlic in oil over medium heat until tender.
3. Add the celery and carrots and cook for a few minutes, stirring occasionally.
4. Add the tomato paste, passata, water, stock concentrate, bay leaf, harder vegetables and lentils.
5. Mix well and cover.

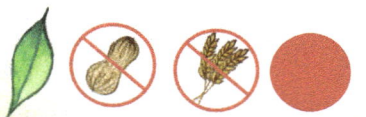

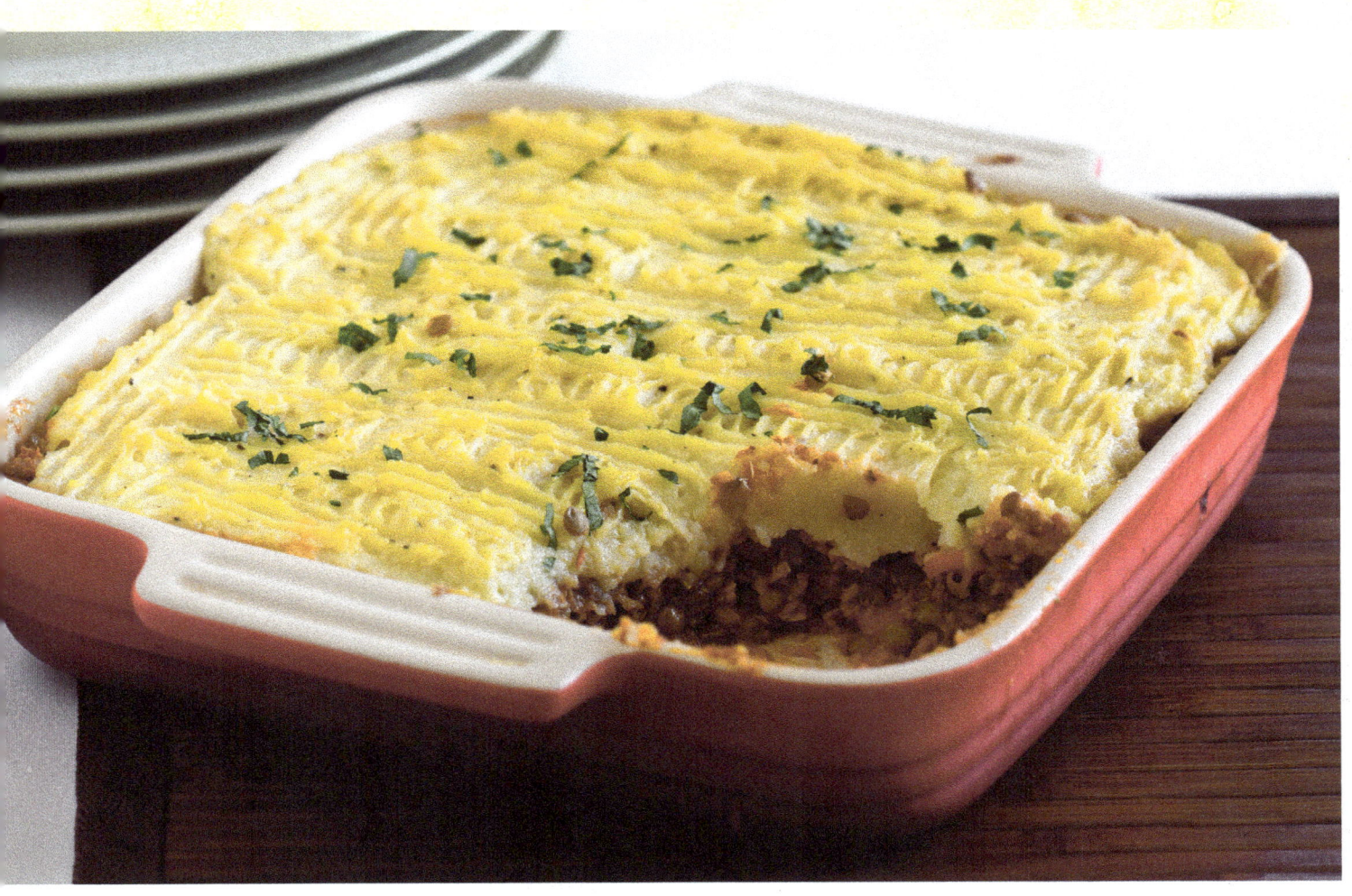

6. Simmer for 15 minutes, stirring occasionally.
7. Preheat oven to 180°C convection or 160°C fan forced.
8. Meanwhile, steam the potato pieces until soft.
9. Using a hand mixer, combine the potatoes, milk, butter or oil, nutmeg, salt and pepper. The potato mix needs to be smooth and quite creamy so that it spreads over the pie filling easily. Add more milk if required.
10. When the lentil mix is cooked, remove from heat and add any faster cooking vegetables, parsley, salt and pepper. These vegetables will cook during the baking time.
11. Pour the lentil mix into your baking dish or dishes and cover with an even layer of mashed potato.
12. If you would like a pattern on top, use a fork to scrape ridges in the potato.
13. Bake for 25-30 minutes and serve hot, garnished with finely chopped parsley.

Play Time!

- For the filling, add different herbs to flavour or even a little soy sauce or red wine!
- For the topping, add some sweet potato or pumpkin to the mix.
- Make little individual servings in large ramekins for that dinner party feel.

Magical Mains

Beautiful Bolognaise

This bolognaise recipe is packed with nutrients and flavour. The orange vegetables are in the mix for their sweetness which complements the acidity of the tomatoes nicely. It may be changed in a multitude of ways to suit what is in your pantry. Have children help with choosing the herbs and vegetables you add. This recipe can easily be made gluten free as there are many suitable pastas on the market now.

Serves 4-5 with pasta

- **1 cup red lentils, soaked for at least 6 hrs***
- **1 onion, finely chopped**
- **3 cloves garlic, crushed**
- **1 tablespoon of oil**
- **1 large red capsicum, finely chopped**
- **1 x 700g bottle of passata**
- **3 tablespoons of tomato paste**
- **1 cup of vegetable stock**
- **⅓ cup of organic red wine (optional: it does add a yummy flavour)**
- **250g pulverised or grated orange vegetables (e.g. pumpkin, carrot or sweet potato)**
- **200g pulverised green vegetables (e.g. beans, broccoli, zucchini)**
- **small bunch of basil leaves, finely chopped**
- **sea salt/pepper to season**

* Red lentils do not require soaking in order to cook quickly. I only soak them for health benefits (see page 64 for more information). If you do not wish to soak them or don't have time, simply add more water to the mix as it cooks to maintain a bolognaise-like consistency.

1. In a large saucepan, stir-fry the onion and garlic in oil until tender.
2. Add the remaining ingredients down to and including the orange vegetables. Mix well.
3. Simmer over medium heat, stirring occasionally to prevent the mix sticking to the bottom of the pan. While the sauce is cooking, prepare your pasta according to package instructions.
4. Once the mixture is thick and the lentils are soft, add the green vegetables and cook for a further 5 minutes.
5. Before serving, stir in the basil and taste for seasoning.

Play Time!

- If you don't want to use red wine in the mix, add some pulverised sun-dried tomatoes.
- If you have plenty of fresh tomatoes, blend 700g to a smooth mix and use this instead of passata.
- Add other herbs such as thyme, oregano or marjoram.

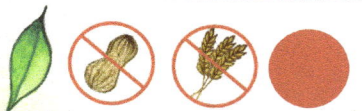

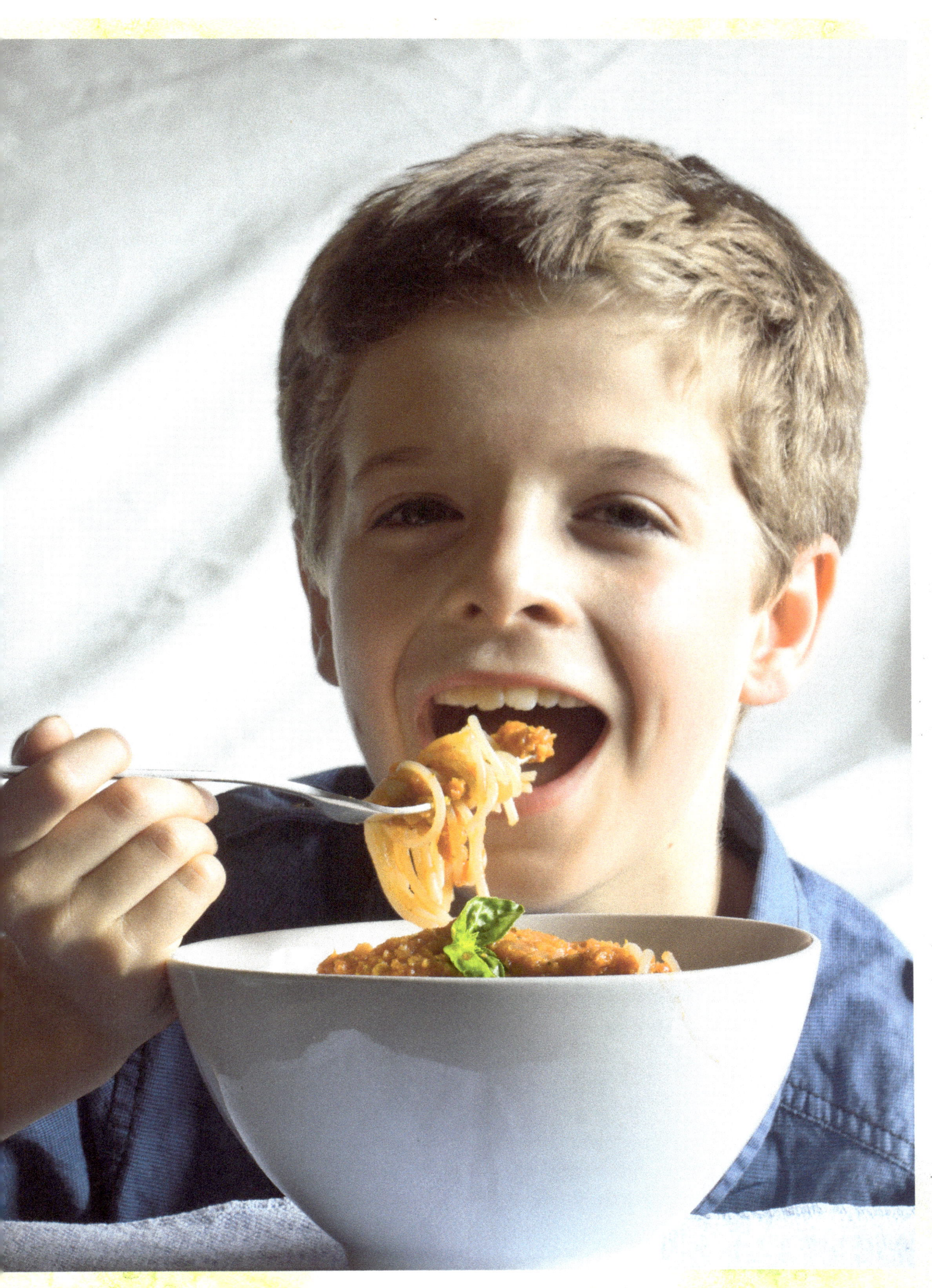
Magical Mains

Tomato Sunrise Slice

This is similar to a quiche recipe, but without pastry. It is lovely as a hot meal with salad, but may also be eaten cold the next day, so is suitable for school lunch boxes. This meal may also be made without the cheese: because of the semi-dried tomatoes and basil it is still very tasty. I sometimes make this slice in a large baking dish as specified below, but at other times I make 2 smaller ones, freezing one for later. Children can be involved in using the food processor and whisking the eggs.

Serves 4-5

1 large onion, grated or pulverised in a food processor.
5 tightly packed cups of grated/pulverised vegetables (e.g. sweet potato, pumpkin, zucchini, cauliflower, spinach, mushrooms, carrots)
1 cup of grated cheese
2 cloves of crushed garlic
1 cup of semi-dried tomatoes
small bunch of basil, leaves only
7 eggs
½ cup of wholemeal wheat or spelt flour
½ teaspoon of baking powder
salt and pepper to season
2 large tomatoes, sliced
paprika to sprinkle (smoked is best)

1. Preheat oven to 180°C convection or 160°C fan forced.
2. Grease and line a 30cm x 21cm baking dish
3. In a large mixing bowl, combine vegetables and most of the cheese (reserve a little for the top of the slice).
4. In your food processor, combine garlic, semi-dried tomatoes, basil, eggs, flour, baking powder and salt and pepper until smooth.
5. Fold the egg mix into the vegetable mix and pour into the baking dish.
6. Top with reserved cheese and slices of tomato. Sprinkle paprika over the top.
7. Bake for 45 minutes or until a skewer comes out clean.

Play Time!

- Use Mediterranean vegetables such as eggplant, mushrooms, capsicums and olives.
- Make it simple: use only one vegetable such as spinach. Add feta and dill to give extra flavour.
- Vary your herbs. Either throw in a mix or use parsley, sage, dill or coriander.

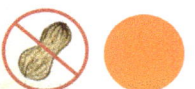

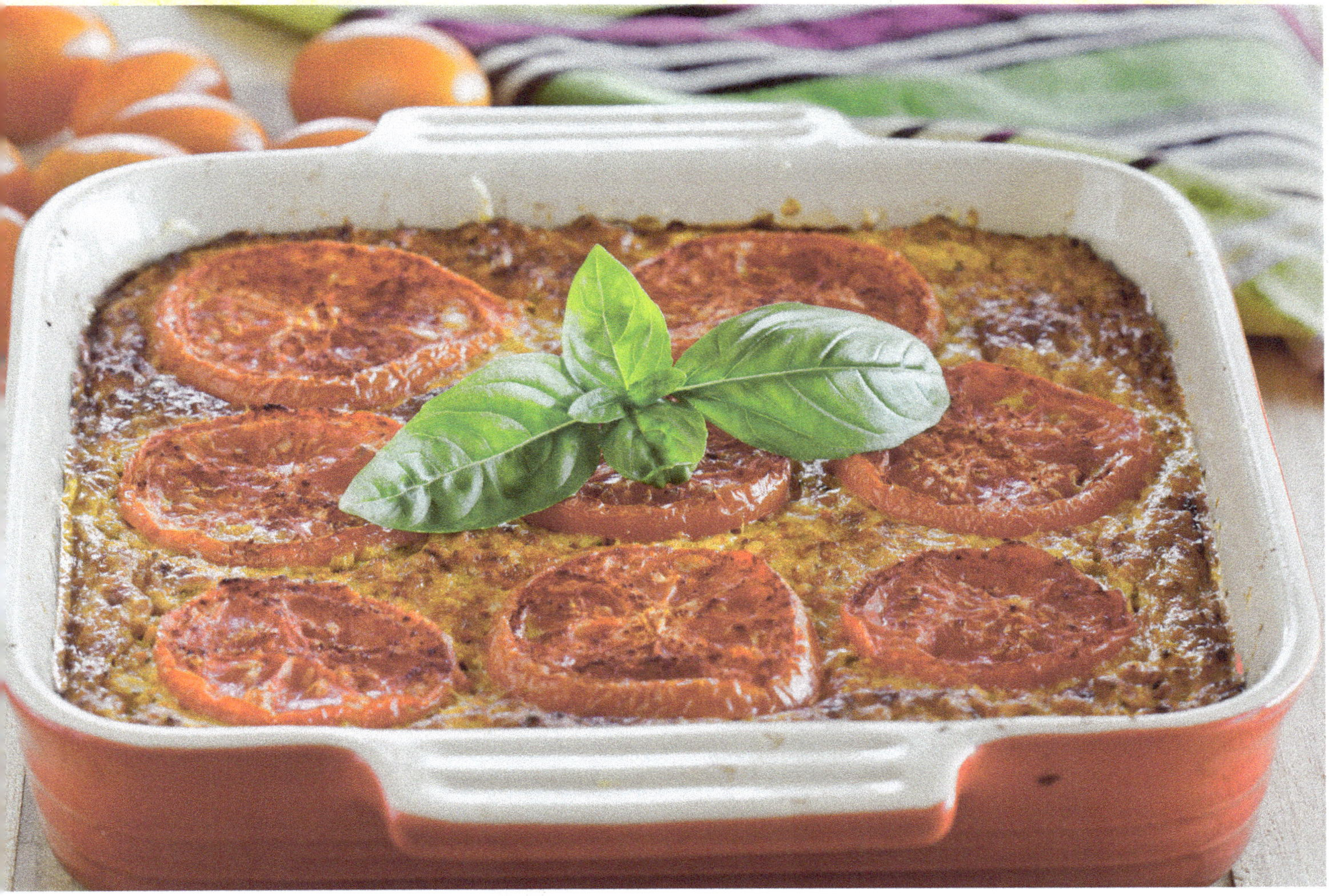

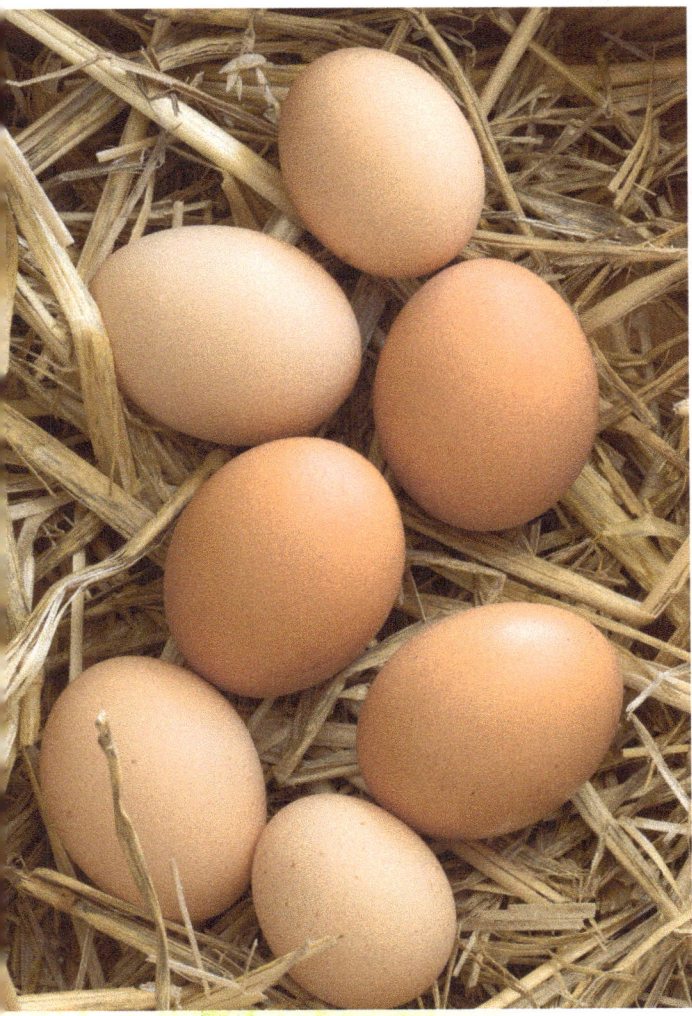
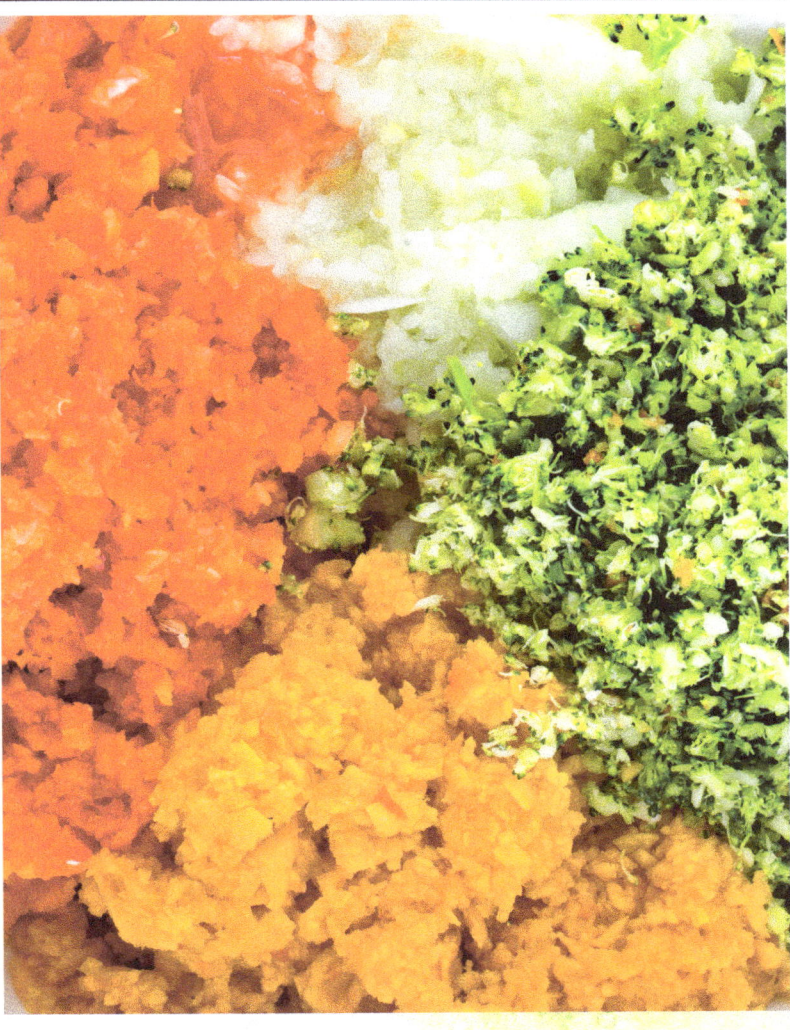

Magical Mains

Better Baked Beans

Canned baked beans are often a favourite with kids and are a quick and easy meal. However apart from the protein in the beans they are of little nutritional value. Full of sugar, salt and thickeners, they are best kept on the supermarket shelf. These baked beans are not only delicious but are a great replacement. Make a large batch and freeze them into smaller portions so you may still enjoy the luxury of that quick and easy meal, but know that you are providing your children with something healthy at the same time.

Serves 4-5

- 2 cups of navy or cannellini beans (soaked overnight) or 5 cups of cooked
- 1 medium-sized onion, finely chopped
- 2 cloves of crushed garlic
- 1 tablespoon of oil
- 1 x 700g bottle of passata
- 4 tablespoons of apple juice concentrate
- 2 teaspoons of blackstrap molasses
- 1 cup of water
- ½ teaspoon of ground nutmeg
- 2 tablespoons of Tamari or soy sauce
- ½ tablespoon of seeded mustard
- pepper and sea salt to taste

1. If you are using dried beans, follow instructions on page 64 for cooking beans.
2. In a large saucepan, stir-fry the onion and garlic in oil until tender.
3. Add the remaining ingredients except for the beans.
4. Simmer covered, over low heat for 10 minutes.
5. Check for taste and adjust seasoning if needed.
6. Add the beans and mix well.
7. Simmer for another 5 minutes before serving.

Play Time!

- Make these beans with 700g of fresh, chopped tomatoes. Add a tablespoon of tomato paste and puree the sauce before adding the beans.
- Add your choice of fresh herbs or vegetables.

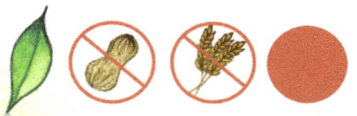

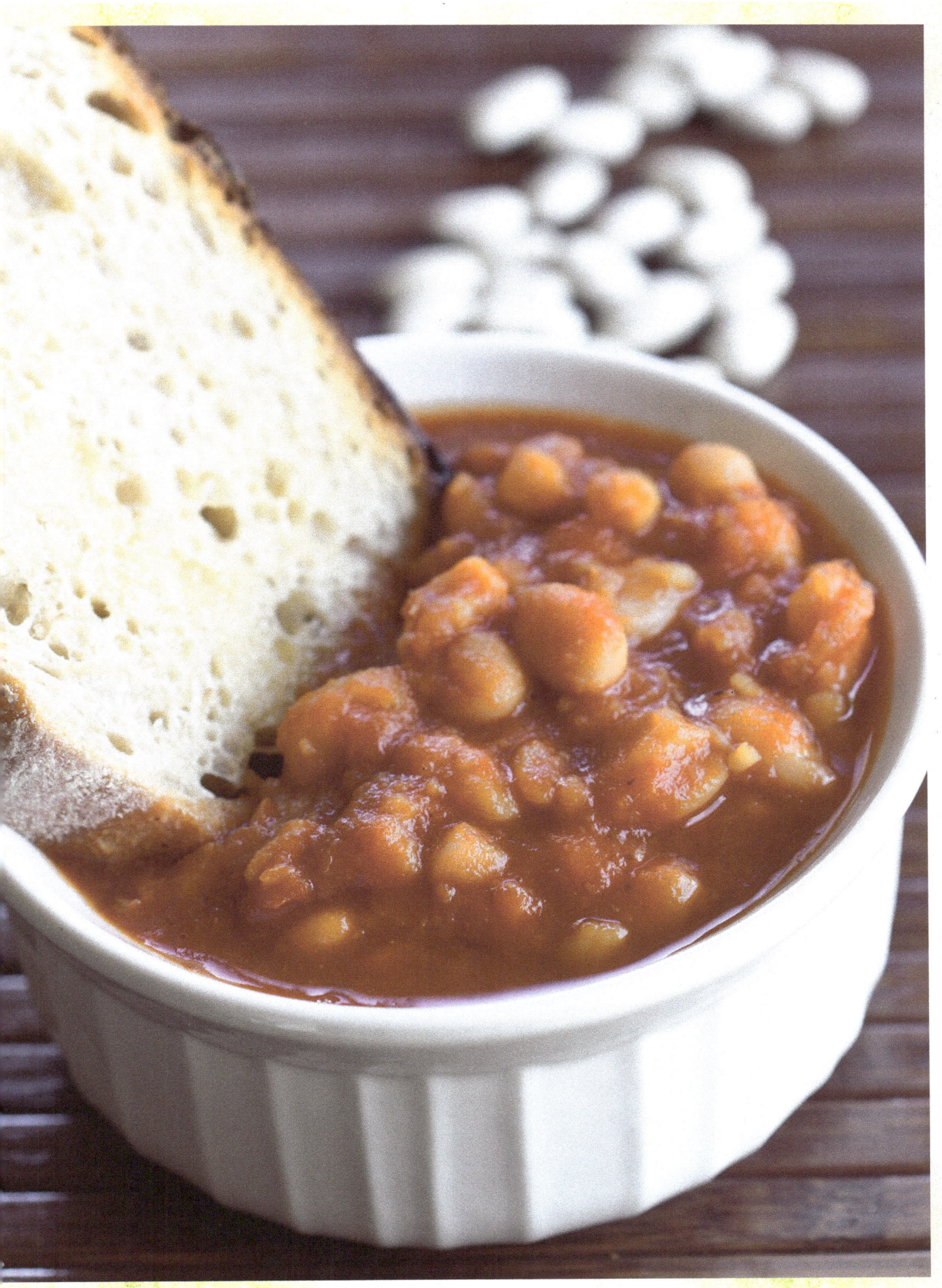

Golden Chickpea Curry

A mild, flavoursome curry, beautiful with bright yellows and greens. I serve it with rice and a salad.

Serves 4-5

1 cup dried chickpeas, (soaked for at least 10 hours) or 2 ½ cups cooked
1 tablespoon of oil or ghee
1 teaspoon of brown mustard seeds
2 teaspoons of fennel seeds
2 teaspoons of nigella seeds
1 large onion, finely chopped
3 cloves of crushed garlic
2 tablespoons of grated ginger
½ teaspoon of mixed spice
1 tablespoon of garam masala
1 x 400g tin coconut cream or equivalent of powdered coconut milk and water
1 cup of water
1 tablespoon of vegetable stock concentrate (for recipe, see page 166)
400g chopped pumpkin, pulverised in the food processor or grated
2 cups of chopped broccoli
sea salt and pepper to taste
½ cup of finely chopped coriander

1. If using dried chickpeas, refer to cooking instructions on page 64.
2. In a large saucepan, heat the oil or ghee and then add your whole spices over medium heat. (i.e. not the powdered ones). Once they become fragrant, add the onion, garlic and ginger and a little water to avoid sticking. Stir until the onion goes soft.
3. Add the remaining spices and stir for a minute.
4. Add the coconut cream, water, stock concentrate, chickpeas and pumpkin. Cover over low to medium heat for 20 minutes, stirring occasionally.
5. Add the broccoli and mix well. Cover for 5 minutes until the broccoli softens.
6. Season with salt and pepper to taste and add the coriander right before serving.

Play Time!

- Puree other vegetables through this curry or use cooked lentils instead of chickpeas.
- Use as a filling for home-made pies.

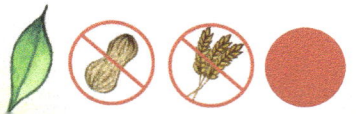

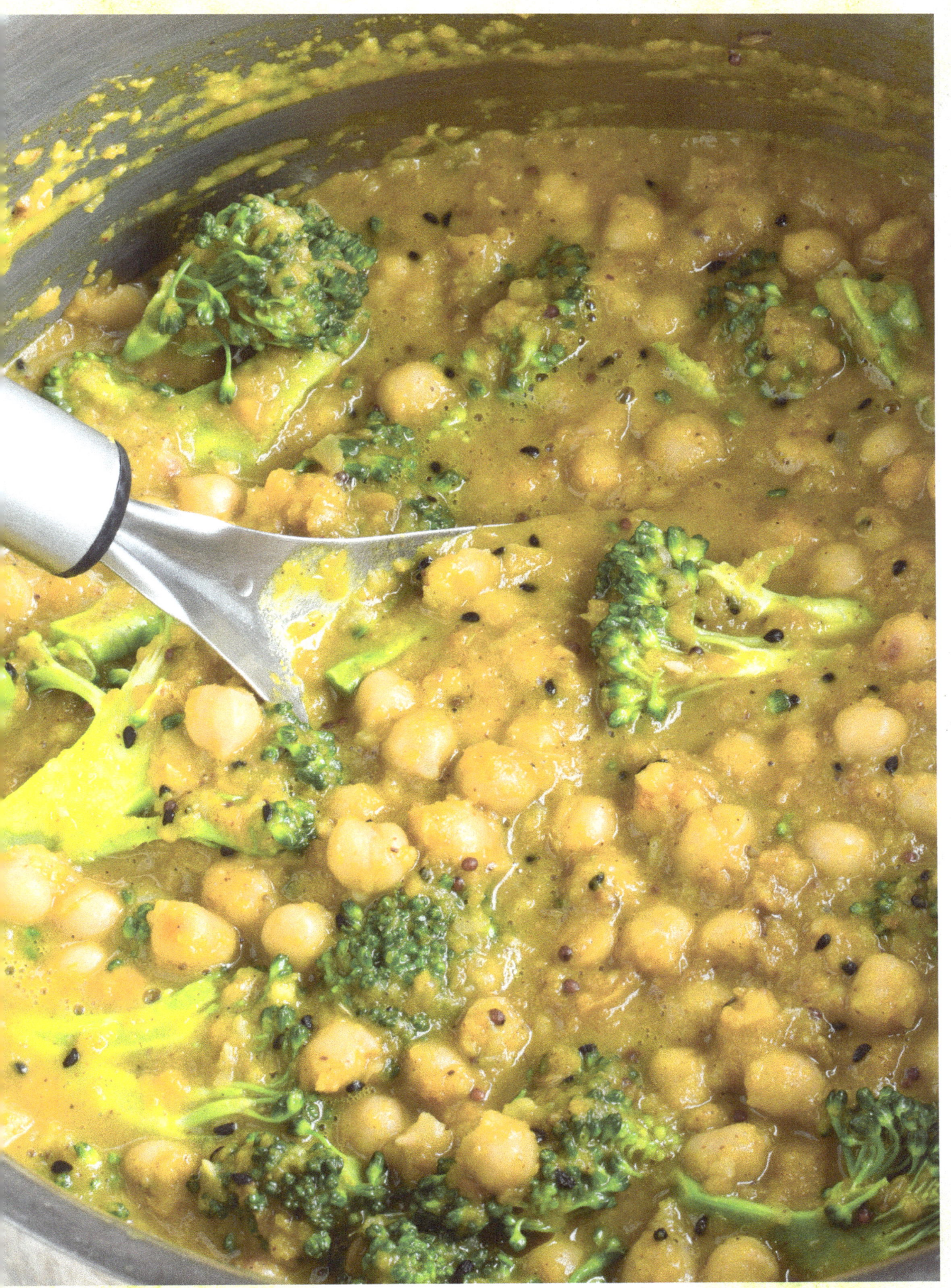

Dreamy Dahl

Dahl is an Indian dish of lentils and spices, usually served with rice or naan bread. You can vary dahl in many ways by using different spice combinations and vegetable additions. Children may enjoy exploring these possibilities and creating their own variations. This is one of our favourites, as it is sweet and mild. I serve it with Crazy Coconut Rice (page 139) and if I have them, a few papadums.

Serves 4-5

1 ½ cups red lentils, soaked for at least 6 hrs*
1 tablespoon of ghee or oil
1 large onion, finely chopped
3 cloves of crushed garlic
1 tablespoon of grated ginger
1 mild chilli – seeds removed (optional)
1 cinnamon stick or 1 teaspoon of ground cinnamon
½ teaspoon of mixed spice

½ teaspoon of turmeric
2 teaspoons of ground cumin
2 teaspoons of garam masala
3 cups of water
250g pulverised or grated sweet potato
1 teaspoon of sea salt
400g of passata or fresh chopped tomatoes
½ cup of finely chopped coriander leaves

* Red lentils do not require soaking in order to cook quickly. I only soak them for health benefits (see page 64 for more information).
If you do not wish to soak them or don't have time, simply add more water to the mix as it cooks to maintain a porridge-like consistency.

1. In a large saucepan, stir-fry the onion, garlic, ginger and chilli in oil until tender.
2. Add the dry spices, including the cinnamon stick and stir for a minute to release the flavours. Add a little water if it starts to stick.
3. Add remaining ingredients except the coriander and mix well.
4. Bring to the boil and then reduce heat to a simmer for about 30 minutes. Cover and stir occasionally to stop the dahl sticking to the bottom of the pan. Dahl is cooked when lentils are soft and the mixture looks creamy.
5. Stir in the coriander and serve hot, with accompaniments mentioned in the description at the top of the page.

Play Time!

- Try other vegetables in this dahl such as pumpkin, capsicum, carrots and zucchinis. Make sure you keep a proportion of the vegetables sweet.
- Once you get used to cooking Indian food, vary your spices.

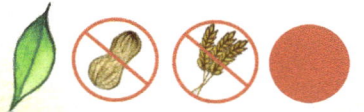

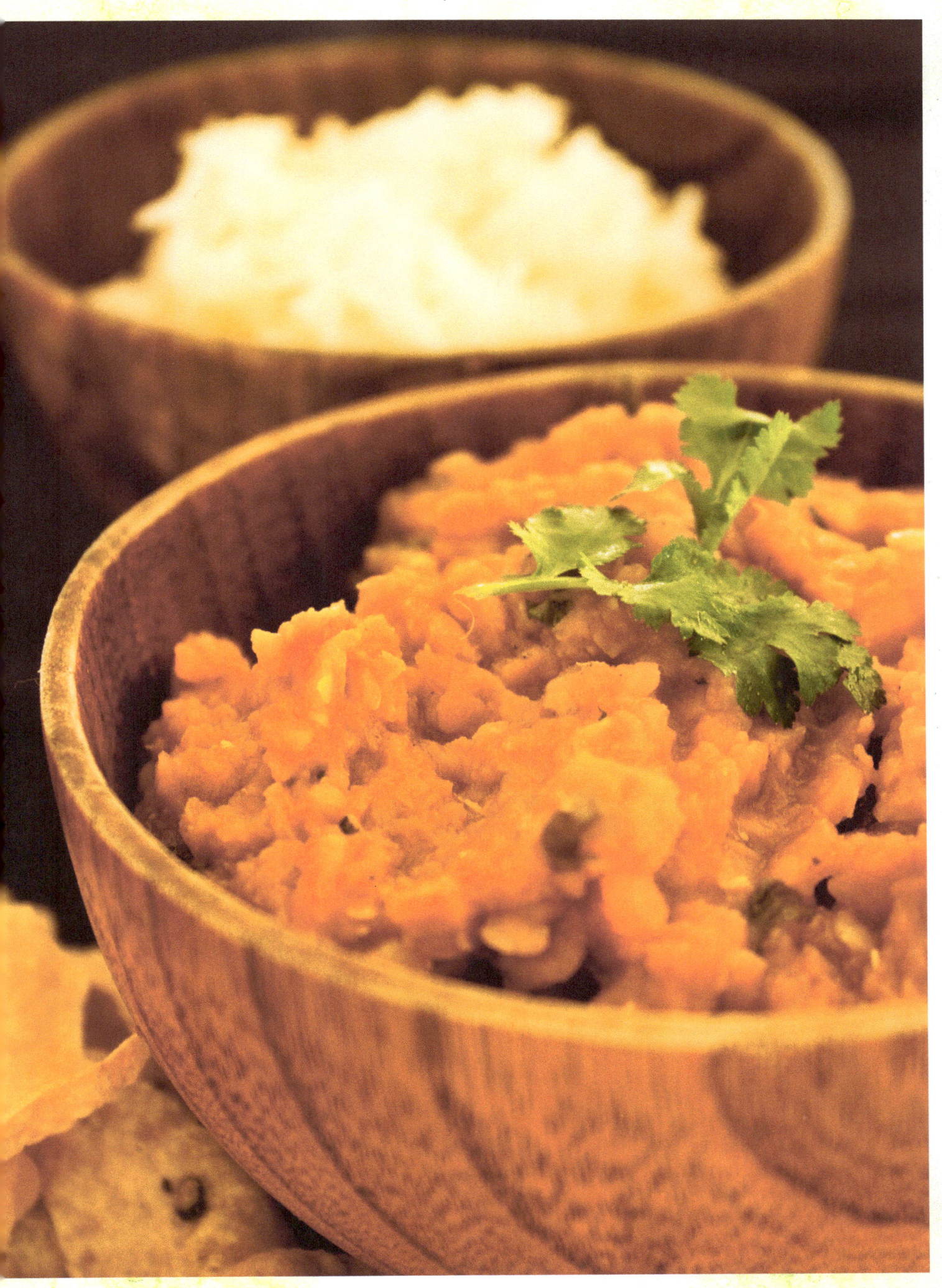

Coconut Dahl

This dahl recipe is sweet and creamy. If you can, squeeze the lime juice over your serving as it really adds something special.

Serves 4-5

- 1 ½ cups red lentils, soaked for at least 6 hrs*
- 1 tablespoon of ghee or oil
- 2 teaspoons of cumin seeds
- 2 teaspoons of fennel seeds
- 1 medium sized onion, finely chopped
- 2 large cloves of crushed garlic
- 1 tablespoon of grated ginger
- 1 mild green chilli, seeds removed, finely chopped
- 2 teaspoons of ground coriander
- 2 teaspoons of garam masala
- ½ teaspoon of ground turmeric
- 2 ½ cups of vegetable stock
- 350g pulverised or grated pumpkin
- 1 x 400g can coconut cream or equivalent of powdered coconut milk and water
- sea salt to taste
- ½ cup coriander leaves, finely chopped
- lime wedges to serve, optional

* Red lentils do not require soaking in order to cook quickly. I only soak them for health benefits (see page 64 for more information). If you do not wish to soak them or don't have time, simply add more water to the mix as it cooks to maintain a porridge-like consistency.

1. Heat the oil in a large saucepan and when it is hot, add the cumin and fennel seeds. Once they become fragrant, add the onion, garlic, ginger and chilli. Mix well.
2. Add the other spices and stir until they become fragrant. Keep your heat to medium-low to avoid burning the mix and add a little water to prevent it from sticking.
3. Add the remaining ingredients, except the salt, coriander and lime. Simmer this mixture over medium heat until it boils and then reduce to low heat and cover. Stir occasionally to make sure the dahl is not sticking to the pan. When the lentils are soft, the dahl is cooked. This will take about 25 minutes.
4. Remove from heat and stir in the salt and coriander leaves. Serve with rice and lime wedges.

Play Time!

- Try other lentils such as puy, green or mung dahl. See the "Cooking Beans and Lentils" section on page 64 for specific soaking instructions.
- Vary the vegetables you add. Use whatever is in your fridge.
- Use the dahl as a filling for homemade pies or pasties

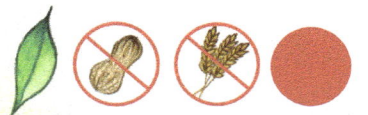

Turkish Casserole

This casserole can be served with rice, quinoa or couscous. It is also delicious accompanied by a green salad.

Serves 4-5

1 cup of dried chickpeas, (soaked for at least 10 hours), or 2 ½ cups of cooked
1 onion, roughly chopped
3 cloves of crushed garlic
2 cups of diced hard vegetables (e.g. pumpkin, sweet potato, carrot, swede)
1 x 700g bottle of passata
½ teaspoon of ground cinnamon
1 teaspoon of sea salt
2 cups chopped faster cooking vegetables
(e.g. capsicum, zucchini, broccoli, cauliflower, mushrooms, squash)
juice of one lemon
freshly ground pepper
2 tablespoons of cold-pressed olive oil
¼ cup of chopped, fresh herbs (mint, parsley, dill- use either or a mix)

1. If you are using dried chickpeas, cook according to directions on page 64.
2. Preheat oven to 180°C convection or 160°C fan forced.
3. In a clay pot or deep casserole dish, combine the chickpeas, onion, garlic, harder vegetables, passata, cinnamon and salt. Fast cooking vegetables such as broccoli, zucchini, and other greens should be added later.
4. With lid on, bake in the oven for 1-1½ hours. The larger your vegetable pieces are, the longer it will take to cook. Halfway through the cooking time, take the casserole out once to stir it. When the harder vegetables are cooked, add the faster cooking vegetables. Bake for a further 10 minutes.
5. Remove from the oven and before serving, stir in the lemon juice, pepper, olive oil and herbs.

Play Time!

- This casserole is delicious pureed and served as a soup. You may need to add a little more water for a thinner soup.
- Use other beans such as cannellini or borlotti instead of the chickpeas.

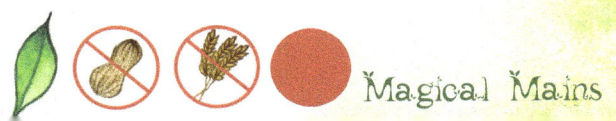

Awesome Adzuki Curry

Adzuki beans are a small, red bean with a very mild flavour. They are an excellent source of protein and are easy to digest. This curry combines them with a mix of vegetables, spices, coriander and lemon. As children gain confidence in the kitchen, meals like this give them an exploring ground for combining different flavours and understanding the difference between faster and slower cooking vegetables.

Serves 4-5

1 ½ cups of adzuki beans, (soaked for 8 hours)
1 tablespoon of ghee or oil
1 medium onion, finely chopped
3 large cloves garlic, crushed
2 tablespoons of grated ginger
1 teaspoon of fennel seeds
1 teaspoon of ground cumin
½ teaspoon of ground turmeric
1 teaspoon of ground coriander
1 x 700g bottle of passata
1 tablespoon of vegetable stock concentrate (recipe on page 166)
1 cup of water
3 cups of diced hard vegetables (e.g. pumpkin, sweet potato, carrot, swede)
2 cups chopped faster cooking vegetables
(e.g. capsicum, zucchini, broccoli, cauliflower, mushrooms, squash)
½ cup of chopped fresh coriander
juice of ½ a lemon

1. Drain adzuki beans and cook according to directions on page 64.
1. In a large saucepan, stir-fry the onion, garlic and ginger in oil until tender. Add a little water if it starts to stick.
2. Add spices and stir. Once they become fragrant, add the passata, stock concentrate, water and harder vegetables. Cover saucepan and simmer for 10-15 minutes, stirring occasionally.
3. When the vegetables are soft, add the remaining fast cooking vegetables and the cooked adzuki beans. Simmer for 5 minutes.
4. Remove from heat and stir in the coriander and lemon juice.

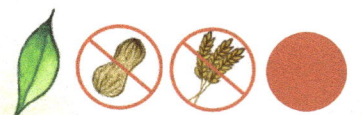

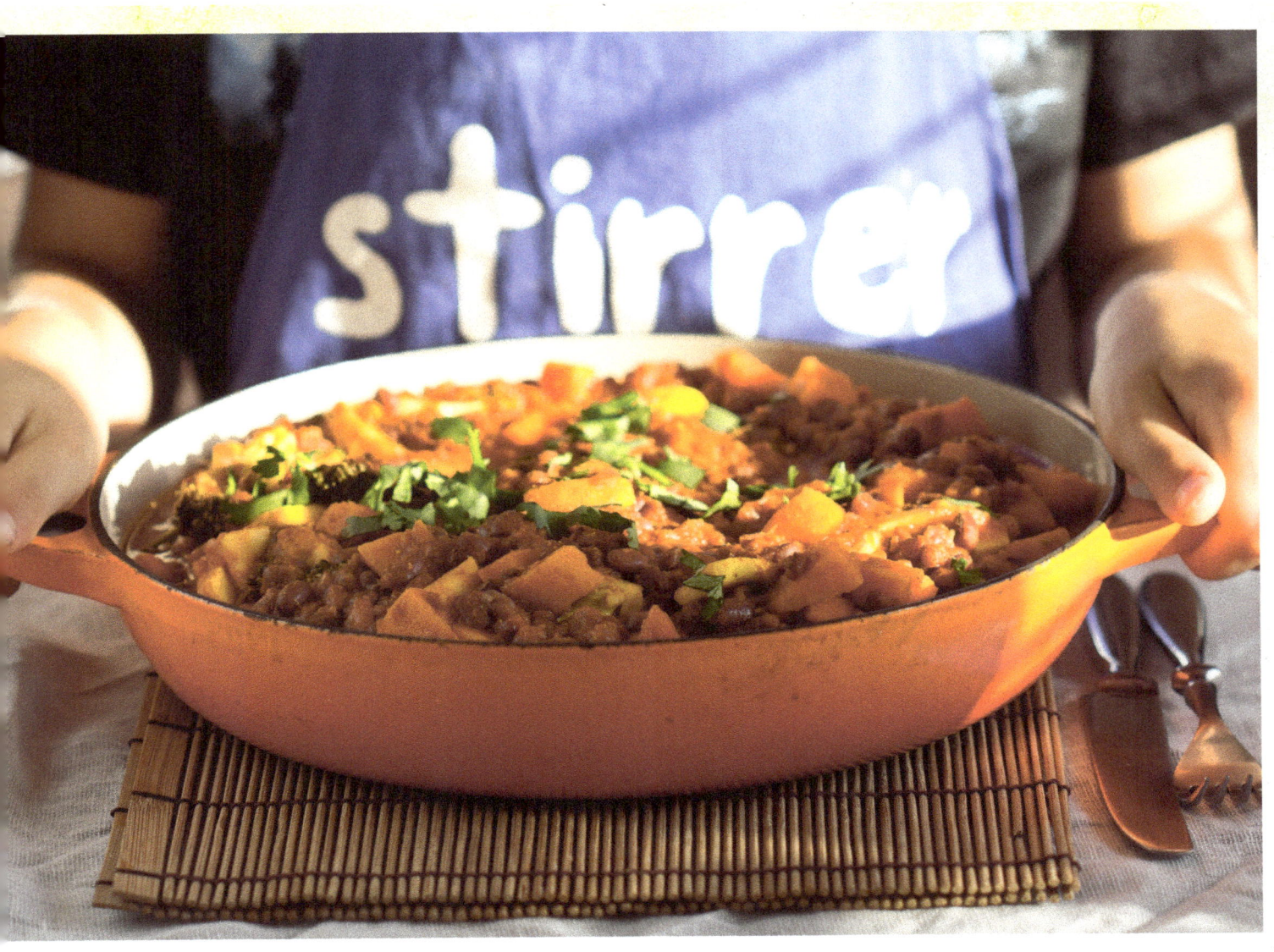

Play Time!

- Vary the vegetables and type of bean you use.
- Use lime juice at the end instead of lemon juice.
- This dish makes a great filling for home-made pies.
- As with any curry, you can add water and puree to make a soup.
- Instead of coriander, use parsley, mint or lemon balm.

Mexican Pie

Mexican food is a big favourite in our house. The combination of spices, beans, avocados and tomatoes is both satisfying and refreshing. This is another way to present these wonderful flavours. I serve this pie with Guacamole and Salsa (recipes on page 98) and fresh greens. Ethan and Ryan like to make the guacamole and salsa themselves. They get to do a lot of taste testing that way!

Serves 5-6

Pastry

3 cups wholemeal wheat or spelt flour
170g cold butter, cubed
1 egg
2-4 tablespoons of chilled water

Filling

1 cup dried pinto or borlotti beans, (soaked for at least 6 hours) or 3 cups of cooked
1 tablespoon of oil
1 large onion, finely chopped
2 cloves of crushed garlic
2 teaspoons of Mexican seasoning (recipe on page 188)
2 tablespoons of tomato paste
1 large capsicum, diced (any colour)
250g of peeled, diced sweet potato or pumpkin
250g of fresh, diced tomatoes
¼ cup finely chopped coriander

1. If you are using dried beans, cook them according to directions on page 64.
2. To make the pastry, place the flour and butter into a food processor and pulse until the mix resembles bread crumbs. If you do not have a food processor, rub the butter into the flour with your fingers.
3. Add the egg and water 1 tablespoon at a time until the dough comes together into a smooth ball. Add more water if necessary.
4. Press dough into a thick square and cover with plastic wrap. Refrigerate for 20-30 minutes
5. Preheat oven to 180°C convection or 160°C fan forced.
6. Divide dough into two pieces, one being double the size of the other. The smaller piece will be your pie top.
7. On a floured board, roll your larger piece of dough out evenly to fit into an 18cm pie dish. To transfer the dough, flour your rolling pin and roll the dough around it. Unroll the dough into the pie dish and press to fit. Trim the edges.

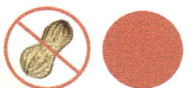

8. Bake for 15 minutes until just browned.
9. Meanwhile, prepare your filling. In a large saucepan, stir-fry the onion and garlic in oil.
10. Stir in the seasoning and mix until fragrant.
11. Add the remaining ingredients except coriander. Mix well and simmer until the vegetables are soft.
12. Remove from heat and stir in the coriander.
13. Roll out the top for the pie and pour filling into the baked shell.
14. Transfer the top to the shell using the rolling pin and press the sides down with the edge of a knife. Punch a couple of air holes in the top with a sharp knife.
15. Bake for 30 minutes or until browned.
16. Serve with suggested toppings.

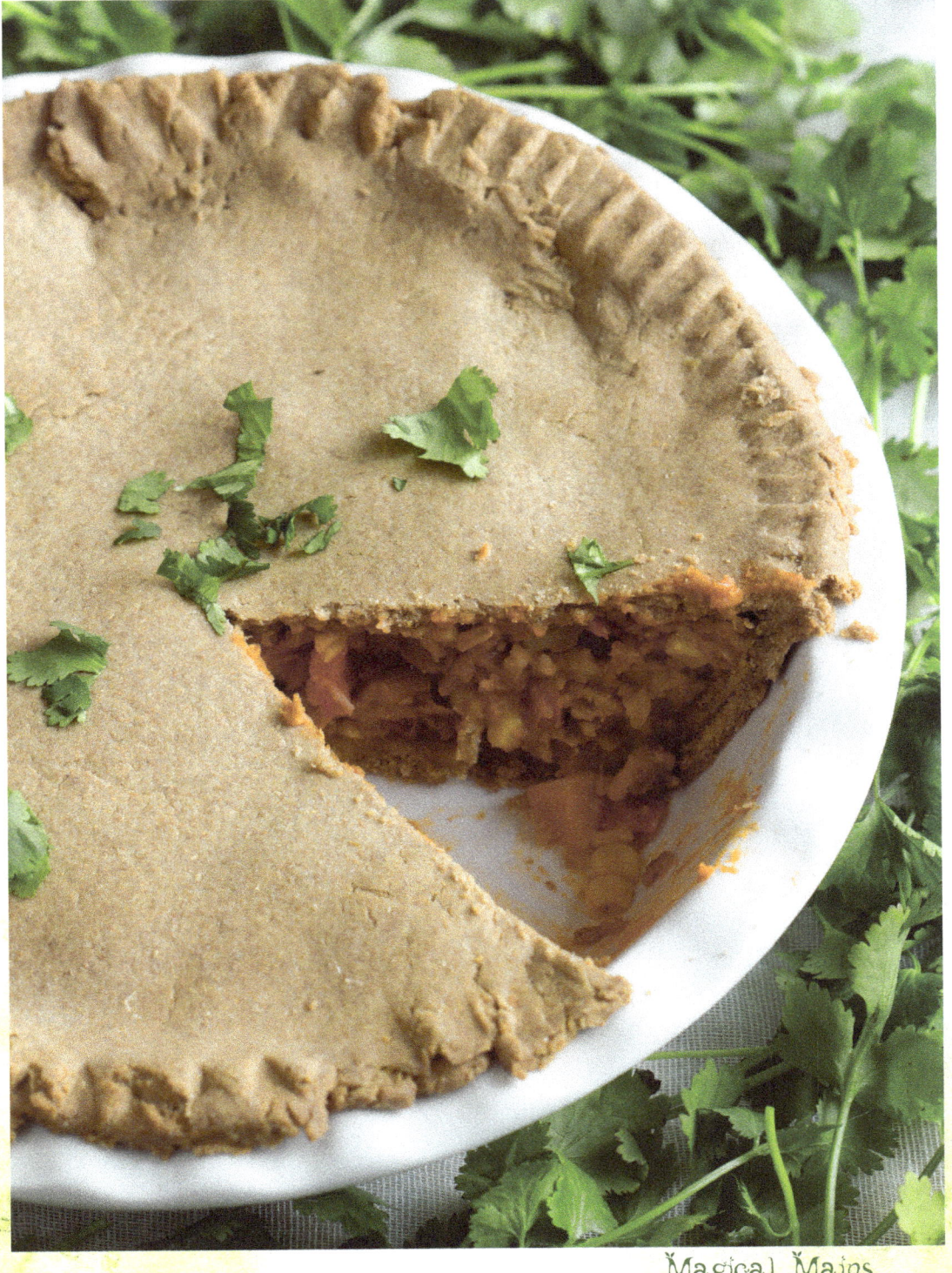

Gado Gado

The great thing about this meal is it is so versatile. As a base, you need your peanut sauce and rice or noodles. Once you have those, create a platter of colour and flavour. You can serve steamed vegetables, salads, tofu, and boiled eggs. I usually keep our platter mostly raw as the peanut sauce is a great contrast to the cooling salads. Sometimes I add steamed broccoli and sweet potatoes and I always serve boiled eggs, compliments of our chooks! Have your children help choose what goes onto the platter. They may like to do some of the preparation and be in charge of presentation.

Makes 2 ½ cups of peanut sauce

Peanut Sauce
1 tablespoon of oil
2 cloves of crushed garlic
1 tablespoon of grated ginger
1 green chilli optional
¾ cup of natural peanut butter
1 x 400g can coconut cream, or equivalent of powdered coconut milk and water
3 tablespoons of soy or Tamari sauce
juice of a lime

Platter ingredients (choose a mix of the following)
steamed vegetables (broccoli, cauliflower, pumpkin, sweet potato, zucchini, cabbage, snow peas, Asian greens, beans, asparagus, corn)
raw salad vegetables/fruits (cucumber, tomato, carrot, zucchini, bean sprouts, avocado, tomatoes, beetroot)
boiled eggs
marinated tofu cubes
Steamed rice or noodles

1. Heat the oil in a small saucepan. Add the garlic, ginger and chilli and stir-fry for a minute.
2. Add remaining sauce ingredients except lime juice.
3. Mix well and simmer gently for 10 minutes.
4. Meanwhile, prepare your rice or noodles and platter.
5. Stir lime juice into sauce just before serving.
6. Present platter with sauce and rice or noodles.

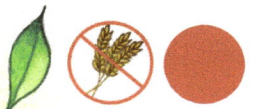

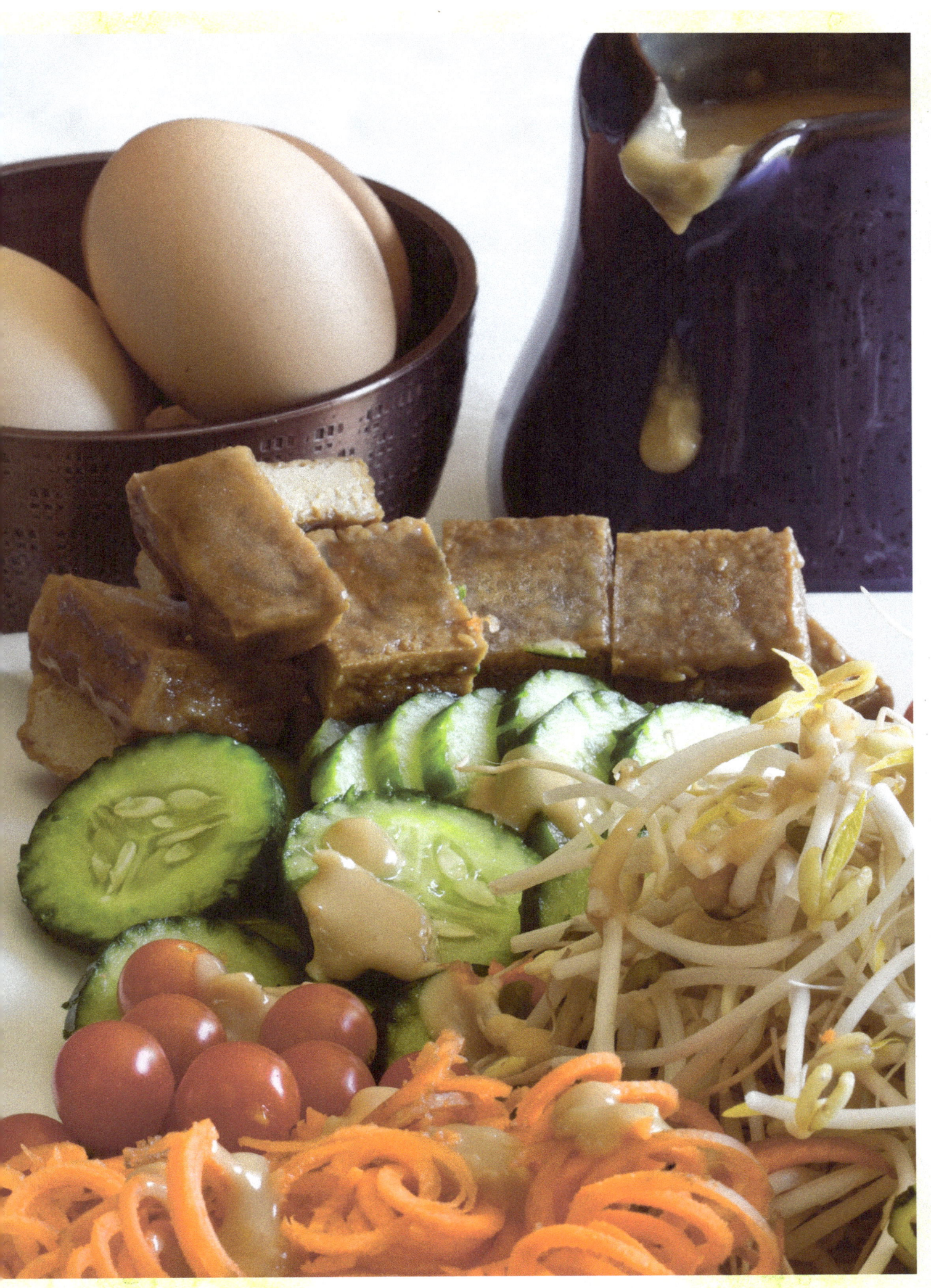

Magical Mains 209

Pumpkin and Sweet Pea Risotto

My youngest son Ryan, doesn't like pumpkin and he is very specific about it, however he does love pumpkin soup and he scoffs this risotto. What he has learned is that often, even if you don't like an ingredient on its own, it tastes very different with other ingredients. With leftover risotto, form into balls and pan fry into little patties. They are great served with a salad in the school lunch box.

1 tablespoon of oil
1 onion or leek, finely chopped
300g arborio rice
½ cup organic white wine
3 cloves of crushed garlic
400g of roughly grated pumpkin (I do this in a food processor)
zest of 1 lemon
2 tablespoons of fresh thyme leaves
900ml vegetable stock
1 cup of fresh or frozen peas
¾ cup of grated Parmesan (optional)
Toasted pine nuts and fresh green leaves to serve.

Note: *I recommend rocket but it may be too spicy for some children. If your children are not up to eating leafy greens yet, serve some sliced cucumber with it. This way they get use to having a salad with their meal which is a great habit to get into.*

1. Bring your vegetable stock to a simmer in a medium-sized saucepan and leave lid on.
2. Add the oil to a separate large saucepan and when it is hot, add the leek or onion. Cook until soft.
3. Add the rice to the pan and stir to coat. Cook for a couple of minutes.
4. Add the wine and garlic and simmer for a minute or so. This cooks off the alcohol.
5. Add pumpkin, half of the lemon zest, thyme and a little of the stock if need be to loosen the mix.
6. Now, add the stock 1-2 ladelfuls at a time, waiting until one lot has absorbed before adding the next. Stir almost constantly as this is how risotto develops its texture. It should take about 15 minutes. Rice texture needs to be a little bit chewy but not crunchy!
7. When all of your stock is used, add the peas and Parmesan cheese. Stir until the peas are tender.
8. Serve your risotto in bowls topped with toasted pine nuts, a little lemon zest and your leafy greens. It should always be served immediately.

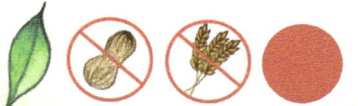

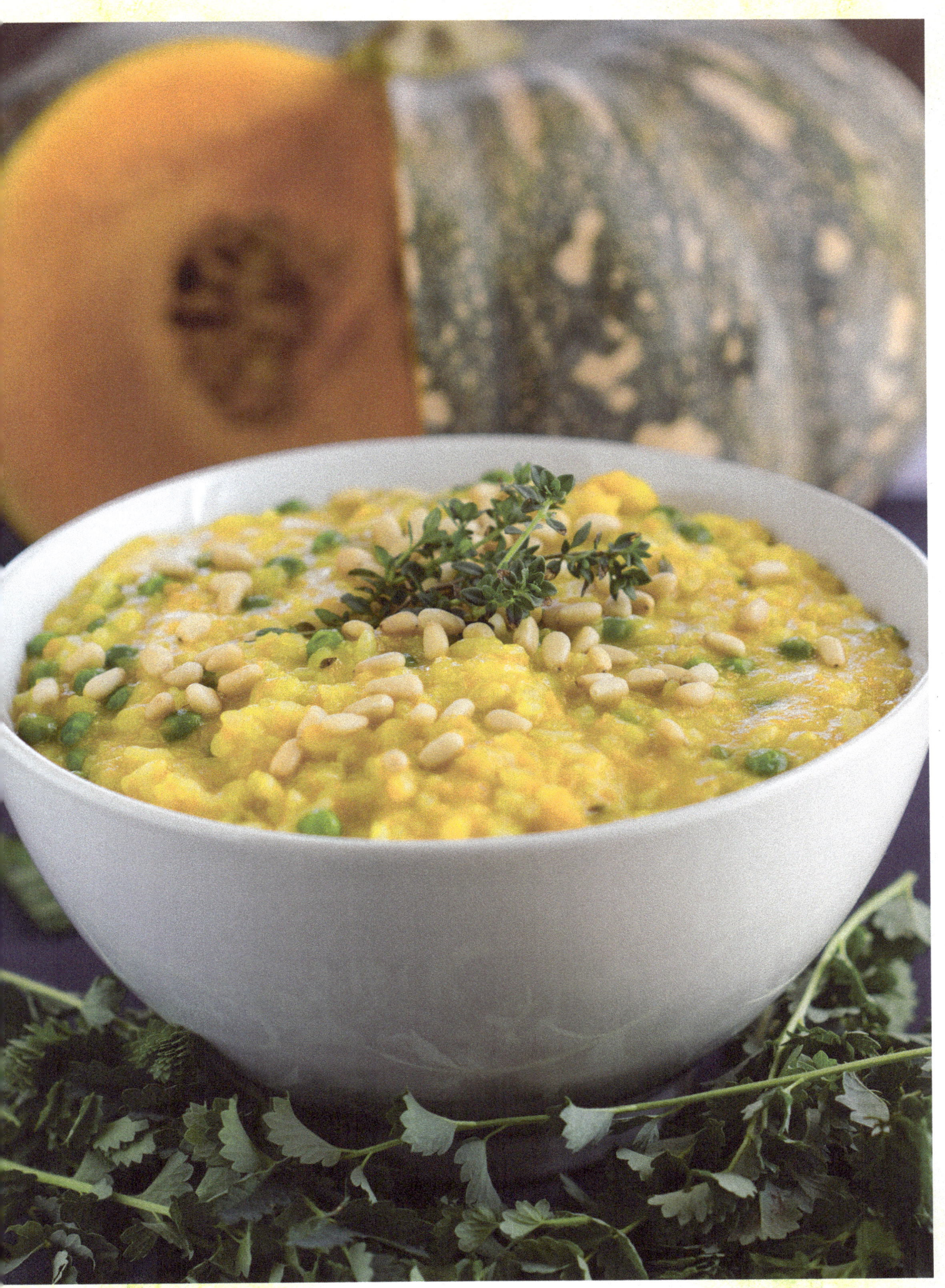

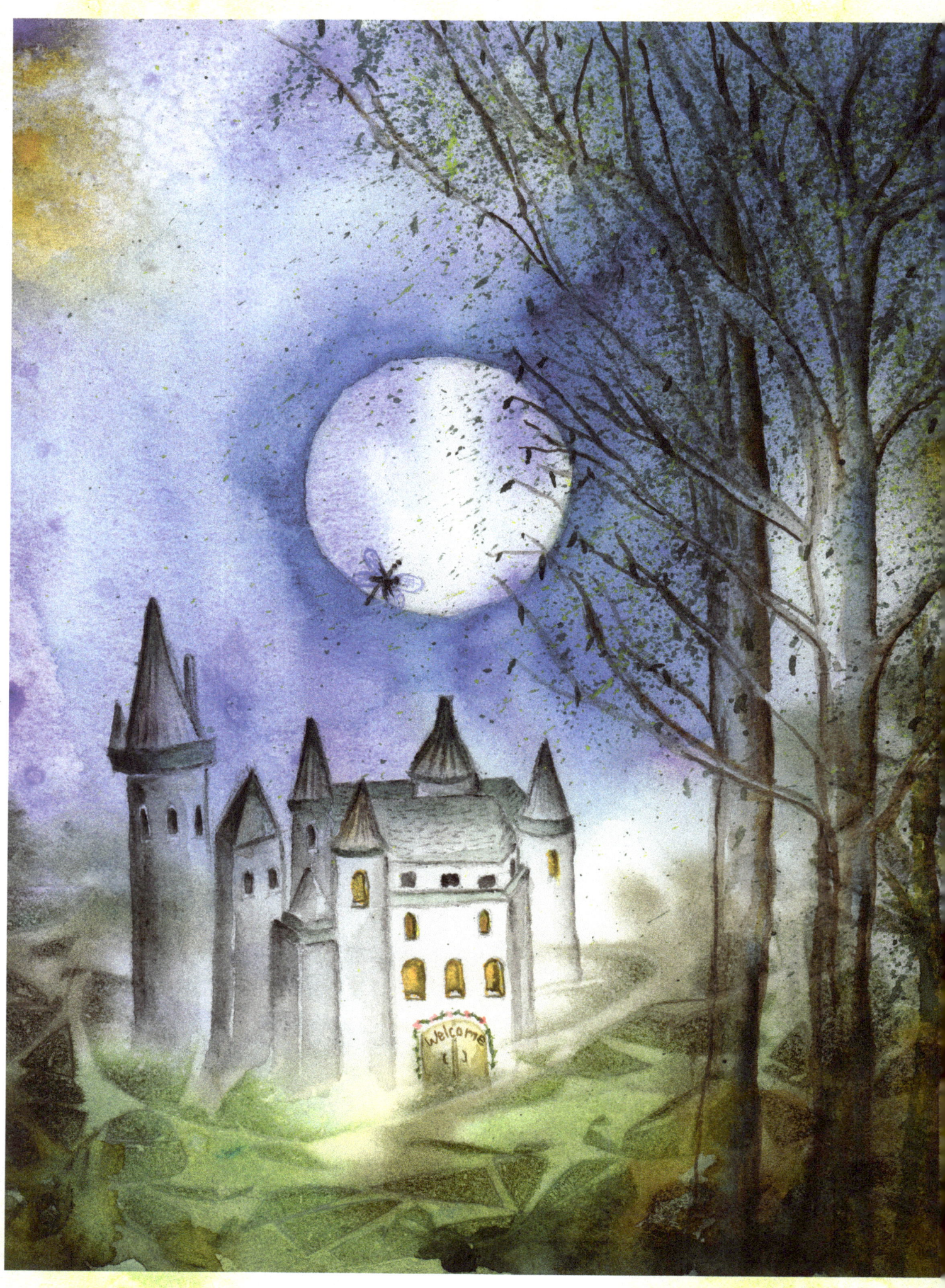

The Land of Sweet

The Land of Sweet

Sweetness, baked and raw, treats for school and much, much more...
Following are a wide variety of recipes including biscuits, cakes, muffins, raw treats, desserts and frozen treats. I did my best to give an idea of the possibilities by using a variety of sweetening products. Please remember the importance of limiting all sweet foods for physical and dental health. Even natural sweeteners are not good for the body in excess. Everything in moderation and balance!

*"Chocolate is the answer.
Who cares what the question is."*
~Author unknown

Wholemeal vs White Flour

When I was testing the baked recipes in this book, I found that the outcome varied greatly depending on where I had sourced my flour. On page 50 there is information about the different types of flour and how they behave in baking, which will give you a full explanation of why this is so. I mostly use organic spelt flours and I found that some of the wholemeal flour was quite course and therefore made the cakes dry. Then again, other wholemeal flour I bought was silky smooth, creating delicious, soft cakes. With this in mind, for the majority of baking recipes, I have specified a half/half approach using both wholemeal and unbleached flour. What I suggest is that you start with this recommendation and then experiment with the flour you find. If you can source a silky wholemeal flour, then by all means use that instead of the less nutritious white flour. In addition to this, when you do use a white flour, it is best to find a brand that is unbleached, as the bleaching is only cosmetic and is not good for us.

A Great Baking Tip

I met a lady once who was a professional baker and she passed on a fantastic baking tip that I would love to share with you. Her advice was, as soon as a cake comes out of the oven, leave it in the tin and wrap it in a large beach towel. Leave it wrapped until it is at room temperature, (a few hours). This will help the cake to retain its moisture and therefore softness that would usually go up in steam. Use this tip for all cakes and muffins and you will notice the difference.

Oven Settings

For baking, the best oven setting is convection. That is the top and bottom elements on with the fan off. However not everyone has this setting. There are some ovens where the fan setting is mandatory. In this case, always cook at a lower temperature, usually 20°C less. Temperatures are indicated for both settings in the recipes that follow.

Cake Tin Sizes

There are so many variations in the sizes of cake tins. It is not essential that you have the exact size. Just make sure that the total area is close. Sometimes it means your cake or slice will be a little thinner or a little higher. If the tin is slightly larger, the mix will cook faster, so keep this in mind when you set your oven timer.

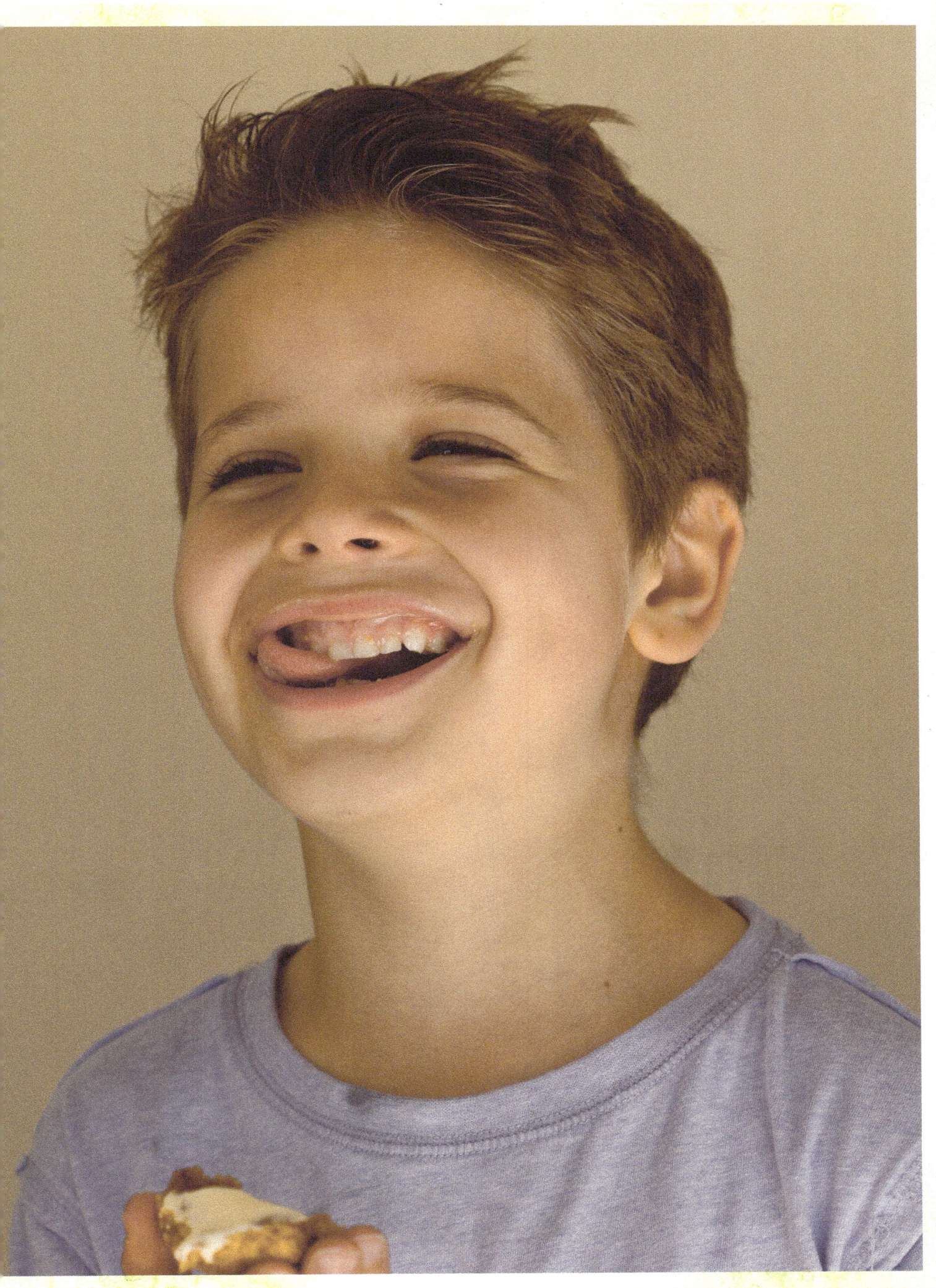

The Land of Sweet

Bliss Balls

Following are a selection of ball recipes. In recent times, health food shops have started selling a similar version of these treats at their counters. They are a great alternative to a chocolate bar, but usually very expensive to buy. They are very easy to make yourself and a great introduction to cooking for children. These recipes involve measuring, adding ingredients to a food processor, blending via a button and then rolling the balls into shape. Apart from the couple of recipes involving the melting of cocao butter or coconut oil, there are no stoves or knives involved that could hurt little hands. We prefer to keep our creations in the freezer, as they don't go completely hard (so can be eaten right away) and keep longer.

Use these as a starting point and then try experimenting with your own flavours. Children love to create their own recipes, although you may want to limit their ingredients a little. Don't want any curry powder thrown in! Some of my recipes are inspired by my favourite chocolate combinations.

Coatings for the balls

Most of the time these balls are rolled in coconut, but here is a more complete list of suggestions:

- Coconut
- Crushed raw nuts
- Crushed roasted nuts
- Sesame seeds
- Crushed raw pepitas (pumpkin seeds)
- Puffed rice cereal (use the smaller cereal for this)

A note on food processors: Some food processors are more powerful than others and so you need to work with what you have. If you have a very powerful machine, you will get away with throwing all of the ingredients in at once. Some may need to grind ingredients separately and then combine them afterwards. In the recipes following, I have written the directions for those with a less powerful machine, however, adjust to your discretion.

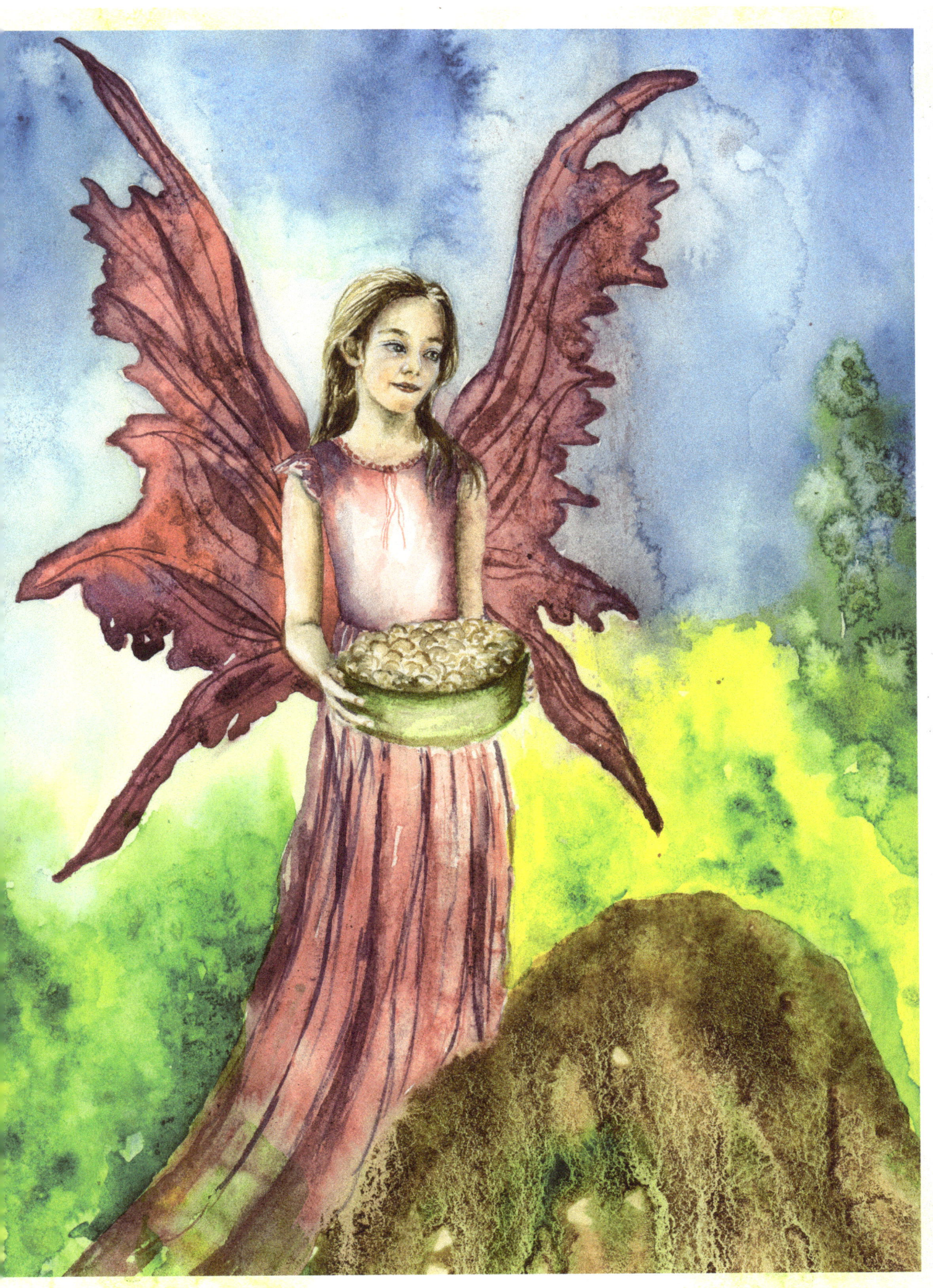

The Land of Sweet

The Original Bliss Ball

This is where it all started. The original Bliss Ball was the first of its type to start selling in health food shops. They are usually made with carob, not a taste for everyone, but some love it as an alternative to chocolate. I think it is a good idea to introduce a child's palate to carob at a young age as it is very high in calcium, so a great food for children. If it isn't for you I have also suggested the use of raw cocao, a nutritious food, rich in antioxidants (see the Superfoods section on page 16 or the glossary, page 284 for more information on raw cacao).

Makes 20 balls

1 cup of mixed nuts and seeds
¼ cup of tahini
¼ cup of honey or rice syrup
¼ cup of carob or raw cocao powder
½ teaspoon of vanilla extract
coatings (see page 216)

1. Place nuts and seeds into a food processor and grind to a fine crumb.
2. Add remaining ingredients and mix on high speed until the mixture is a thick paste.
3. Roll mixture into balls and coat.
4. Freeze or refrigerate and they will become firmer.

Play Time!

- Try peanut butter in place of the tahini.
- Use just one type of nut for a dominant flavour. Macadamias, almonds, cashews and hazelnuts are all great choices.
- Add some puffed rice or puffed quinoa cereal.

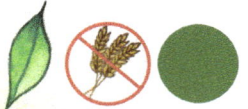

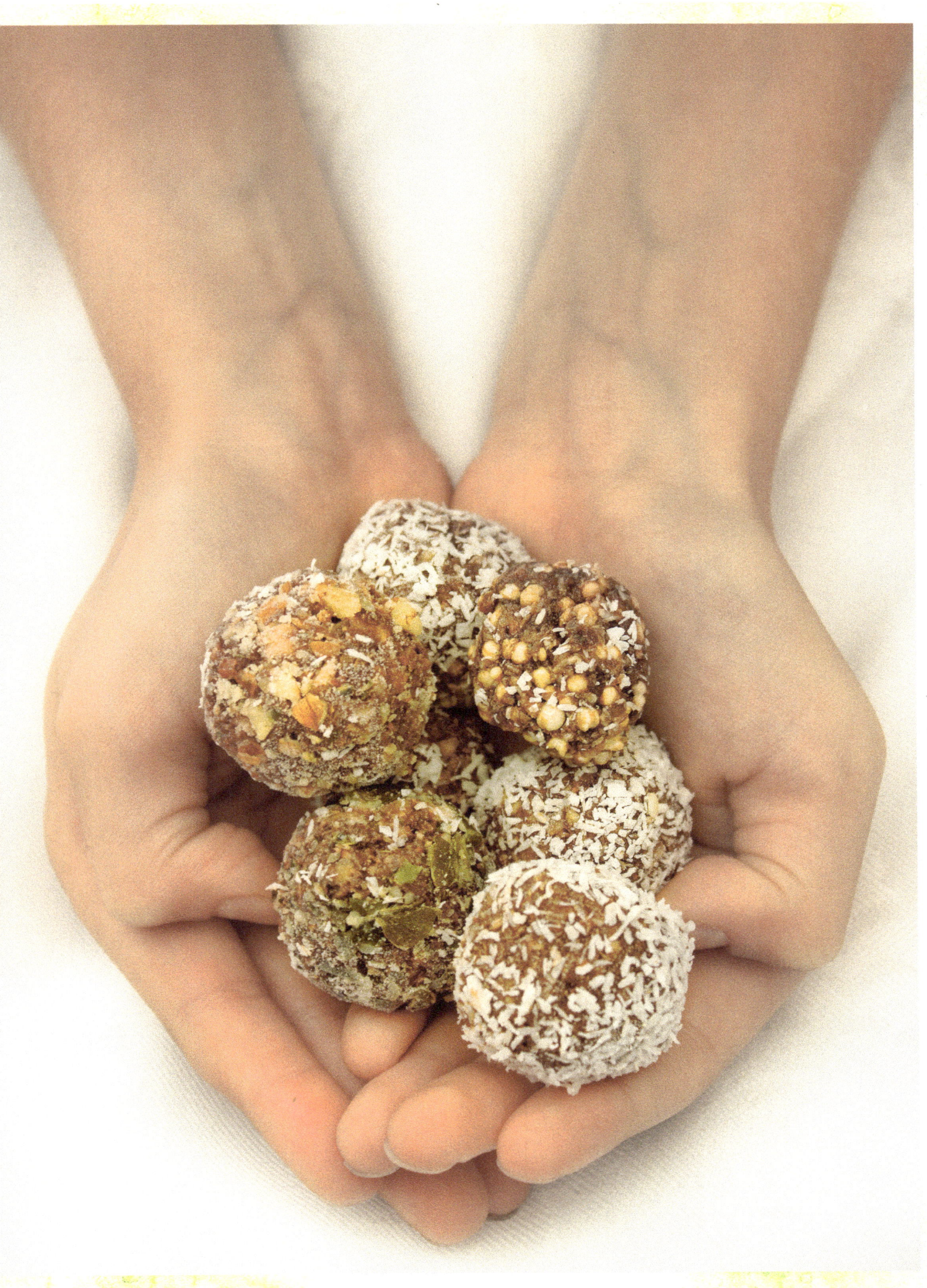

Chocolate Goji Balls

Goji berries are sweet, chewy, dried berries, rich in vitamins and anti-oxidants. They complement the chocolate and nuts beautifully to make a treat that is just as delicious as it is healthy.

Makes 28 balls

1 cup of mixed nuts

½ cup of sunflower seeds or pepitas (or a mix of both)

½ cup of goji berries

⅓ cup of raw cocao powder

½ cup desiccated coconut

40g coconut oil or cocao butter, melted over low heat.

⅓ cup of raw honey or maple syrup

coatings (see page 216)

1. Place nuts and seeds into a food processor and grind to a fine crumb.
2. Add remaining ingredients and mix on high speed until the mixture is a thick paste.
3. Roll mixture into balls and coat.
4. Freeze or refrigerate and they will become firmer.

Play Time!

- Use cranberries instead of goji berries. Cranberry and chocolate is a yummy combination.
- Use just one type of nut for a dominant flavour. Macadamias, almonds, cashews and hazelnuts are all great choices.

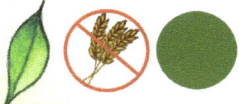

Almond and Cashew Balls

This recipe was inspired by something I once purchased in a health food shop. I loved the taste but the price was excessive and I endeavoured to come up with my own version with the help of the ingredients list. Enjoy!

Makes 20 balls

½ cup of almonds

½ cup of cashews

¼ cup of sunflower seeds

¼ cup of sesame seeds

¼ cup of sultanas

¼ cup of barley malt

1 teaspoon of vanilla extract

¼ cup of walnut oil (or other cold pressed nut/seed oil)

⅓ cup of puffed amaranth or puffed quinoa

coatings (see page 216)

1. Place nuts and seeds into a food processor and grind to a fine crumb.
2. Add remaining ingredients and mix on high speed until the mixture is a thick paste.
3. Roll mixture into balls and coat.
4. Freeze or refrigerate and they will become firmer.

Play Time!

- Use other dried fruits instead of the sultanas.
- Use honey instead of the barley malt.

Chocolate Mint Balls

Mint grows easily almost anywhere and there are so many different types. These include spearmint, peppermint, chocolate mint and lemon mint. Experiment with what is available for a refreshing chocolate treat.

Makes 30 balls

1 cup of raw mixed nuts
½ cup of seeds (e.g. sunflower, hemp and or pepitas)
1 cup of pitted medjool dates
½ cup of raw cocao powder
1 small bunch (or large handful) of fresh mint leaves
2-3 tablespoons of milk to form paste. (Amount will depend on the moistness of your dates)
coatings (see page 216)

1. Place nuts and seeds into a food processor and grind to a fine crumb.
2. Add remaining ingredients, making sure the milk is added gradually. The mix should be of a consistency that will hold its shape.
3. Roll mixture into balls and coat.
4. Freeze or refrigerate and they will become firmer.

Play Time!

- Instead of the mint, add a chilli - seeds removed. Chilli chocolate is now gaining popularity.
- Instead of the mint, use the grated zest of an orange for chocolate orange flavoured treats.

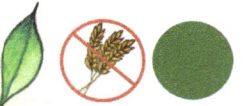

222 The Land of Sweet

Almond and Apricot Balls

Almonds are a lot better for you if soaked before you eat them. See page 64 for more information. If you soak your almonds, omit the fruit juice or milk from this recipe.

Makes 25 balls

½ cup of raw almonds
½ cup of sunflower seeds
½ cup of dried apricots
½ cup of desiccated or shredded coconut
1 tablespoon of rice or maple syrup
¼ cup of sultanas
¼ cup of oil (use a good cold pressed nut or seed oil)
1 teaspoon of vanilla extract (optional)
coatings (see page 216)

1. Place nuts and seeds into a food processor and grind to a fine crumb.
2. Add remaining ingredients and mix on high speed until the mixture is a thick paste.
3. Roll mixture into balls and coat.
4. Freeze or refrigerate and they will become firmer.

Play Time!

- Use other dried fruit in place of the apricots, e.g. cranberries, peaches or pineapple.
- Use ½ cup of chopped, fresh coconut in place of the desiccated coconut. Add the fruit juice gradually if you do this as you will need less.

Chocolate, Honey Almond Balls

This recipe is very simple, and one of my favourites.
Makes 28 balls

60g coconut oil
2 cups of raw almonds
⅓ cup of cocoa
⅓ cup of raw honey
coatings (see page 216)

1. Melt coconut oil over very low heat until it is liquid.
2. Meanwhile, grind almonds to a meal in your food processor.
3. Add the coconut oil to the almonds with remaining ingredients, and blend until well mixed.
4. Roll mixture into balls and coat.
5. Freeze or refrigerate and they will become firmer.

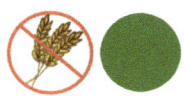

Cranberry and Apple Balls

This recipe uses fresh coconut meat and it gives new meaning to the phrase "fresh is best".
To extract the coconut from the shell, I use the point of a knife to separate chunks and then a potato peeler to remove the woody husk.
Makes 35 balls

1 cup of dried, unsweetened cranberries
1 cup of raw almonds
1 cup of sunflower seeds
200g raw coconut meat
⅓ cup of apple juice concentrate
coatings (see page 216)

1. Place nuts and seeds into a food processor and grind to a fine crumb.
2. Add remaining ingredients and mix on high speed until the mixture is a thick paste.
3. Roll mixture into balls and coat.
4. Freeze or refrigerate and they will become firmer.

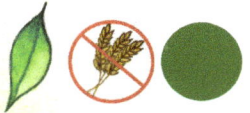

The Land of Sweet

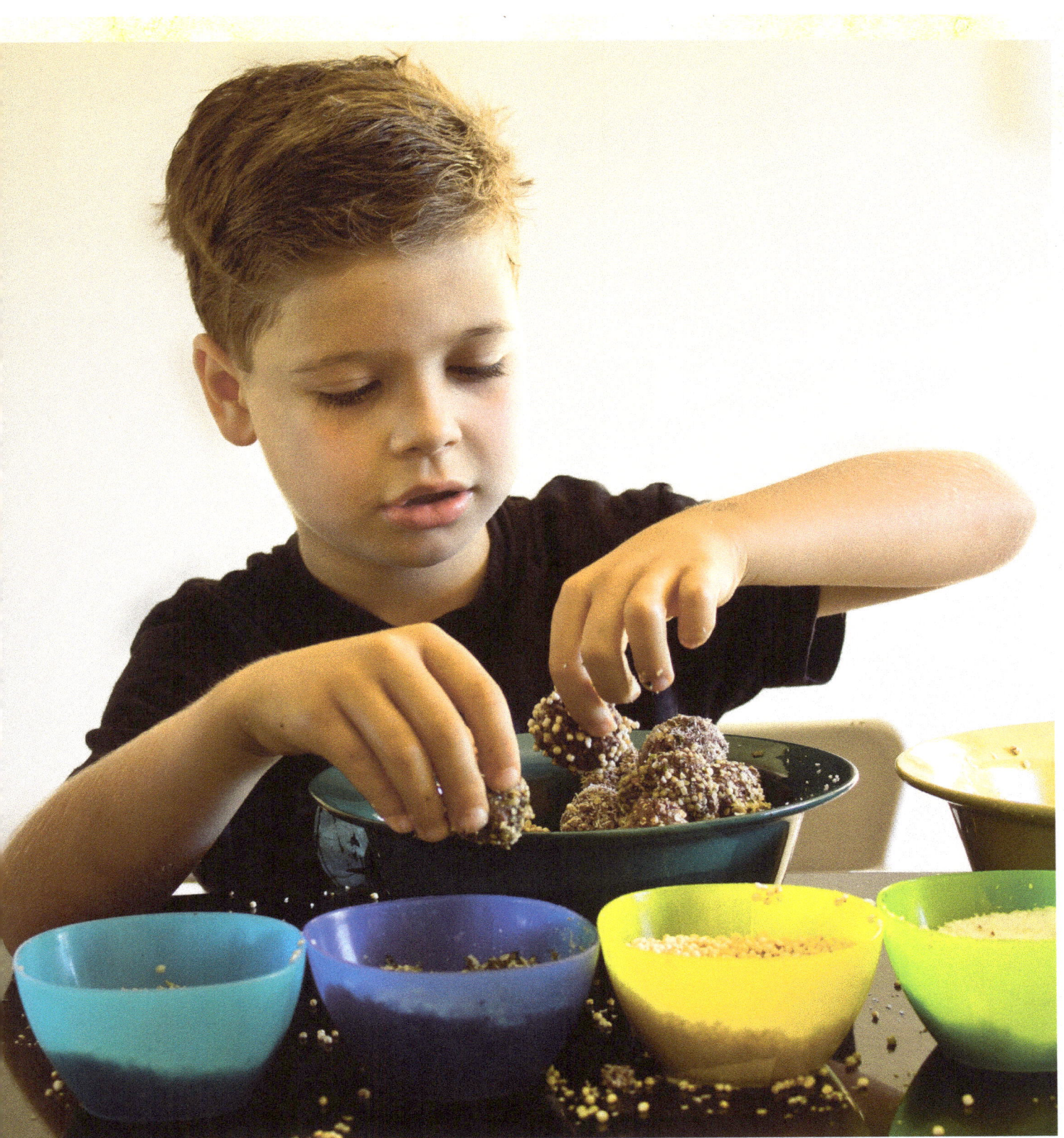

Play Time!

- Use other dried fruit in place of the cranberries, e.g. goji berries, apricots or peaches.
- Use another sweetener in place of the apple juice concentrate, e.g. pear juice concentrate, maple syrup, rice syrup or honey.

Gingerbread Biscuits

These biscuits are rich with the flavour of gingerbread, but also more wholesome than the average biscuit. With wholemeal flour and rapadura sugar, both you and your children can enjoy making and eating these healthy treats with piece of mind.

Makes 20-25

¼ **cup of oil**

½ **cup of rapadura sugar**

1 beaten egg

1 tablespoon of blackstrap molasses

½ **teaspoon of fresh lemon juice**

1 teaspoon of ground ginger

¼ **teaspoon of ground cinnamon**

⅛ **teaspoon of ground cloves**

¾ **cup of wholemeal wheat or spelt flour**

¾ **cup of unbleached wheat or spelt flour**

½ **teaspoon of baking powder**

1. Preheat oven to 180°C convection or 160°C fan forced.
2. Line a baking tray with baking paper.
3. In a medium sized mixing bowl, mix together all of the ingredients except the flour and baking powder. You can do this with beaters or by hand.
4. Add remaining ingredients and mix well.
5. To make them into biscuits you have a couple of options. You can do the quick way and just put teaspoonfuls onto the baking sheet, or if you like your biscuits to be neat and professional looking, roll into balls and either leave them as balls or press down with a fork for a flatter biscuit. All will look and taste good. If you do leave them as balls, cook for a few minutes longer.
6. Bake for 12-15 minutes or until slightly browned and firm to touch.
7. When they come out of the oven, carefully transfer to a cooling rack. They will be soft and fragile while hot but once cool they will become firm.

Tip: *If you have decided to shape your mixture into balls, wet your hands first and then leave a small bowl of water next to you so that you can re-wet your hands whenever they become sticky again. This will work whenever you need to handle a sticky dough.*

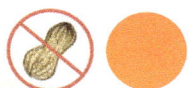

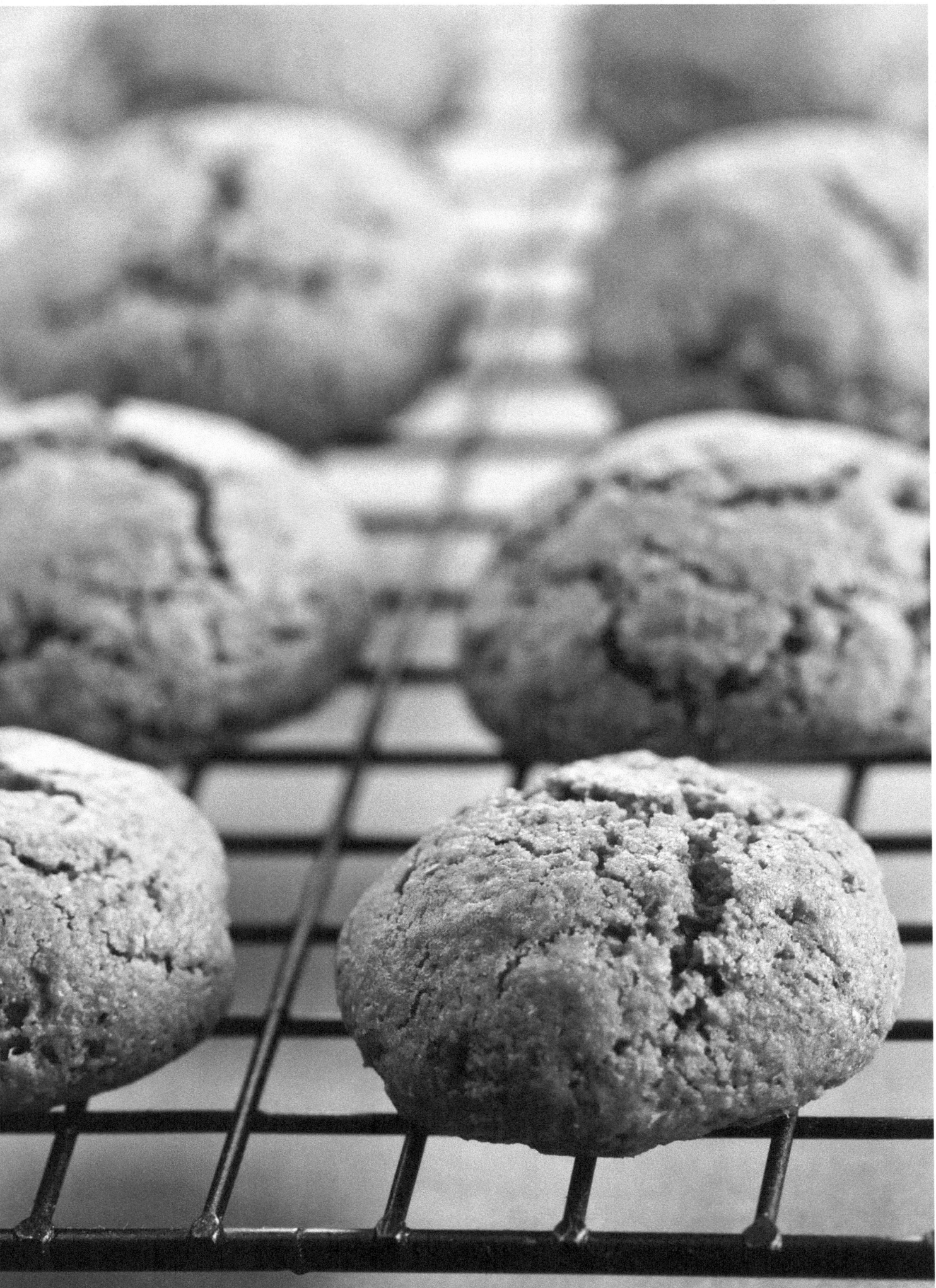

Chocolate Chip Pecan Biscuits

In this recipe, there is the option of using rice or coconut flour. I discovered this by accident one day when I was out of rice flour and had to substitute. The result was so yummy I had to include the option. Of course many people will not yet have access to coconut flour and so will have to use the rice flour in the meantime. Most biscuits are easy for children to make and these are no exception. Just make sure you have some chocolate left for the biscuits.

Makes 20-25

½ **cup of unbleached spelt flour**

½ **cup of brown rice flour or coconut flour**

½ **teaspoon of baking powder**

2 **tablespoons of ground arrowroot**

½ **cup of crushed pecans**

½ **cup of chocolate chips or blocked chocolate broken into chunks**

⅓ **cup of oil**

½ **cup of maple syrup**

1 **teaspoon of vanilla extract**

1. Preheat oven to 180°C convection or 160°C fan forced.
2. Prepare a baking tray by greasing or laying out baking paper.
3. In a mixing bowl, combine the flours, baking powder, arrowroot, pecans and chocolate.
4. In a smaller bowl, whisk the oil, syrup and vanilla together.
5. Add the wet to dry ingredients and mix well.
6. Put teaspoonfuls of the biscuit mixture onto the baking tray or, if you prefer your biscuits to be smooth, roll mix into small balls. Press lightly onto the baking tray leaving a 5cm gap between each biscuit.
7. Bake for 10-12 minutes, or until golden.
8. Gently move biscuits to a cooling rack to harden.

Play Time!

- Use walnuts or almonds in place of the pecans.
- Add ½ a cup of sultanas or chopped dried apricots.
- Add the grated zest of an orange in place of the vanilla extract.
- To make a vegan version, use vegan chocolate.

The Land of Sweet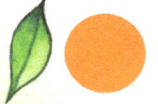

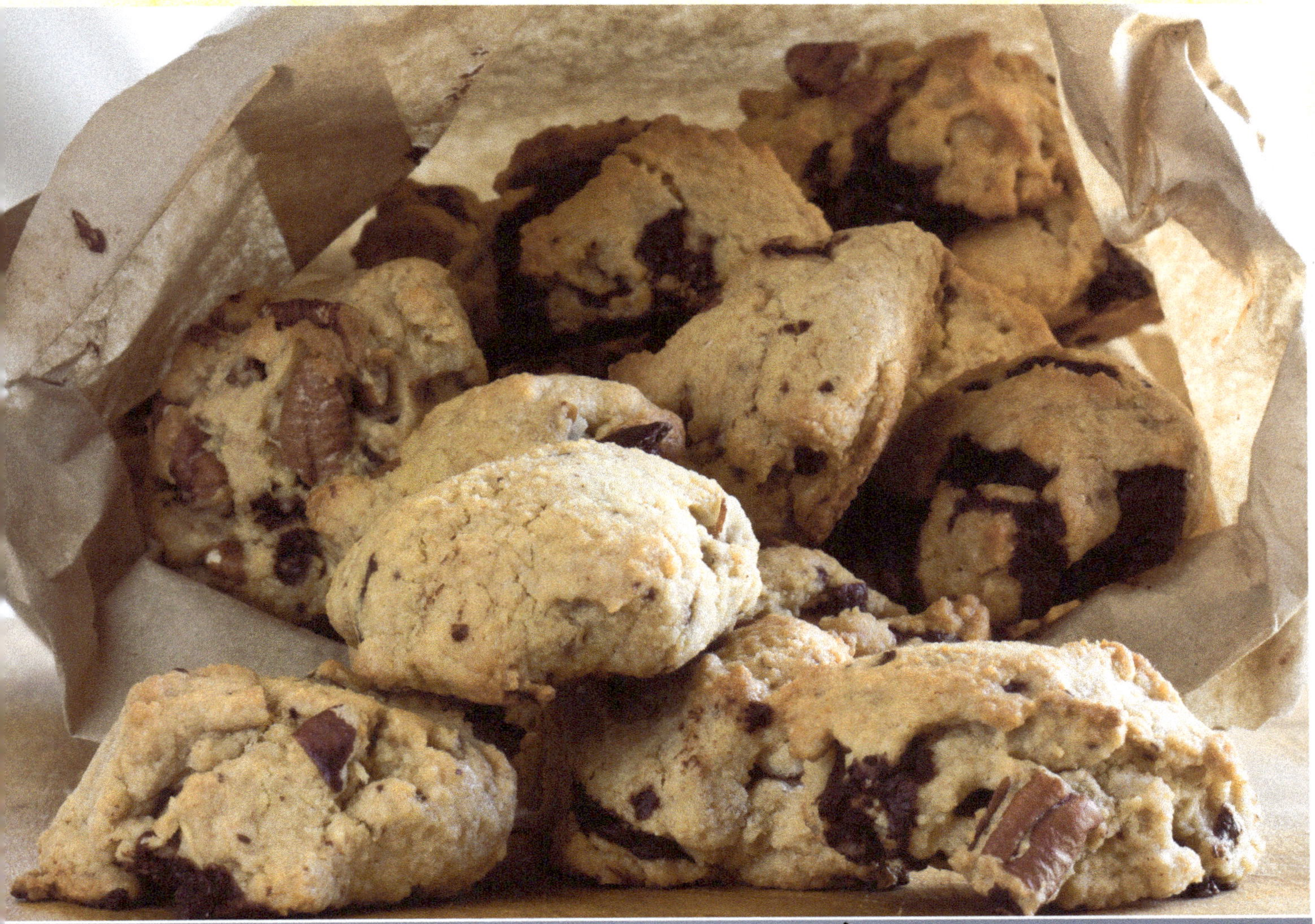

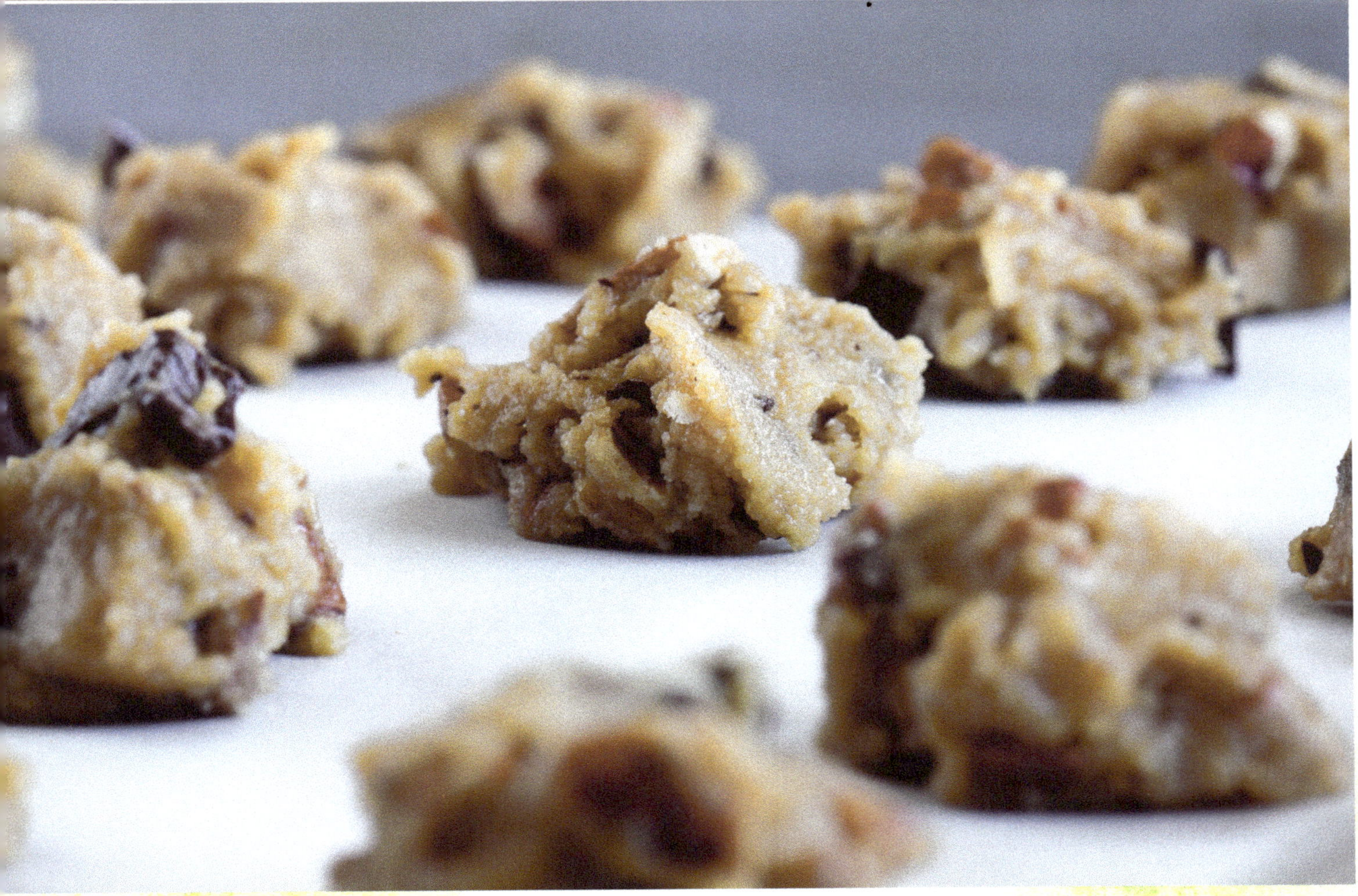

The Land of Sweet 229

Jam Drops

These biscuits are sweet and crunchy. They are pretty as a gift too and very easy for children to make.

Makes 20-25

1 cup of unbleached spelt flour
½ cup of brown rice flour
½ teaspoon of baking powder
2 tablespoons of ground arrowroot
⅓ cup of oil
⅓ cup of maple syrup
3-4 tablespoons of fruit spread (jam made without the sugar)
maple syrup to glaze

1. Preheat oven to 180°C convection or 160°C fan forced.
2. Prepare a baking tray by greasing or laying out baking paper.
3. In a mixing bowl, combine the flours, baking powder and arrowroot.
4. Add the oil and syrup to dry ingredients and mix well.
5. Roll biscuit mixture into small balls and press lightly onto the baking tray leaving a 5cm gap between each biscuit.
6. Using the end of a teaspoon, daub a small amount of the fruit spread onto the top of each biscuit.
7. Bake for 10-12 minutes, or until golden.
8. Brush drops with extra syrup and gently move to a cooling rack to harden.

Play Time!

- Use coconut flour in place of the rice flour.
- Add the grated zest of an orange or lemon.

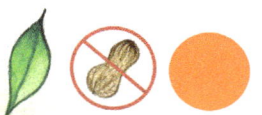

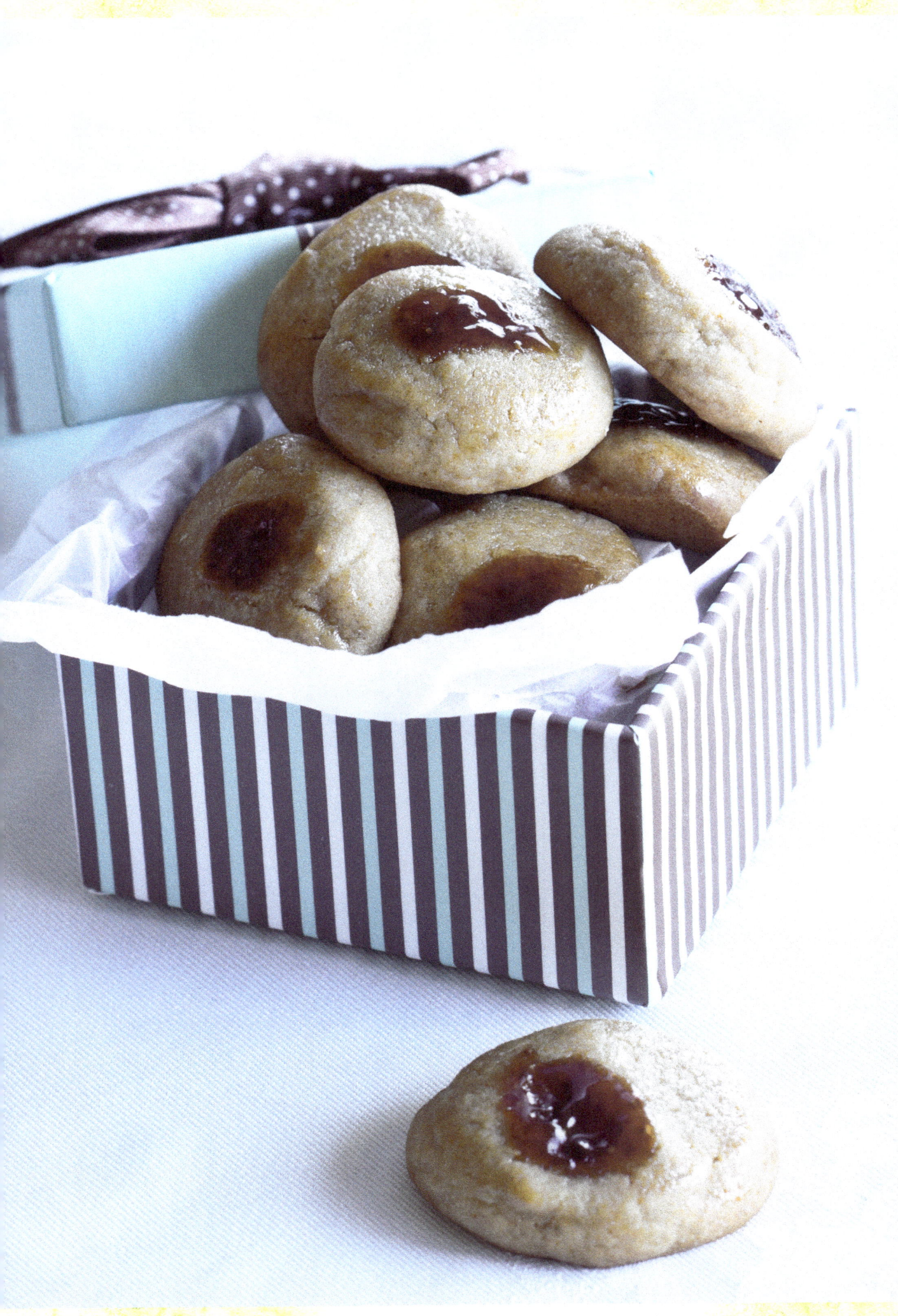

The Land of Sweet 231

Muesli Bars

These are a lunch box staple in our house hold. They freeze really well and taste better than the bought muesli bars. See the creative tips at the bottom of the page for the many ways you may adjust this recipe to suit your family's tastes. Children are bound to come up with interesting combinations!

1½ cups of rolled oats
2 cups of puffed rice cereal
½ cup of brown rice flour
1 cup of sunflower seeds
1 cup of desiccated coconut
100g dried apricots
200g pitted dates
⅓ cup of oil
2 large eggs
3 tablespoons of honey or rice syrup

1. Preheat oven to 180°C convection or 160°C fan-forced.
2. Line base and sides of a 21cm x 30cm baking pan with baking paper, allowing a 2cm overhang on 2 of the opposing sides.
3. Now you need to decide whether or not you want chunky fruit in your bars or if you would like it to be very finely chopped. If you want chunky fruit bars, then chop up your dates and apricots by hand. If not, add these two fruits to the food processor in the next step.
4. In a food processor, mix oil, eggs and honey together until smooth.
5. Combine dry ingredients in a large mixing bowl and then add the wet ingredients. Mix well.
6. Transfer to prepared pan. Using the back of a large metal spoon, press mixture evenly into the pan. Bake for 20 minutes or until lightly browned. Cool in pan, then cut into squares.

Play Time!

- Replace the dried apricots with other dried fruit. Keep the dates for sweetness, but try cranberries, sultanas, dried apple, pear or figs.
- Replace the puffed rice cereal with puffed quinoa
- Use nuts instead of sunflower seeds or a mix of both!
- Add other nutritious seeds such as pepitas, sunflower, hemp or linseeds.
- Add a teaspoon of mixed spice or cinnamon. (You could make an apple and cinnamon version using dried apple and ground cinnamon)
- Add the grated zest of an orange or lemon for tang.

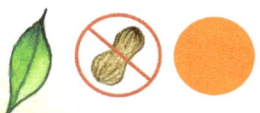

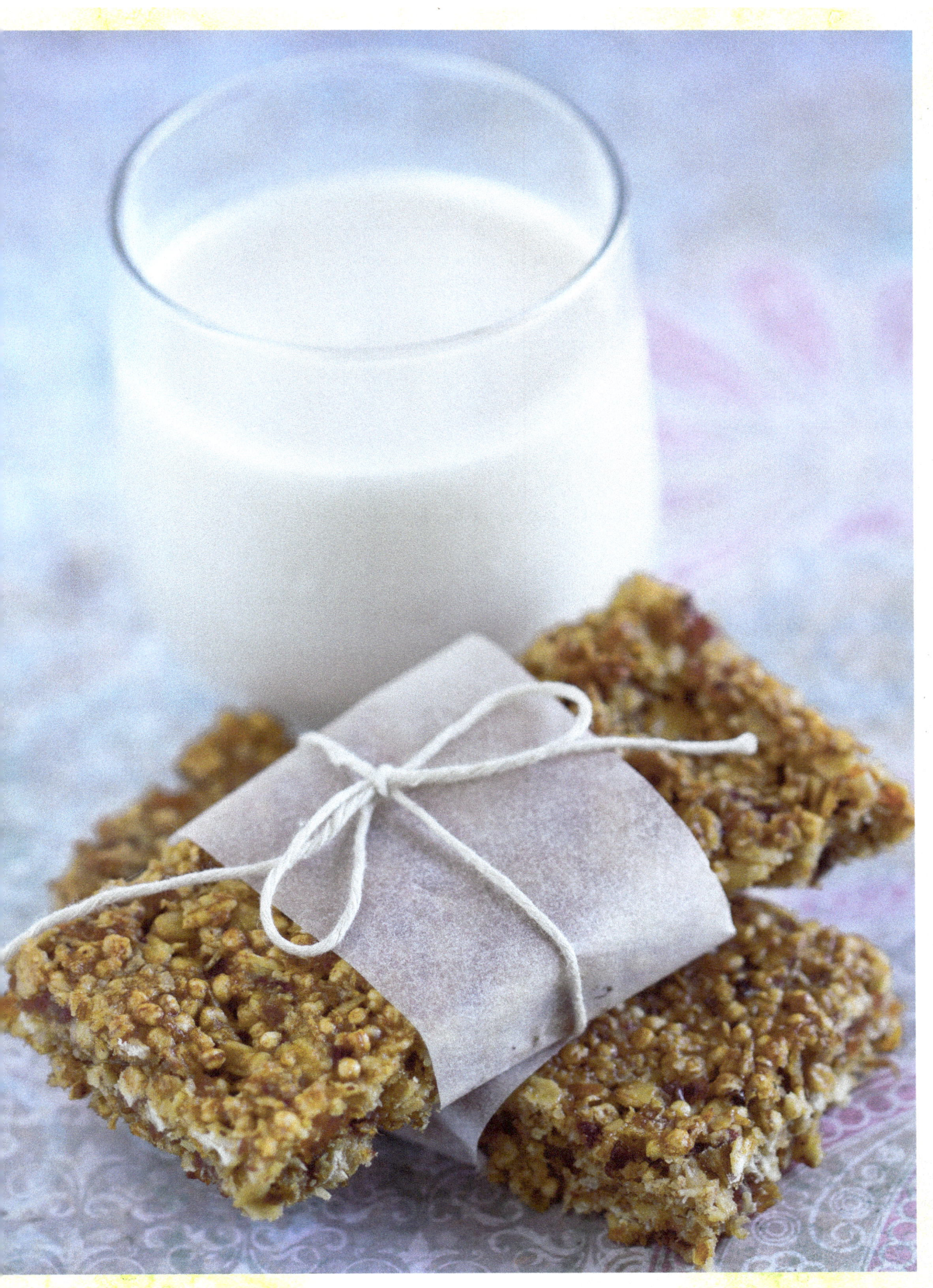

Basic Scone

You can make these as is and jazz them up with some lovely fruit spread or honey, or you can add a variety of different accessories to the dough. For ideas, see "Play Time" below. Children can follow most of the steps in scone making with very little help.

Makes 15 medium-sized scones

1 ½ cups of wholemeal wheat or spelt flour
1 ½ cups of unbleached wheat or spelt flour
¼ teaspoon of sea salt
3 teaspoons of baking powder
85g butter, cut into cubes
3 tablespoons of honey
175ml milk
squeeze of lemon juice (this will aid the raising agents)
milk, to brush on top

1. Preheat oven to 200°C convection or 180°C fan-forced. Grease or line a baking tray.
2. In a large bowl, combine the flour, baking powder and salt.
3. Add the butter, then rub in with your fingers until the mix looks like fine crumbs. As you do this, raise your hands high to aerate the mixture. You can use a food processor to do the mixing, however if you do, aerate it with your fingers afterward.
4. Slightly warm your milk and add the honey, vanilla and lemon juice. Mix well.
5. Make a well in the dry mix, then add the liquid and combine it quickly with a cutlery knife. Do not over-mix.
6. Sprinkle some flour evenly onto the work surface and tip the dough out. Cover the dough and your hands with a little more flour, and pat into a round shape about 3cm in height.
7. Take a 5cm cutter (I use a glass) and dip it into some flour. Plunge into the dough, then repeat until you run out of space. By this point you'll probably need to press what's left of the dough back into a round shape to cut out more. Carefully place scones onto the baking tray so that they are just touching and brush the tops with milk.
8. Bake for 20 minutes until risen and golden on the top. Leave to stand for 10 minutes before serving. Eat warm or cold on the day of baking.

Play Time!

- For sweet scones, add dried fruit such as sultanas, apricots, cranberries or dates. Or add fresh fruit such as blueberries, raspberries or grated apple.
- For a savoury scone, add grated cheese, herbs and or sun-dried tomatoes.

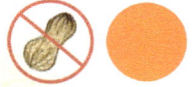

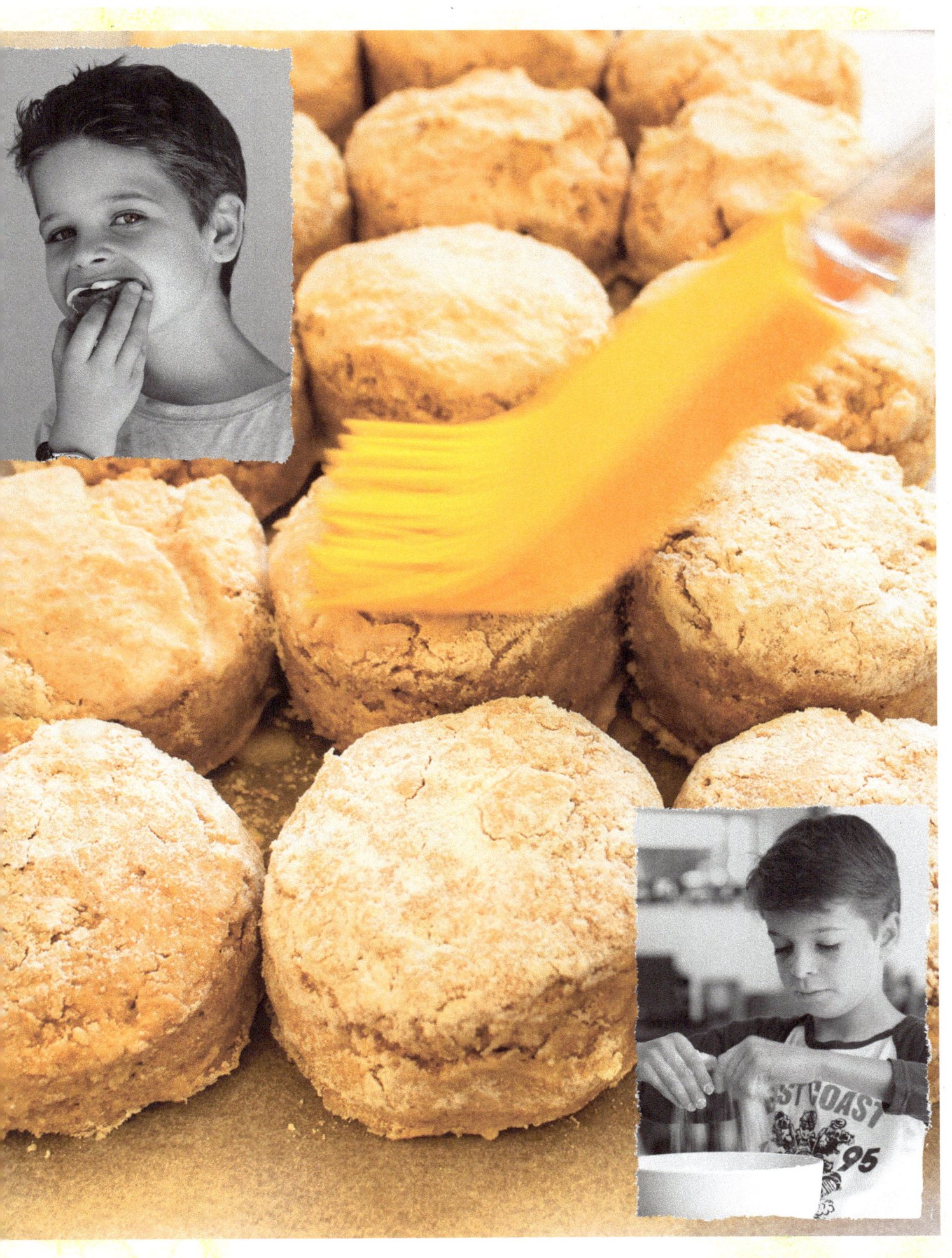

Lime and Coconut Scones

These scones are naturally sweet and the hint of lime complements the coconut flavour.

Makes 15 medium-sized scones

1 ½ cups of wholemeal wheat or spelt flour
1 ½ cups of unbleached wheat or spelt flour
3 teaspoons of baking powder
1 tablespoon of finely grated lime zest
80g butter, cut into small cubes
3 tablespoon of maple syrup*
½ - ¾ cup of coconut milk
milk, to brush on top

* An alternative to maple syrup is to add 2 tablespoons of rapadura or coconut sugar. You will need a little more coconut milk in its place.

1. Preheat oven to 200°C convection or 180°C fan-forced. Grease or line a baking tray.
2. Combine the flour, baking powder and lime zest into a large bowl.
3. Add the butter, then rub in with your fingers until the mix looks like fine crumbs. As you do this, raise your hands high to aerate the mixture. You can use a food processor to do the mixing, however if you do, aerate it with your fingers afterward.
4. Add the liquid sweetener and ½ cup of coconut milk. Gently mix with a knife until just combined. Depending on the flour you use, you may need more coconut milk, but add it gradually so that you don't make your mixture too wet. The mixture should be firm enough to form into a large ball without sticking to your fingers, but not too dry.
5. Sprinkle some flour evenly onto the work surface and tip the dough out. Lightly coat the dough and your hands with a little more flour and pat into a round shape about 3cm in height.
6. Take a 5cm cutter and dip it into some flour. Plunge into the dough, then repeat until you have run out of room. By this point you'll probably need to press what's left of the dough back into a round shape to cut out another set.
7. Place them onto a baking tray so that they are just touching one another and brush the tops with milk.
8. Bake for 20-25 minutes until risen and golden on the top. Leave to stand for 10 minutes before serving. Eat warm or cold on the day of baking.

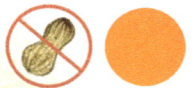

The Land of Sweet

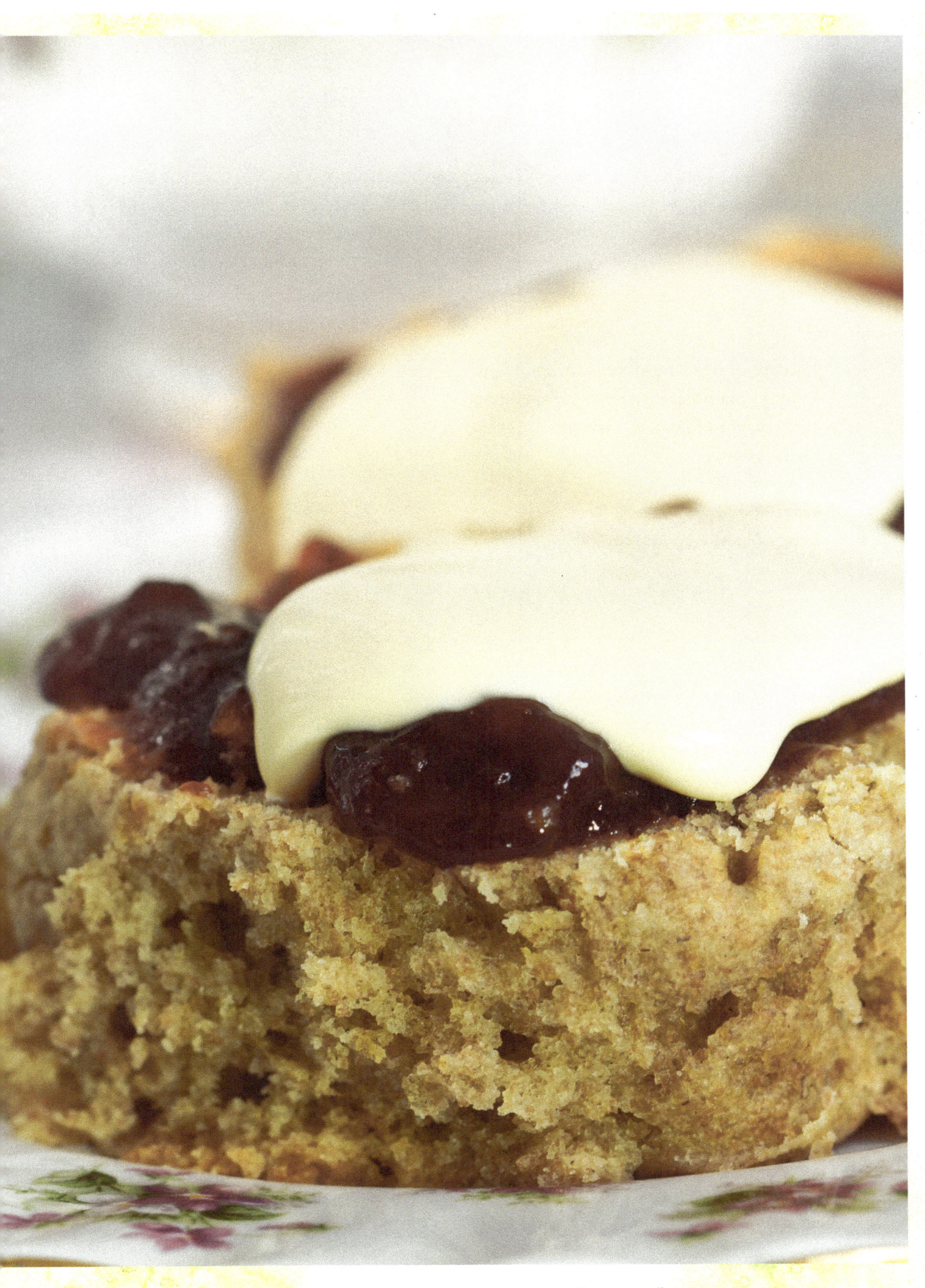

Pumpkin Scones

These are a moist and delicious scone with a beautiful orange colour. You can be creative with this recipe. Add mixed spice and you can also substitute maple syrup for the honey which will give you a pumpkin pie flavour. Another option is to substitute the mashed pumpkin with stewed apple (apple sauce) to make apple scones. You may need to sprinkle a little more flour on to make up for the increased moisture in the apple.

Makes 15 medium-sized scones

- 1 ¼ cups of wholemeal wheat or spelt flour
- 1 ¼ cups of unbleached wheat or spelt flour
- 2 ½ teaspoons of baking powder
- 55g soft butter
- ¼ cup of milk
- 3 tablespoons of honey
- 1 cup of mashed pumpkin

1. Preheat oven to 200°C convection or 180°C fan-forced. Grease or line a baking tray.
2. Combine the flour and baking powder in a large bowl.
3. Add the butter, then rub in with your fingers until the mix looks like fine crumbs. As you do this, raise your hands high to aerate the mixture. Be aware that if you use a food processor your scones will not be as light.
4. Slightly warm your milk and add the honey, then the pumpkin.
5. Make a well in the dry mix, then add the liquid and combine it quickly with a cutlery knife. Do not over mix.
6. Sprinkle some flour evenly onto the work surface and tip the dough out. Lightly coat the dough and your hands with a little more flour and pat into a round shape about 3cm in height.
7. Take a 5cm cutter and dip it into some flour. Plunge into the dough, then repeat until you run out of space. By this point you'll probably need to press what's left of the dough back into a round shape to cut out more scones.
8. Place them onto a baking tray so that they are just touching one another and brush the tops with milk.
9. Bake for 25 minutes until risen and golden on the top.
10. Leave to stand for 10 minutes before serving. Eat warm or cold on the day of baking.

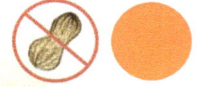

Cranberry and Vanilla Cake Bars

These are a cross between a slice and a cake. They are sweet and slightly tangy because of the cranberries. Children can participate by measuring and blending.

1 cup of dried, unsweetened cranberries
2 eggs
½ cup of maple syrup
¾ cup of oil
2 teaspoons of vanilla extract or one vanilla bean, seeds only
1 cup of wholemeal wheat or spelt flour
1 cup of unbleached wheat or spelt flour
2 teaspoons of baking powder
⅓ cup of semolina
3-4 tablespoons of chopped almonds (for topping)

1. Preheat the oven to 180°C convection or 160°C fan-forced.
2. Lightly grease and line a 16cm x 25cm rectangle cake tin.
3. Blend cranberries and all other wet ingredients in a food processor.
4. Combine flour, baking powder and semolina in a mixing bowl.
5. Add wet ingredients to dry and combine gently until just mixed.
6. Pour into tin and top evenly with nuts.
7. Bake for 30-35 minutes or until cake skewer comes out clean.
8. Cool in tin and then cut into bars and serve.

Play Time!

- Replace the cranberries with goji berries or dried apricots.
- Add cinnamon or mixed spice.
- Vary the nuts used on top or for a nut free version, top with coconut.

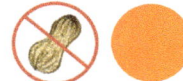

The Land of Sweet

Honey and Apple Cake

This cake is moist, delicious and naturally sweetened with honey. Regarding the apple sauce, I buy apples when they are in season and stew/puree a whole lot. I then freeze them into small portions so that I have apple sauce on hand when I need it. Should you find yourself without any, the cake will work just as well using ¾ cup of oil (instead of ¼ cup) and ¼ cup of water.

- **1 cup of honey**
- **1 egg**
- **¾ cup of apple sauce or stewed apple**
- **¼ cup of oil**
- **1 teaspoon of ground cinnamon**
- **1 teaspoon of mixed spice**
- **½ teaspoon of nutmeg**
- **1 cup of wholemeal spelt or wheat flour**
- **1 cup of unbleached spelt or wheat flour**
- **2 teaspoons of baking powder**
- **1 large apple peeled and sliced thinly**

1. Preheat the oven to 180°C convection or 160°C fan-forced.
2. Grease and line a loaf tin or 19cm round tin.
3. Using electric beaters, beat the honey until it is creamy. This will take 2-3 minutes.
4. Add the egg, apple sauce, oil and spices. Beat until well combined
5. Sift in flour and baking powder, then gently fold the mix until just combined.
6. Pour into the prepared pan and top with sliced apple.
7. Bake 45 minutes or until a cake skewer comes out clean. Follow the baking tip on page 214 for an exceptional cake.

Play Time!

- Use stewed pear and sliced pear on top instead of the apple.
- Leave out the spices and add lemon zest or 2 teaspoons of vanilla extract.
- Make into muffins.

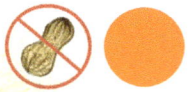

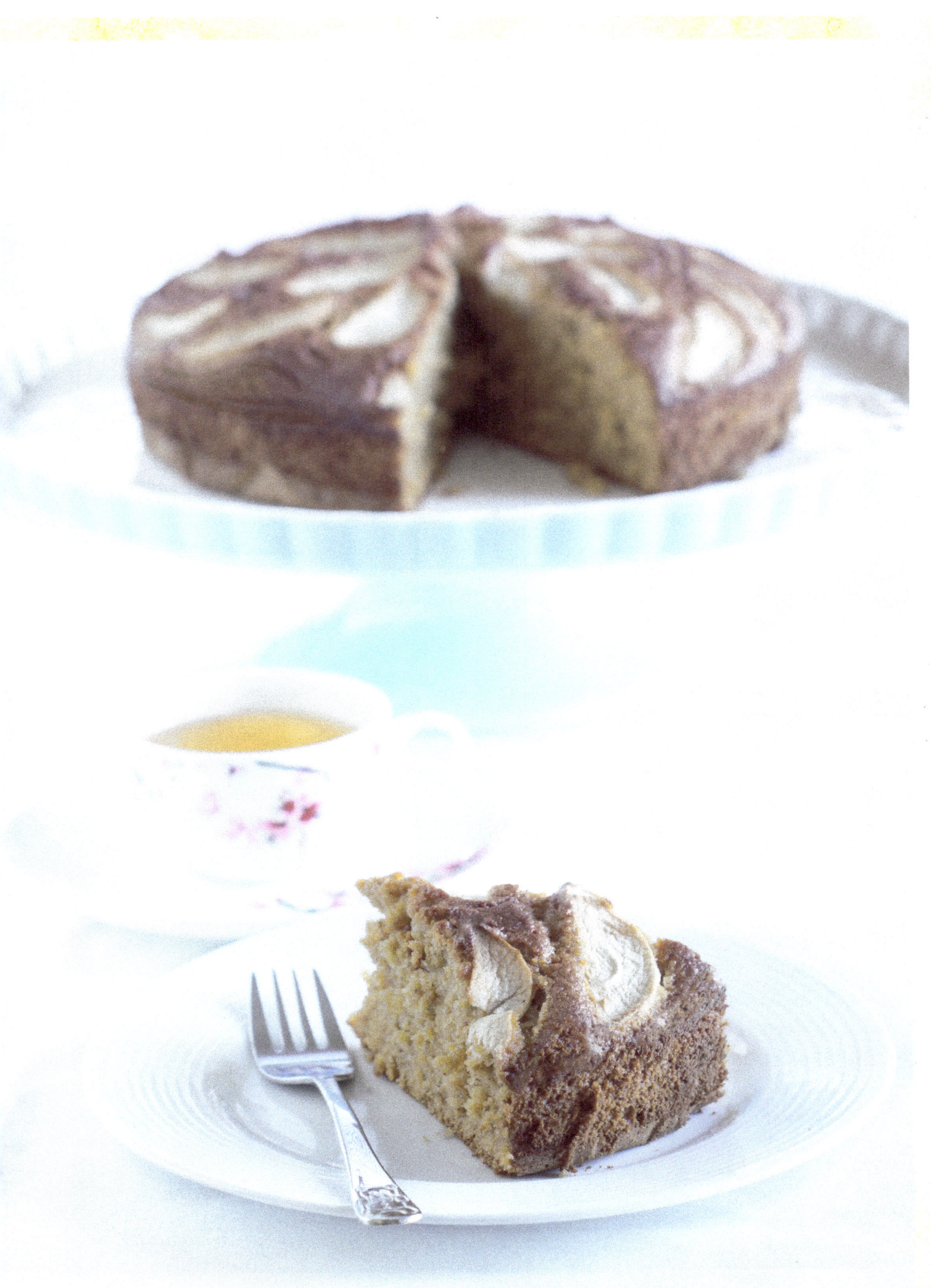

Carrot Cake

This cake is very moist and flavoursome. We like the flavour of the coconut oil, however you can use other oils in its place. I have indicated that this cake can be nut-free as it is just as good without the walnuts.

1 cup of wholemeal wheat or spelt flour
1 cup of plain unbleached wheat or spelt flour
2 teaspoons of baking powder
1 teaspoon of mixed spice
1 ½ teaspoons of ground cinnamon
¾ cup of coconut oil
¼ cup of milk
3 eggs, beaten
1 cup of rapadura or coconut sugar
½ cup of grated apple
1 ½ cups of grated carrot
1 cup of chopped walnuts (leave out for a nut free version)

Cream-Cheese Topping

200g cream-cheese, softened: out of the fridge
2 tablespoons of raw honey
2 tablespoons of lemon juice
crushed walnuts to top (leave off for a nut free version)

1. Preheat the oven to 180°C convection or 160°C fan-forced.
1. Grease and line a 19cm square cake tin.
2. Place flour, baking powder and spices into a large bowl and mix well.
3. In a separate, smaller bowl, whisk the oil, milk, eggs and sugar. Stir in the apple, carrot and walnuts.
4. Pour the wet ingredients into the dry and mix until it all comes together, being careful not to over-mix.
5. Pour batter into the cake tin and bake for 35-40 minutes or until a cake skewer comes out clean.
6. Follow the baking tip on page 214 for an exceptional cake.
7. Meanwhile, to make the icing, combine the cream-cheese, honey and lemon juice with a fork or in a food processor.
8. Spread over the cake and top with crushed walnuts.

The Land of Sweet

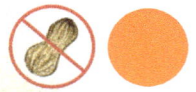

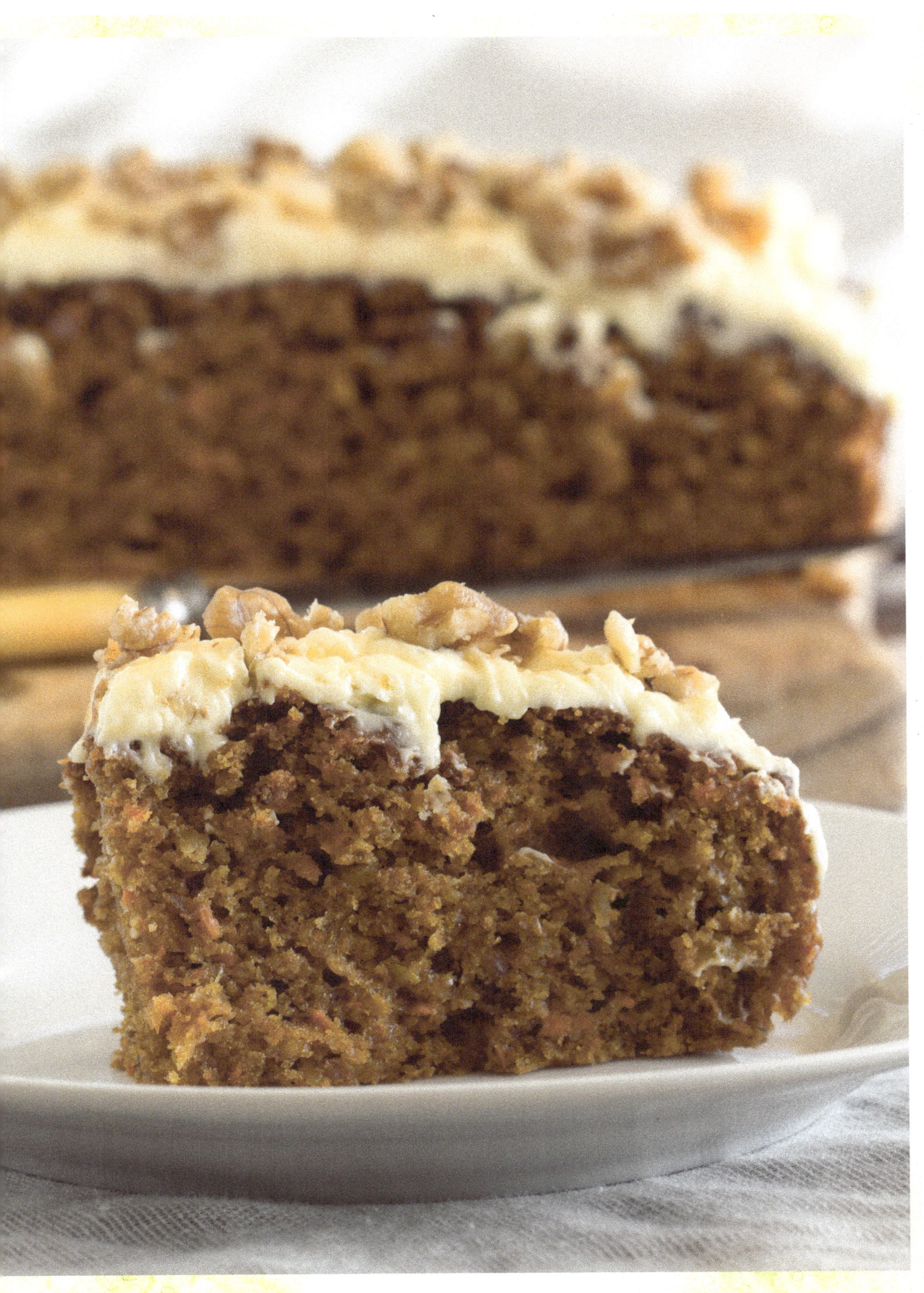

Chocolate Cupcakes

Thanks to the zucchini in this recipe, these little cakes are moist and soft. Even better, once it cooks the zucchini becomes invisible! If you can, use Dutch cocoa which has a smoother taste and darker colour.

Makes 21 cakes

½ cup of oil

3 eggs

1 cup of rapadura or coconut sugar

½ cup of cocoa

2 cups grated or pulverised zucchini (squeeze the excess liquid out)

1 cup of wholemeal wheat or spelt flour

1 cup of plain unbleached wheat or spelt flour

2 teaspoons of baking powder

Icing

100g cream cheese

3 tablespoon of raw cacao

2 tablespoon of maple syrup

45g fresh or frozen raspberries

1. Preheat the oven to 180°C convection or 160°C fan-forced.
2. Prepare a patty cake pan with cases.
3. With and electric mixer or whisk, combine the oil, eggs, sugar and cocoa.
4. Stir in the zucchini until evenly mixed.
5. Gently stir in the flour and baking powder.
6. Spoon into the patty cases and bake for 20 minutes or until a cake skewer comes out clean.
7. Follow the baking tip on page 214 for exceptional cakes.
8. While your cakes are cooling, make the icing. Combine all icing ingredients in a food processor or with a hand mixer until smooth.
9. Either pipe the icing onto the cakes or spread with a knife. An easy way to pipe the mix is to put it into a "zip-lock back" and cut a small corner off. Squeeze the icing through the small hole in a circular pattern onto the top of each cake.

Play Time!

- Add other flavours to your icing mix instead of raspberries, e.g. blueberries, strawberries, orange zest or peppermint leaves.

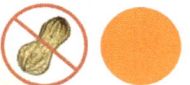

The Land of Sweet

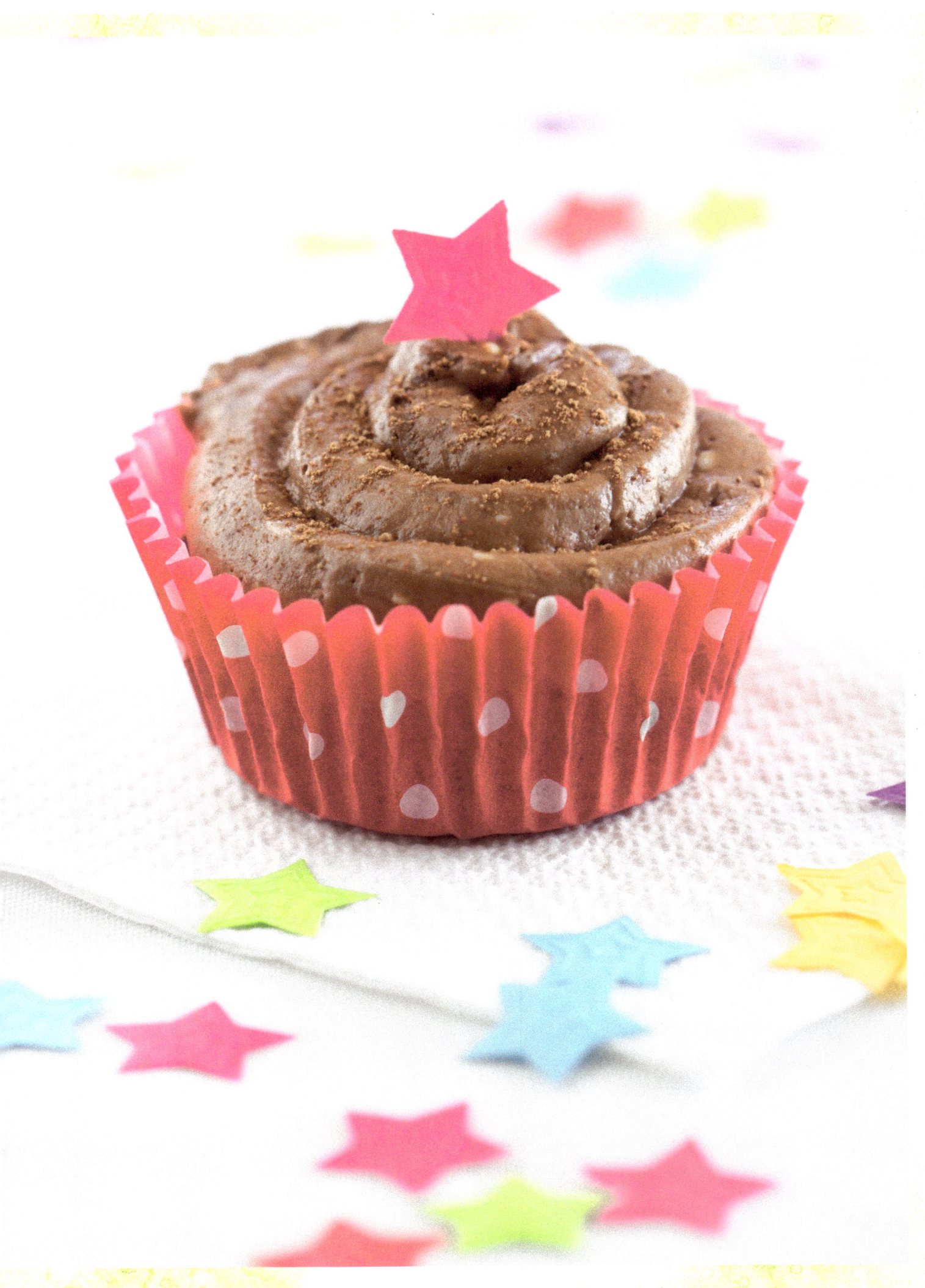

Once Upon a Time Muffins

These muffins are lovely and moist. They don't actually taste like sweet potato, they just taste sweet with a hint of coconut. I highly recommend the pumpkin version mentioned in the playtime below.

Makes 12 muffins

½ cup of coconut oil

1 cup of rapadura or coconut sugar

2 eggs

1 cup of mashed sweet potato (275g of raw sweet potato equals 1 cup of cooked/mashed)

½ cup of milk

1 cup of wholemeal wheat or spelt flour

1 cup of unbleached wheat or spelt flour

2 teaspoons of baking powder

1. Preheat the oven to 180°C convection or 160°C fan-forced.
2. Prepare a muffin tin with cases or by greasing the muffin holes.
3. With a hand mixer or food processor, combine all ingredients except the flour and baking powder.
4. Fold in the flour and baking powder.
5. Spoon into muffin cases and bake for 20-25 minutes, or until a skewer comes out clean.
6. Follow the baking tip on page 214 for exceptional muffins.

Play Time!

- For a sweet, spicy muffin, add 2 teaspoons of cinnamon, ½ teaspoon of nutmeg and 2 teaspoons of mixed spice.
- For a pumpkin pie flavoured muffin, replace the sweet potato with pumpkin and add 1 teaspoon of cinnamon and 1 teaspoon of mixed spice. Reduce the milk to ¼ cup as pumpkin is wetter than sweet potato.
- Add a cup of blueberries or chopped apple for a fruity flavour.
- Walnuts or pecans are also a lovely addition to this muffin.

246 The Land of Sweet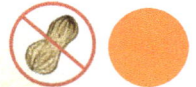

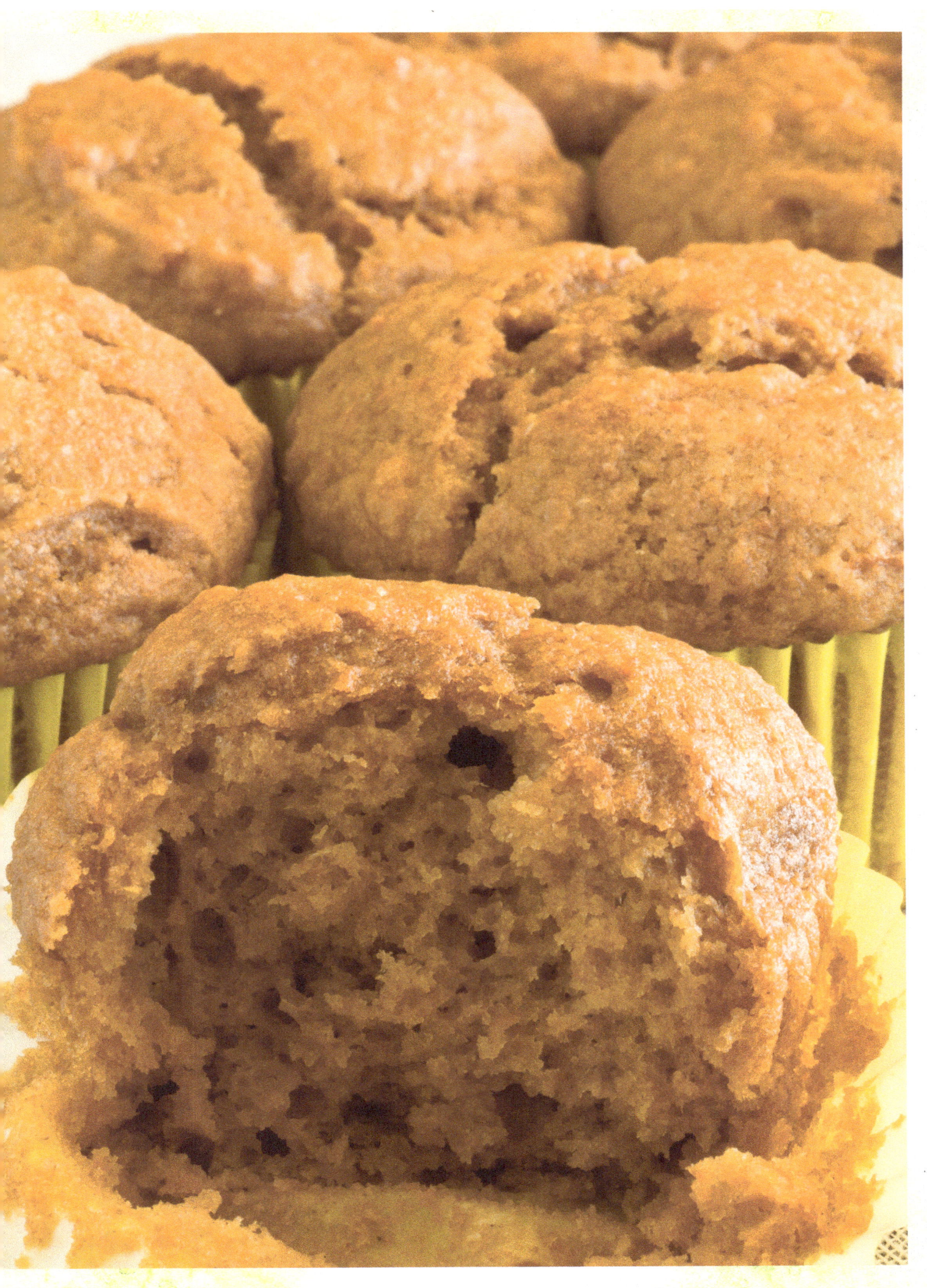

Lemon Syrup Muffins

If you like lemon and coconut, these are for you. They are a variation on the traditional lemon syrup cake and are in a convenient serving for one size. Children will love making these and then pouring the syrup over after they are cooked. If you do not have coconut sugar, rapadura is a suitable replacement.

Makes 12 muffins

2 eggs
1 cup of coconut sugar
¾ cup of coconut milk
½ cup of milk
grated zest of one lemon
1 cup of wholemeal spelt or wheat flour
1 cup of unbleached spelt or wheat flour
2 teaspoons of baking powder

Syrup
juice of one lemon
2 tablespoons of water
2 tablespoons of coconut sugar

1. Preheat the oven to 180°C convection or 160°C fan-forced.
2. Prepare a muffin tin with cases or by greasing the muffin holes.
3. Whisk eggs, sugar, coconut milk, milk and lemon zest.
4. Fold in dry ingredients and spoon into muffin cases
5. Bake for 20 minutes or until a skewer comes out clean.
6. Meanwhile, make the lemon syrup by combining all of the syrup ingredients over low heat. Once the syrup starts to bubble, remove from heat.
7. Poke holes in the muffins and pour the syrup over the top. It will sink into the cake making it lemony and sticky. Perhaps one to eat outside!

Play Time!

- Use lime instead of lemon for a lime and coconut flavoured muffin.
- Sprinkle desiccated coconut over the syrup topped muffin.

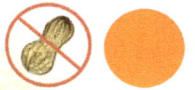

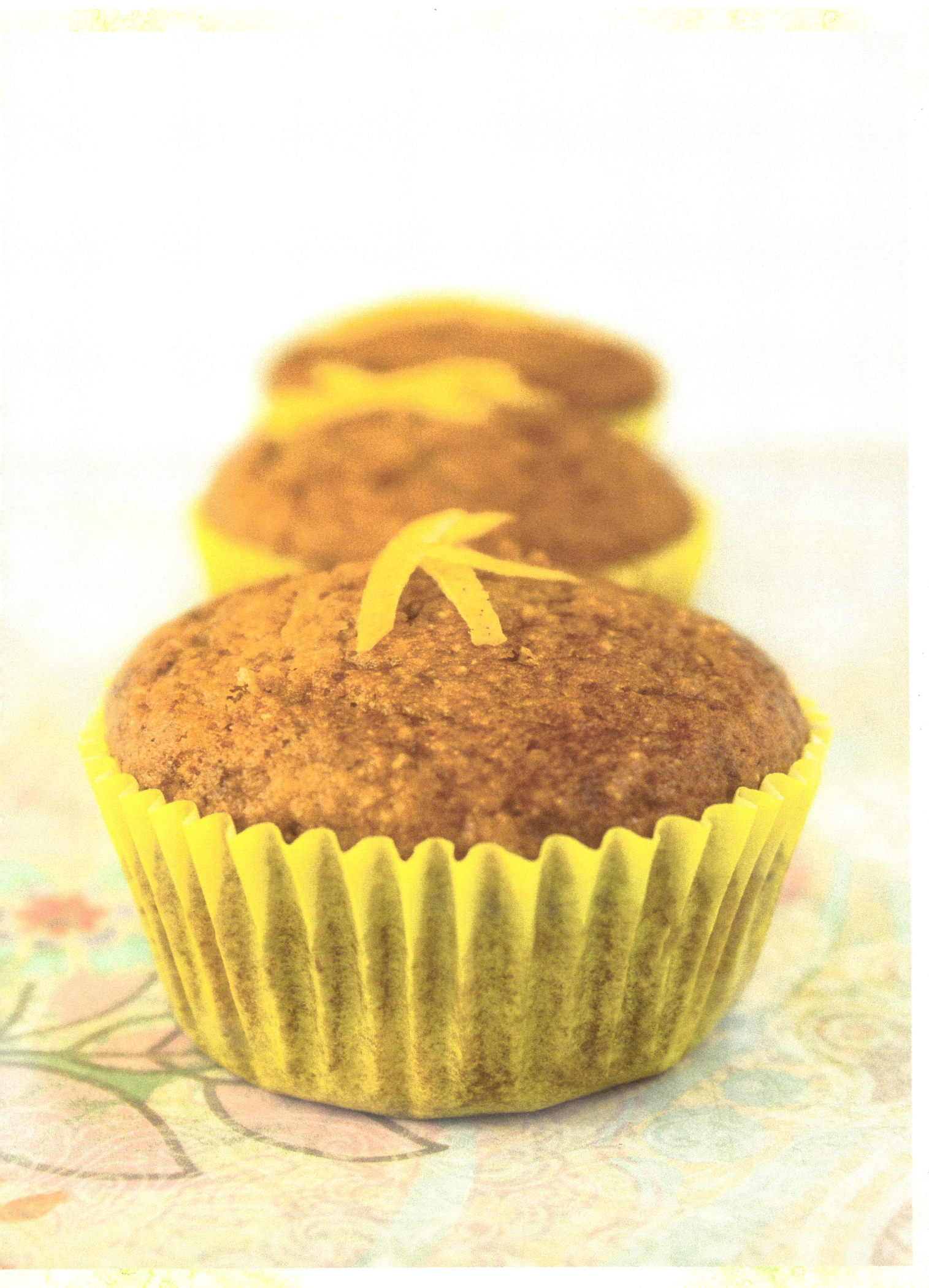

Blueberry and Apple Muffins

These muffins are sweet with fruity flaovur. The apple sauce replaces a large quantity of the oil that would otherwise be needed to make them moist.

Makes 12 muffins

¾ cup of rapadura or coconut sugar

2 eggs

½ cup of apple sauce or pureed stewed apple

¼ cup of oil

½ cup of milk

1 teaspoon of vanilla extract

1 teaspoon of cinnamon (optional)

1 cup of wholemeal wheat or spelt flour

1 cup of unbleached wheat or spelt flour

2 teaspoons of baking powder

1 cup of fresh or frozen blueberries

1. Preheat the oven to 180°C convection or 160°C fan-forced.
2. Prepare a muffin tin with cases or by greasing the muffin holes.
3. In a medium-sized mixing bowl, whisk the wet ingredients and cinnamon.
4. Add the flour and baking powder and mix gently, taking care not to over mix.
5. Add blueberries and stir in gently.
6. Spoon into muffin cases and bake for 20-25 minutes (until cake skewer comes out clean).
7. Follow the baking tip on page 214 for exceptional muffins.

Play Time!

- Use other berries in place of the blueberries.
- Omit the cinnamon and add the grated zest of a lemon.
- Use stewed pear instead of apple sauce.

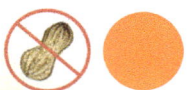

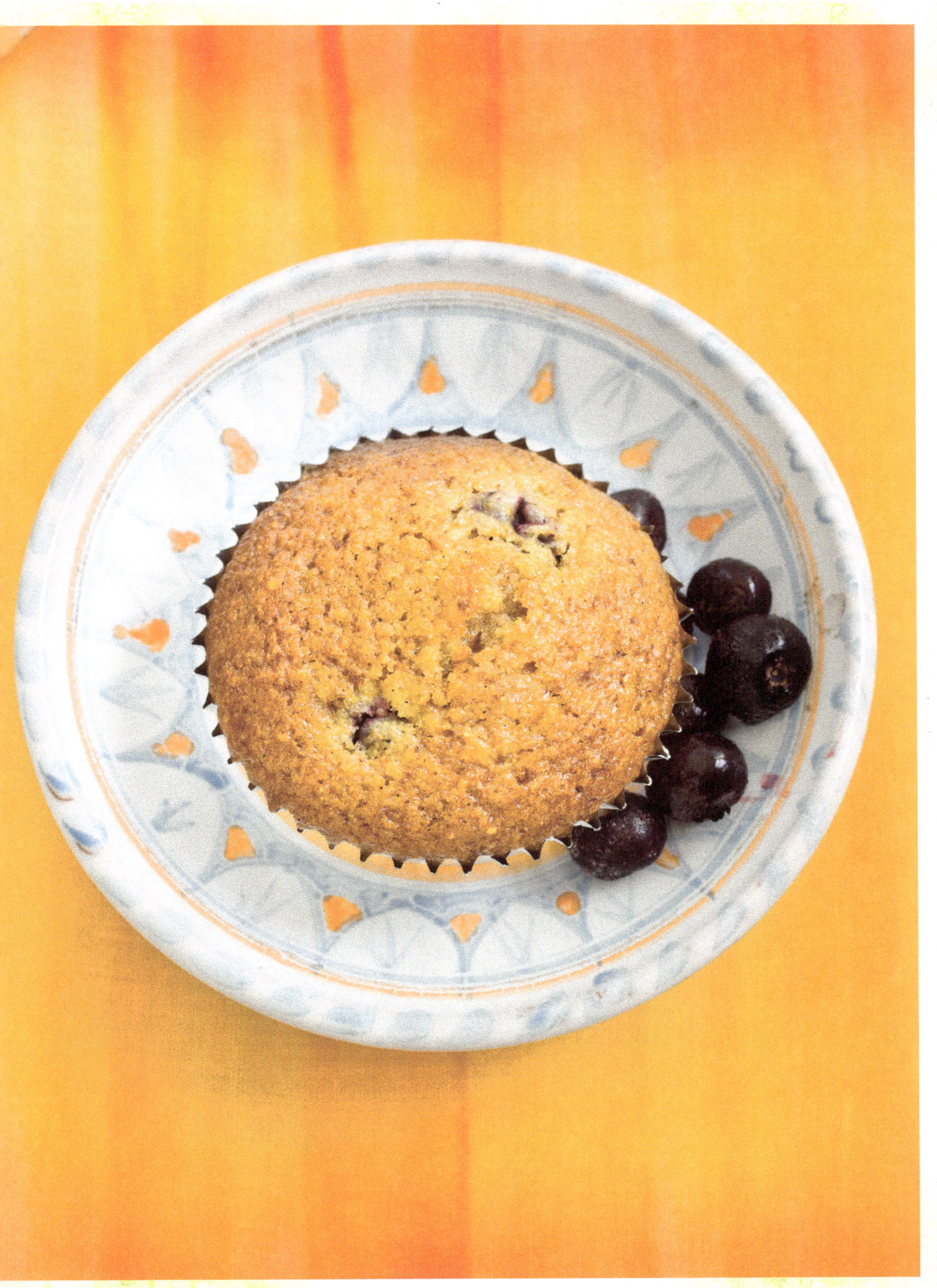

Happily Ever After Muffins

Like the Once Upon a Time Muffins, these don't actually taste of vegetable. The flavour of the spices, nuts and molasses in the sugar are the dominant tastes, making them a delicious healthy treat.

Makes 12 muffins

1 large egg

¾ cup of rapadura or coconut sugar

½ teaspoon of mixed spice

½ teaspoon of cinnamon

¼ teaspoon of ground nutmeg

⅔ cup of oil

1 teaspoon of vanilla extract

150g (1 cup) of grated zucchini

100g crushed pecans

2 teaspoons of baking powder

¾ cup of wholemeal wheat or spelt flour

¾ cup of unbleached wheat or spelt flour

1. Preheat the oven to 180°C convection or 160°C fan-forced.
2. Prepare a muffin tin with cases or by greasing the muffin holes.
3. With your beaters or food processor, combine egg, sugar, spices, oil and vanilla until well mixed.
4. Stir in the zucchini and nuts until well mixed.
5. Gently stir in the flour and baking powder until just combined.
6. Spoon into muffin cases and bake for 20-25 minutes or until cake skewer comes out clean.
7. Follow the baking tip on page 214 for exceptional muffins.

Play Time!

- Replace the zucchini with carrot.
- Leave out the spices and replace with the zest of an orange or lemon.
- Use walnuts instead of pecans.

The Land of Sweet

Crispy Cashew Rice Treats

*This is a **slice** which I cut into squares. It is sweet and slightly sticky and best served from the fridge or freezer. You can change the nuts you use, or even use puffed quinoa instead of the rice cereal. For those with peanut allergies, other nut butters will work as well.*

½ cup of rice syrup

¾ cup of natural peanut butter (or another nut butter)

¾ cup of cashews, roughly chopped

2 cups of brown rice cereal

1. Oil a 16cm x 25cm baking dish.
2. Bring rice syrup to the boil then lower heat and simmer for 2 minutes.
3. Add peanut butter and turn heat to low.
4. Mix thoroughly for about 3 minutes.
5. Combine cashews with rice crisp cereal in mixing bowl.
6. Add peanut butter mix and combine.
7. Press into the baking dish and let it cool in the fridge.
8. Cut into squares and serve.

Play Time!

- Use puffed quinoa instead of puffed rice.
- Add dried cranberries, goji berries or chopped dried apricots.
- Use almonds or macadamia nuts instead of cashews.
- Add ½ cup of LSA (recipe on page 86).
- Add 3 tablespoons of raw cacao powder.

The Land of Sweet

Divine Raw Brownies

These brownies have a rich chocolate flavour, made with pure ingredients and are a treat that you can enjoy knowing that you are eating well. The children I have tested these on always asked for seconds, even the ones who are usually fussy!

Base

1 cup of pecans, soaked for 6 hours
1 cup of walnuts, soaked for 6 hours
⅓ cup of sultanas
100g chopped medjool dates - seeds removed
⅓ cup of raw cocao powder
1 teaspoon of vanilla extract

Icing

20g raw cacao butter
⅓ cup of raw cocao powder
¼ cup of maple syrup

1. Grease and line a 16cm x 25cm baking dish with baking paper.
2. Process the base ingredients in a food processor until well combined and crumbly.
3. Wet your hands and then press the mixture into the base of the prepared dish.
4. Melt cocao butter over low heat and whisk with remaining icing ingredients.
5. Spread evenly over the prepared base and cover with plastic wrap.
6. Chill for at least 2 hours.
7. Cut into squares and serve.

Play Time!

- Add goji berries or dried cranberries.
- Use cashews in place of either pecans or walnuts.
- Add cinnamon or the zest of an orange.
- Top with desiccated coconut.
- If cacao butter is not available, use coconut oil as a substitute.

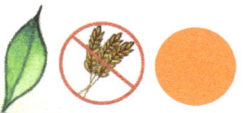

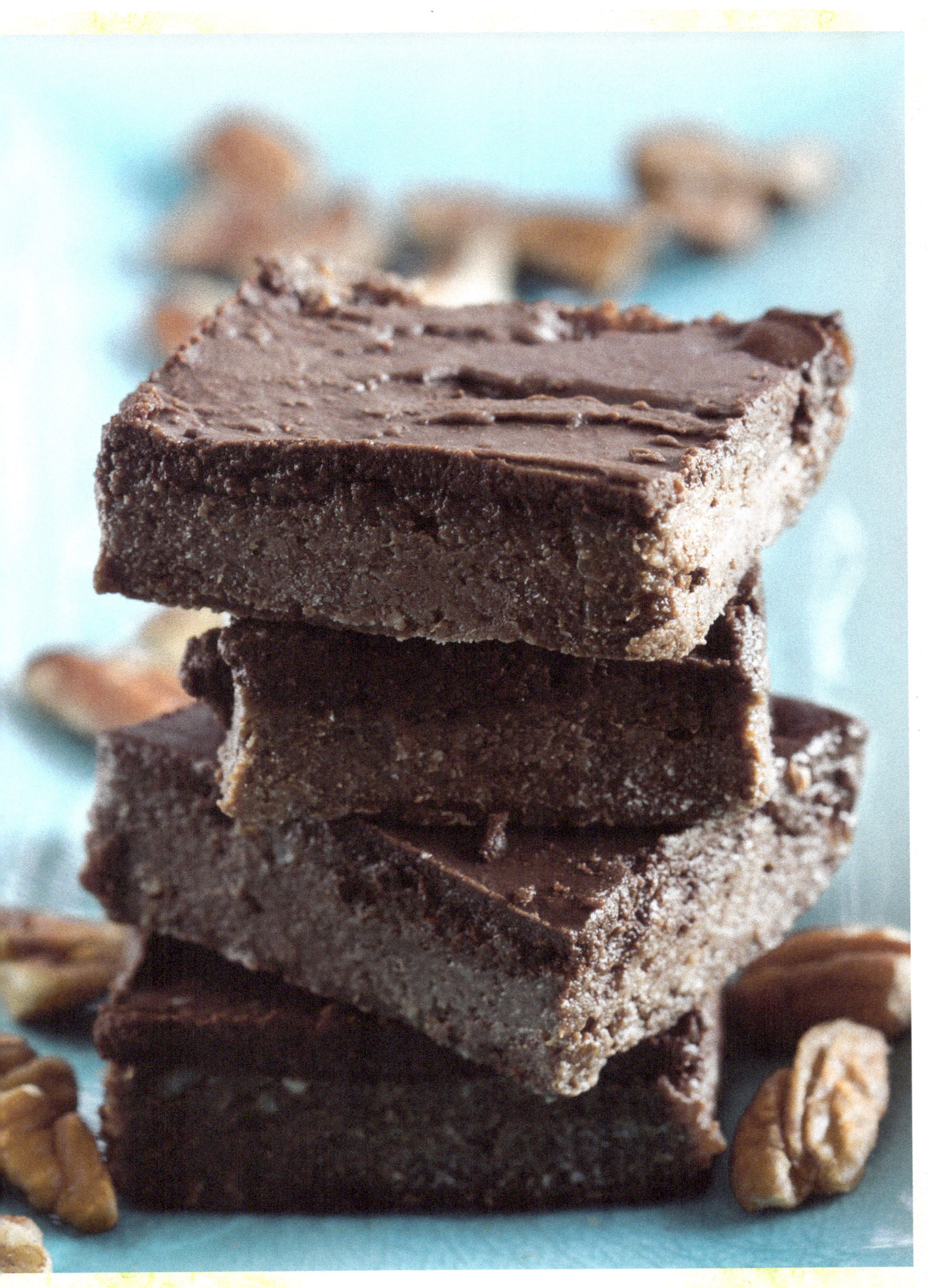

Raw Coconut Rough

This is a recipe for raw chocolate. That's right, it is chocolate and it is good for you because it contains so many healthy ingredients. It stores well in the freezer.

½ cup of raw almonds
½ cup of pepitas (pumpkin seeds)
½ cup of sunflower seeds
1 cup of desiccated coconut
¾ cup of raw cacao powder
½ cup of coconut oil
½ cup of maple syrup

1. Grease and line a 16cm x 25cm baking dish with baking paper.
2. Place almonds and seeds into a food processor and process to a fine crumb.
3. In a medium-sized mixing bowl, combine the nuts and seeds with the coconut and cacao.
4. If your coconut oil is not already liquid, melt over very low heat.
5. Add oil to the dry mix with the syrup and mix well.
6. Press evenly into your dish and cover with plastic wrap.
7. Refrigerate until hard. This will take a few hours. If you can't wait, put it into the freezer.

Play Time!

- Add dried fruits such as goji berries, cranberries, sultanas or apricots.
- Use shredded coconut to add more texture.
- Add cinnamon or the zest of an orange.

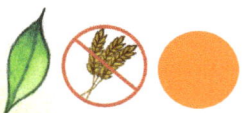

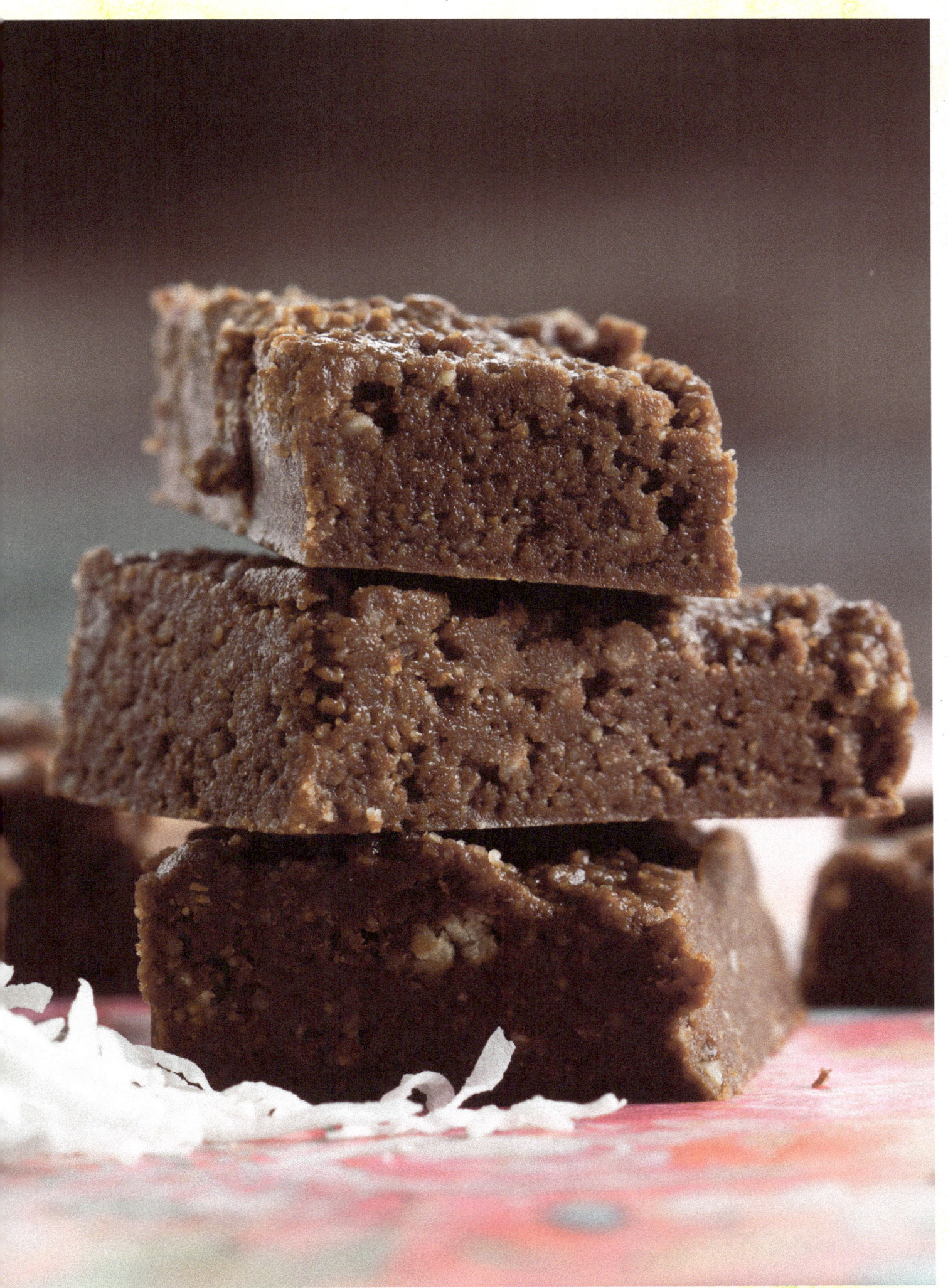

Frozen Fruit

In many cases, nature has made fruit sweet enough. I am thinking of pineapple, oranges, grapes, blueberries, home-grown strawberries, bananas, mangoes, paw paw, and for those in tropical areas, an even wider range of less known fruits. One of the simplest ways to pacify that sweet tooth is to freeze pieces of fruit and eat them as an ice block. Grapes and other smaller berries may be frozen as they are. Pineapple of course, needs to be peeled and cut into pieces and oranges can be quartered and left with skins on, providing a nice handle when eating. Bananas need to be peeled and a paddle pop stick makes it easier to eat.

Home-Made Ice Blocks

Buy yourself some of those ice block makers from your local department store or kitchen shop and you can make a variety of different flavours, from simple to more complex. See below for ideas:

Fresh juice

Fresh juice with pieces of fruit in

Pureed mango, pineapple and coconut milk (my children's favourite)

Pureed raspberries and orange juice

Pureed fruit such as berries, bananas or mango and yoghurt. (Basically make a smoothie)

Pureed bananas, cocoa or carob and cashews

Passion fruit, banana and yoghurt. (Remember not to put passion fruit into your food processor or you will have pureed seeds!)

Passion fruit, mango and pineapple

Yoghurt, honey and berries

When you have chosen your combination and pureed or mixed the ingredients, decanter into your moulds and freeze. Remember liquid expands as it freezes so don't fill the moulds right to the top.

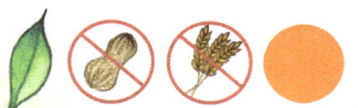

Multicoloured Ice blocks

These ones are a little more work but still quite simple

Choose a couple of different flavours (making sure they go well together) and then do your ice blocks in stages. For example, make up a mixture of pureed pineapple and mango, half fill your containers and freeze. Then top up with orange juice and return to the freezer. The kids will love the two tones and different flavours in one ice block.

Quick Ice Creams

Ice cream doesn't have to be made in an ice cream maker with loads of sugar and cream, you can make a faster version with frozen fruit. Below are some of my combinations. Once you taste them, try creating your own: you can even add ingredients such as dried fruit and shredded coconut.

Tropical Bliss

Mango, pineapple and coconut: such a great combination. You can also add mint and/or ginger which add something extra special.

Serves 4

3 frozen mango cheeks
1 cup of frozen, chopped pineapple
½ cup of coconut cream
Passion fruit to serve on top (optional)

1. Mix mango, pineapple and coconut cream in the blender until smooth.
2. Serve immediately topped with passion fruit.

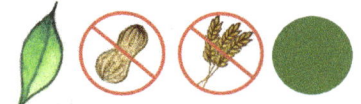

Banana and Berry Fluff

A creamy, banana and berry flavoured dessert.
Serves 4

3 frozen bananas
1 cup of frozen berries
½ cup of coconut cream

Mix all ingredients in your food processor or blender until smooth and serve immediately.

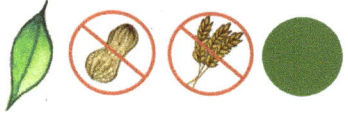

Chocolate Banana Cream

This dessert is rich. Only a small portion is needed to feel satisfied.
Serves 4

3 frozen bananas
2 tablespoon of raw cocoa powder
1 tablespoon of honey or rice syrup
½ cup of cashews

Mix all ingredients in your food processor or blender until smooth and serve immediately.

Play Time!

- Try macadamias instead of the cashews.
- Use carob instead of cocao.
- Add raspberries for a tangy contrast.

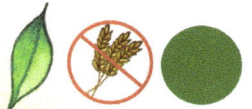

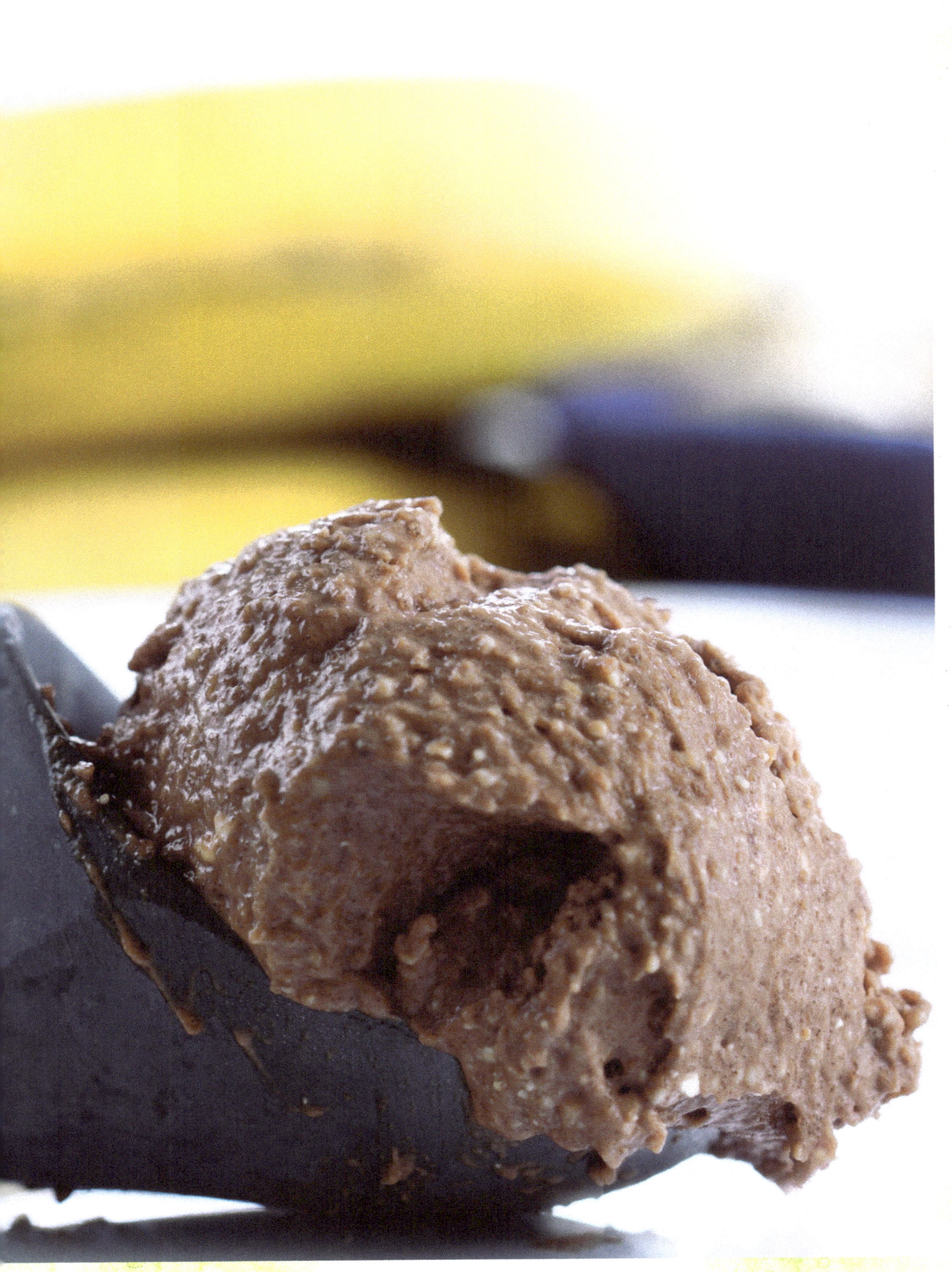

Saucy Banana Pudding

This is a self-saucing pudding which tastes a bit like banana and butterscotch.

Serves 5-6

¼ cup rapadura or coconut sugar
160g of peeled bananas
2 eggs, lightly beaten
½ cup oil
1 teaspoon of vanilla extract
¾ cup wholemeal wheat or spelt flour
¾ cup unbleached wheat or spelt flour
1 ½ teaspoons of baking powder

Sauce

1 ½ cups of boiling water
2 tablespoons of barley malt
¾ cup of rapadura or coconut sugar
Cream, custard or ice cream to serve

1. Preheat the oven to 180°C convection or 160°C fan-forced.
2. With an electric mixer or food processor, blend the sugar, bananas, eggs, oil and vanilla until smooth.
3. Gently mix the dry ingredients into the wet.
4. Pour into an un-greased small loaf tin. It will seem like there is not enough of the cake mix but don't worry, there is. It will expand with the sauce. Spread it evenly over the bottom of the tin.
5. Mix the sauce ingredients together until the sugar and malt have dissolved. Pour over the top of the cake mix, It will look funny with bits floating around. This is the way it is suppose to be. The cake will rise to the top and the sauce will sink to the bottom.
6. Bake in the oven for 40-50 minutes or until a skewer comes out clean.
7. Serve warm with cream, custard or ice-cream.

Play Time!

- Add fresh or frozen berries to the cake mix.
- Add some dark chocolate chips to the cake mix.
- Grate the zest of a lemon or orange into the cake mix.

The Land of Sweet

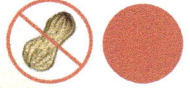

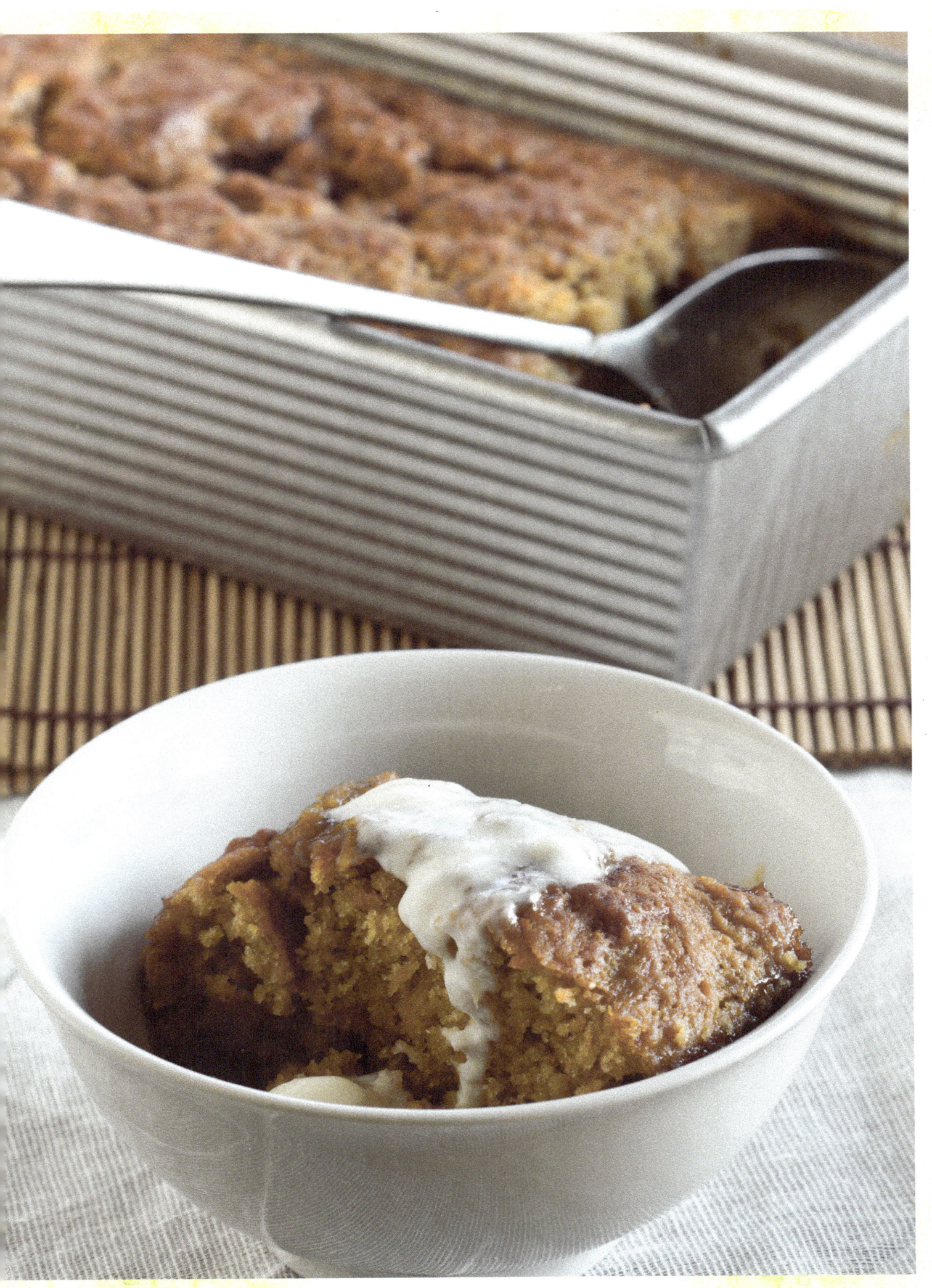

Cinderella Custard

This custard tastes like the filling from a pumpkin pie.

Serves 4-5

2 cups of milk

1 teaspoon of ground ginger

½ teaspoon of ground cinnamon

½ teaspoon of ground nutmeg

200g mashed butternut pumpkin (approx. 250g raw)

1 teaspoon of vanilla extract

4 eggs

½ cup of maple syrup

1. Place milk and spices into a medium saucepan and heat but don't bring to the boil.
2. With an electric beater, beat the pumpkin, vanilla, eggs and maple syrup until smooth.
3. While whisking the milk mix, slowly add the egg mix to your saucepan.
4. Return to heat and stir for 8-10 minutes, until thick and coats the back of a spoon.
5. Serve warm or cold.

Play Time!

- Leave out the spices and add the grated zest of a lemon or orange.
- Leave out the spices and add ¼ cup of cocoa powder.

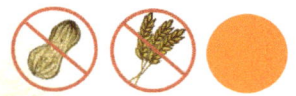

Peach Pie

*When stone fruit is in season, indulge in this yummy pie.
It is also great with half peaches and half apple in the filling.*
Serves 7-8

Crust
1 ½ cups of wholemeal spelt or wheat flour
1 ½ cups of unbleached spelt or wheat flour
½ cup of rapadura or coconut sugar
170g butter, chilled and chopped
1 egg, lightly beaten
2-3 tablespoons of chilled water (may need more depending on the absorbency of the flour)

Filling
700g peach flesh (this measurement is without the stones and skin)
1 teaspoon of ground cinnamon
1 teaspoon of vanilla extract
⅓ cup of maple syrup
⅓ cup of wholemeal spelt or wheat flour

1. Place the flour, sugar and butter into a food processor and pulse until the mix resembles bread crumbs. Otherwise rub the butter into the flour and sugar with your fingers.
2. Add the egg and water then mix until the dough comes together into a smooth ball. Add more water if necessary.
3. Press dough into a thick square and cover with plastic wrap. Refrigerate for 20-30 minutes.
4. Preheat oven to 180°C convection or 160°C fan forced.
5. Divide dough into two sections, one being slightly larger than the other.
6. On a floured board, roll the larger piece out evenly to fit into an 18cm pie dish. To transfer the dough, flour your rolling pin and roll the dough around it. Unroll the dough into the pie dish and press to fit. Trim the edges..
7. Bake for 15 minutes until just browned.
8. Meanwhile, prepare your filling. Combine the peach slices with the cinnamon, vanilla and maple syrup, then stir in the flour.
9. Roll the remaining piece of dough into a top for your pie.
10. Pour the filling into the baked shell and transfer the pie top the same way you did with the shell. Press the sides down with the flat of a butter knife and poke a couple of holes in the top to allow air to escape.
11. Bake for 30 minutes and serve warm or cold.

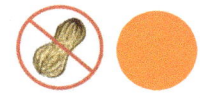

The Land of Sweet

Chocolate Chia Pudding

This is a "Super Food" dessert! With chia seeds, goji berries and raw cacao it doesn't get much better for taste or nutrition and because it is healthy, it doesn't have to be limited as much as the average chocolate pudding. It can be served as a dessert or morning or afternoon tea snack. Alter it any number of ways. Check out the "Play Time" for ideas.

Serves 4-5

2 cups of milk
1 cup of raw cashews
2 tablespoons of goji berries
2 tablespoons of raw cacao powder
5 tablespoons of maple syrup
4 tablespoons of chia seeds

1. In a blender, combine all of the ingredients except the chia seeds. Blend until the mix is smooth. At this point, taste for sweetness and add more maple syrup if it is not sweet enough for you.
2. Stir in the chia seeds and then pour into a container.
3. Refrigerate for a couple of hours. Stir a couple of times before the time is up in order to stop the chia from clumping together. When it is ready, it will be the consistency of a thick custard. Serve in any number of ways: see "Play Time".

Play Time!

- Instead of sweetening with maple syrup you can use honey or rice syrup.
- Add other flavours such as vanilla, cinnamon, orange zest, peppermint leaves, pineapple sage or raspberries. Choose one of these flavours rather than adding them all.
- Use other nuts such as almonds or macadamias.
- There are many ways to serve this pudding: 1. in a small glass topped with coconut or fresh fruit. 2. In a tall glass using layers of pudding and banana. 3. As a side to a fruit pie. 4. Use as a filling in a tart but use double the quantity of nuts. 5. Throw a small container into lunch packs for morning tea. 6. A replacement for cream or ice-cream.

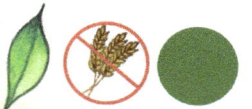

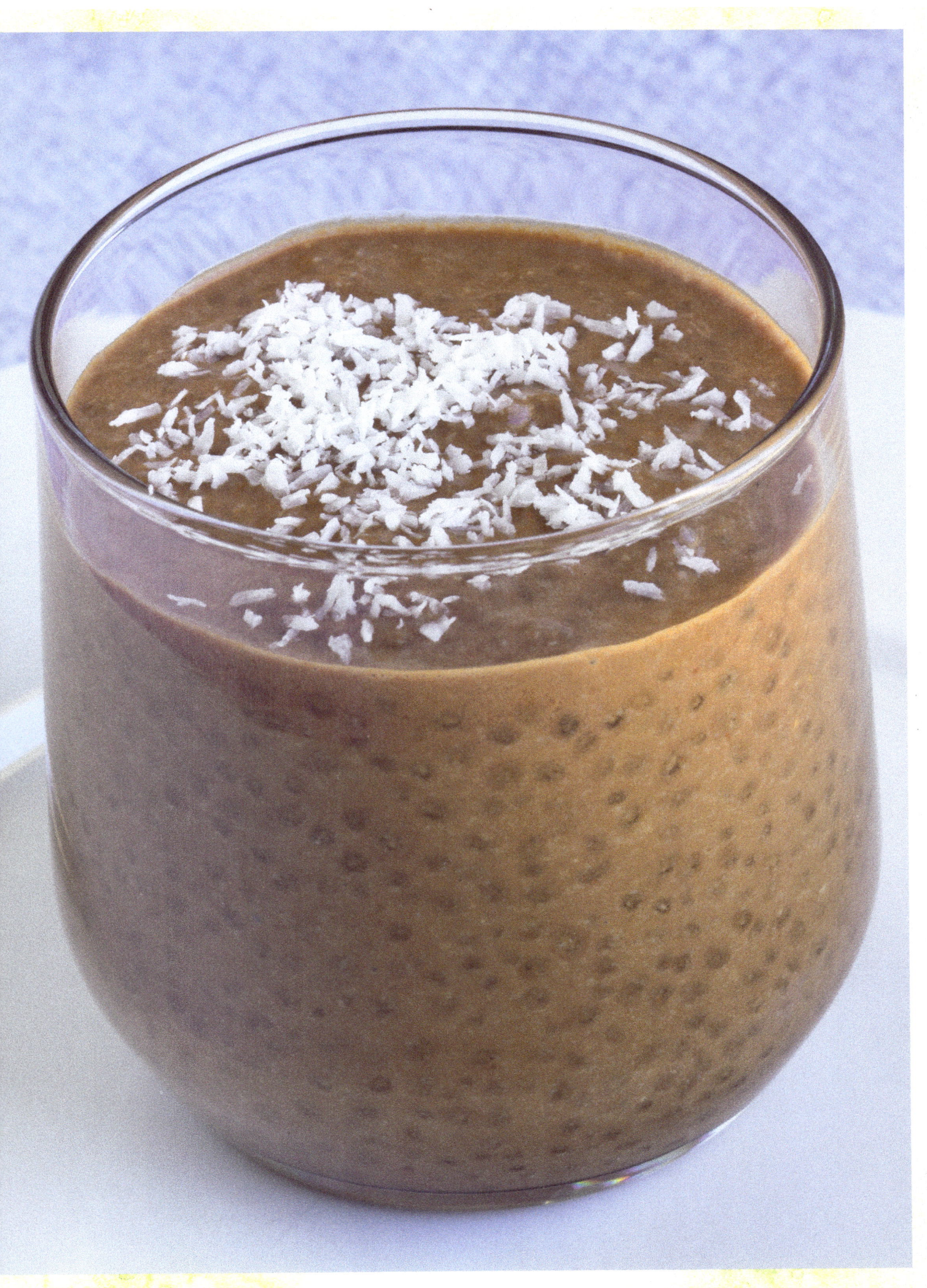

Apple Crumble

Apple crumble is one of the most versatile desserts you can make. There are so many fruits and flavours you can add to the bottom layer and many varieties for the top as well. This is a gluten-free version with vegan options in the playtime.

Serves 4-5

900g apples, peeled and diced

150g almond meal

50g cold butter

2 tablespoons of rapadura or coconut sugar

1 teaspoon of mixed spice

2 tablespoons of maple syrup

1 teaspoon of vanilla extract

1. Preheat the oven to 180°C convection or 160°C fan-forced.
2. Lightly grease a 16cm x 25cm rectangle baking dish.
3. In a large saucepan, place the apples and a couple of tablespoons of water. Cover and steam over medium heat until the apples are tender.
4. Meanwhile, in a mixing bowl, rub the butter into the almond meal until it resembles bread crumbs. I do this in the food processor with the pulse button.
5. Stir in the sugar.
6. Remove apples from heat and add the mixed spice, maple syrup and vanilla extract. Mix well.
7. Pour into the baking dish.
8. Spread crumble evenly over the top of the fruit and place into the preheated oven.
9. Bake for 20-25 minutes.

Play Time!

- For a vegan version, replace the butter with coconut oil.
- Add fresh or frozen berries. They go very well with apple.
- Leave out the mixed spice and add a tablespoon of ground ginger. It goes very well with the apple.
- If you like rolled oats, replace half the almond meal with them.

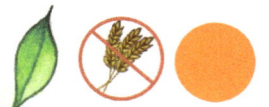

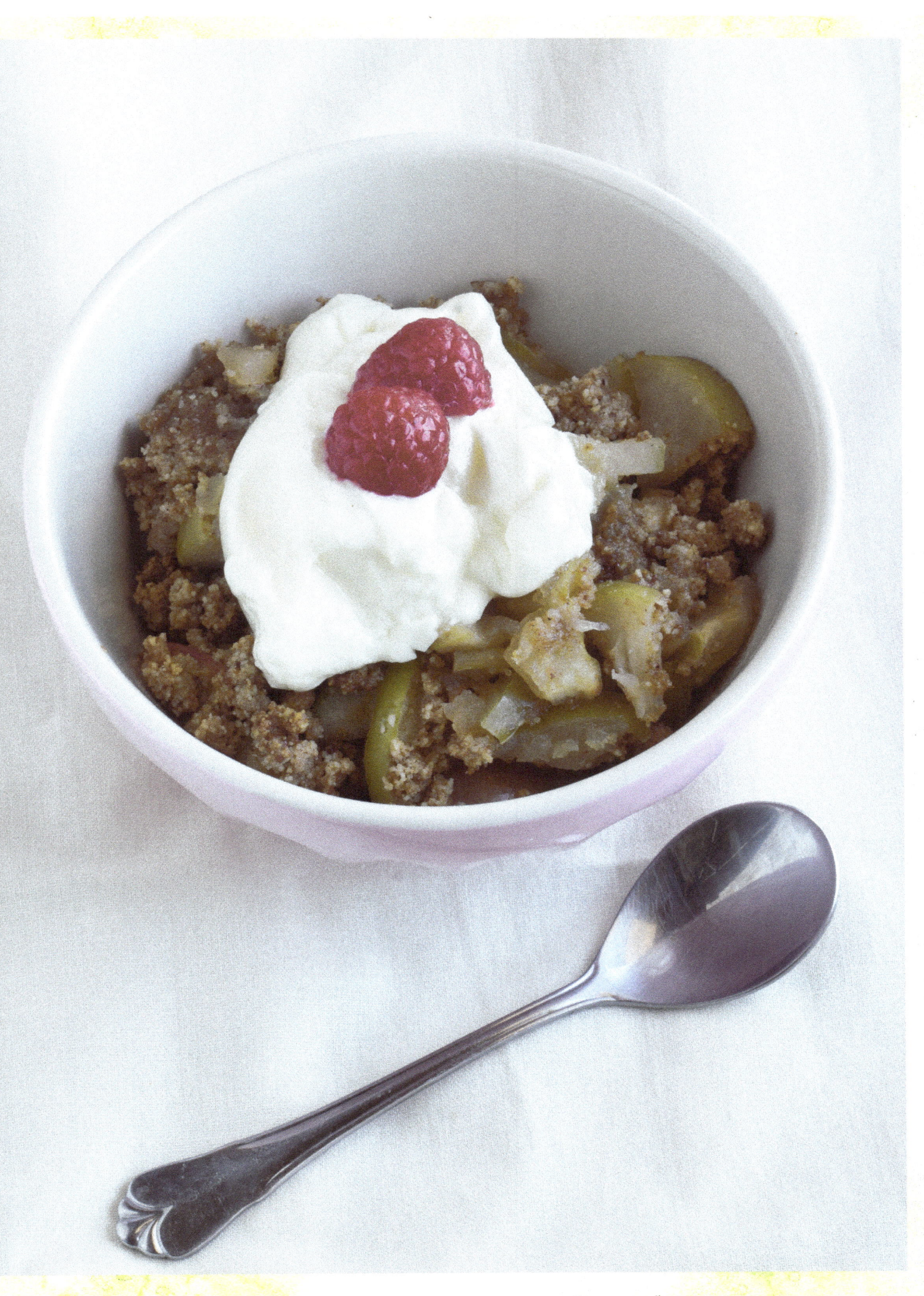

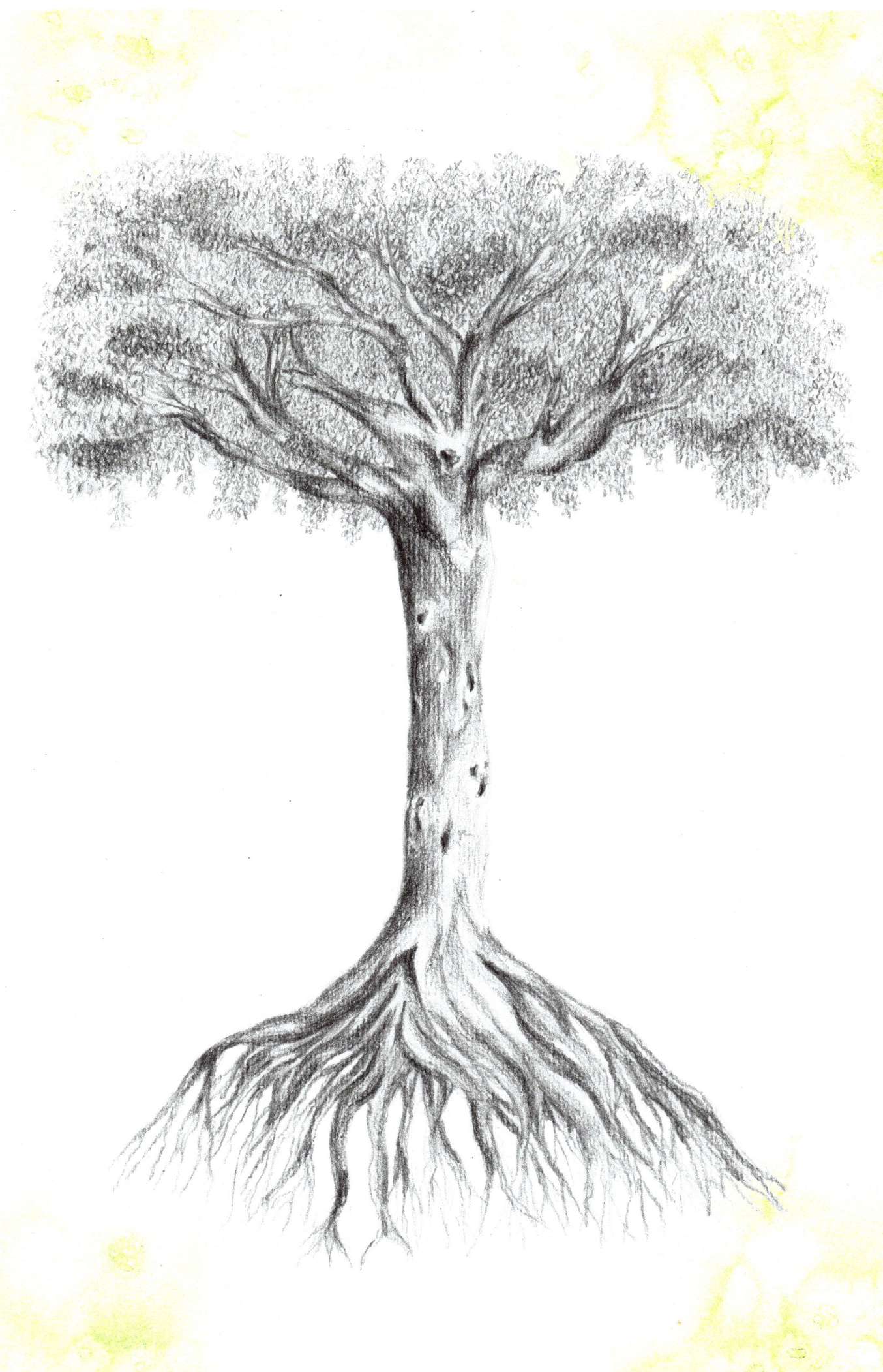

The Roots of Health: Information for Parents

A child who feels good in the morning and has the energy and nutritional requirements needed to get through the day will naturally be happier. Adults of course are the same. Humans feel better, look better and are smarter with good nutrition. Childhood is a time of play and creativity, imagining and discovery. What better gift can you give your child than the space to experience this magic without the setbacks that poor health will inevitably bring.

"We are indeed much more than what we eat, but what we eat can nevertheless help us to be much more than what we are".
~Adele Davis

The Roots of Healthy Eating

If you look at the habits and personal choices of people when it comes to food, common sense will tell you that obesity is NOT genetic. If your mum and dad are obese, it does not mean that you have to end up this way. It will however, take education to move away from your parent's food choices.

There is a group of people who live on an island called Okinawa, off the Japanese mainland. Okinawans live longer than most other people around the world. Their diet is simple and consists of mostly fresh vegetables and whole grains with a little fish. They exercise daily and possess a reverence for the earth and it's cycles. They are slim, agile and radiant with health, well into old age. However recent generations of these people have adopted a more westernised diet, including a lot of fast and convenience foods. As a result, the newer generations are showing higher numbers of obese people. Just as being obese is not genetic, being slim, agile and healthy requires certain dietary and lifestyle choices.

Being Healthy Is Not Just About What We Eat...

More and more people are realising that health is related not just to the state of the body, but also the state of the mind and spirit. It is for this reason that this book deals with more than just recipes. Nourishing foods are a big part of health, but so too is a connection to the earth and a sense of where our food comes from. If we are more aware of the journey our food has made from garden or pasture to table, we are more likely to make wiser choices and feel better for it.

Also a feeling of well being in the kitchen and around meal times will aid healthy digestion. Of course there are many facets of lifestyle and child rearing that affect happiness and therefore health. This book does not deal with them all, but I will do my best to encompass all that is related to food, its preparation and how we consume it.

Inspiring Children's Choices

Feeding your child a healthy diet is more likely to become an adult habit if you provide education along the way. Point out the benefits of one food over the drawbacks of another in terms of how their bodies will be affected. You need to speak in terms that will motivate your child to choose healthy foods. Help the child to understand the causes of different diseases, such as heart disease, cancers, diabetes and many colds that can result from a poor immune system. I used the metaphor of a war and armies to explain the immune system to my boys. They have their own personal armies inside their bodies who protect their health. Certain foods make their armies strong and others weaken the soldiers, allowing enemy bugs to attack: thus resulting in a cold, flu or other bugs. When children understand how their food choices affect them, then they are more likely to rejoice in their healthy diet and be proud of the choices they are able to make themselves.

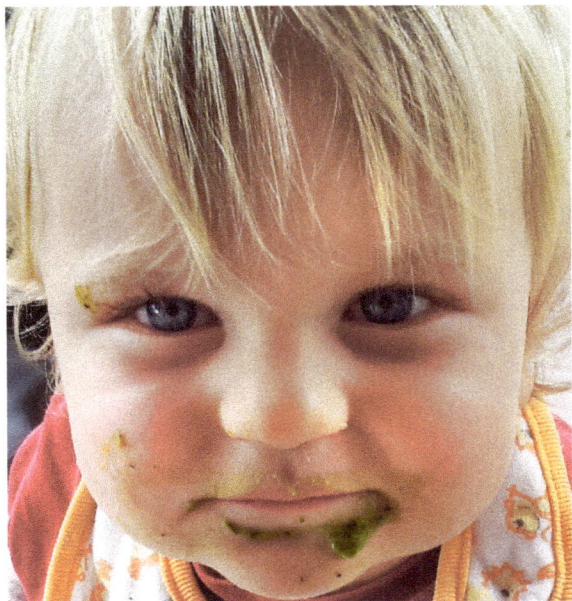
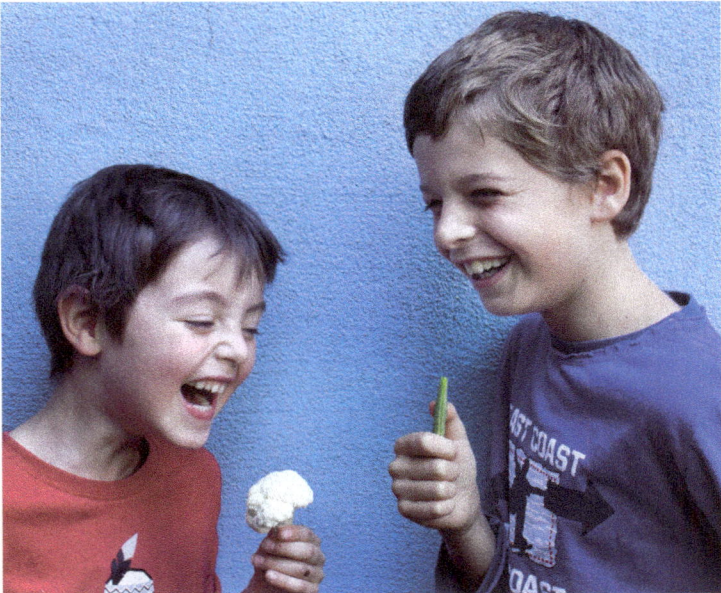

Diversifying Your Child's Palate

Have you ever wondered about the differences in food likes and dislikes culturally? How can a Korean relish the taste of Kim chi, an Australian love Vegemite and an Eskimo sit down to a meal of Walrus or Bearded Seal? I believe it is all about what we are exposed to as children. My kids love lentils, beans, tofu, salad and vegetables, but those foods have been a part of their diet from the time they were babies. Likewise, some children are fed fast food from a young age. These foods are loaded with salt, sugar and fat. It is little wonder that they say no to a healthy salad or stew if offered this choice at a later stage.

As a child grows, their palate adapts to what they have been fed. Children who are given very sugary foods over a period of time will need more sugar in order to taste the sweetness in foods. Something naturally sweetened with honey or maple syrup may not taste sweet enough. In this way, it is more challenging to change the eating habits of a child raised on nutritionally redundant foods such as white flour products and sugary sweets. However, it is not impossible. In fact it is never too late, even when we are adults, and it is worth the change. See page 26 for instructions on how to train stubborn taste buds. Once your palate is re-educated, junk foods that were desirable in the past, no longer taste so good.

Here is a finding released by an Australian research team from the Baker IDI Heart and Diabetes Institute in Melbourne:

" genes remember a sugar hit for two weeks. What's more, continued poor eating habits can permanently alter your DNA and potentially pass the genetic damage onto your descendants."

These results give truth to the popular phrase "You are what you eat." You may not feel the effects of bad diet right away, but unless you change your eating habits, with time various health problems such as diabetes, heart disease and others will develop. Even if you don't have a disease, ask yourself how you feel on a daily basis. Are you full of energy? Is it easy to get up in the morning? Is your sleep restful? Does your body feel good? Is it easy to go to the toilet and do you go every day? If you answered no to any of these questions, then you are not living to your health potential. If you don't want to pass along potentially unhealthy genes to your children and grandchildren, then a healthy diet is of great importance.

So give your family's palates the opportunity to relearn. Did you know that if you eat enough of a food that you dislike, you will end up developing a taste for it? My son didn't like broccoli as a toddler. So every time we had broccoli I put a very small piece on his plate which he was obliged to eat. I wasn't force feeding him broccoli, merely asking him to try it over and over. I counted and it took twenty tries for him to start enjoying it. Now he asks for seconds.

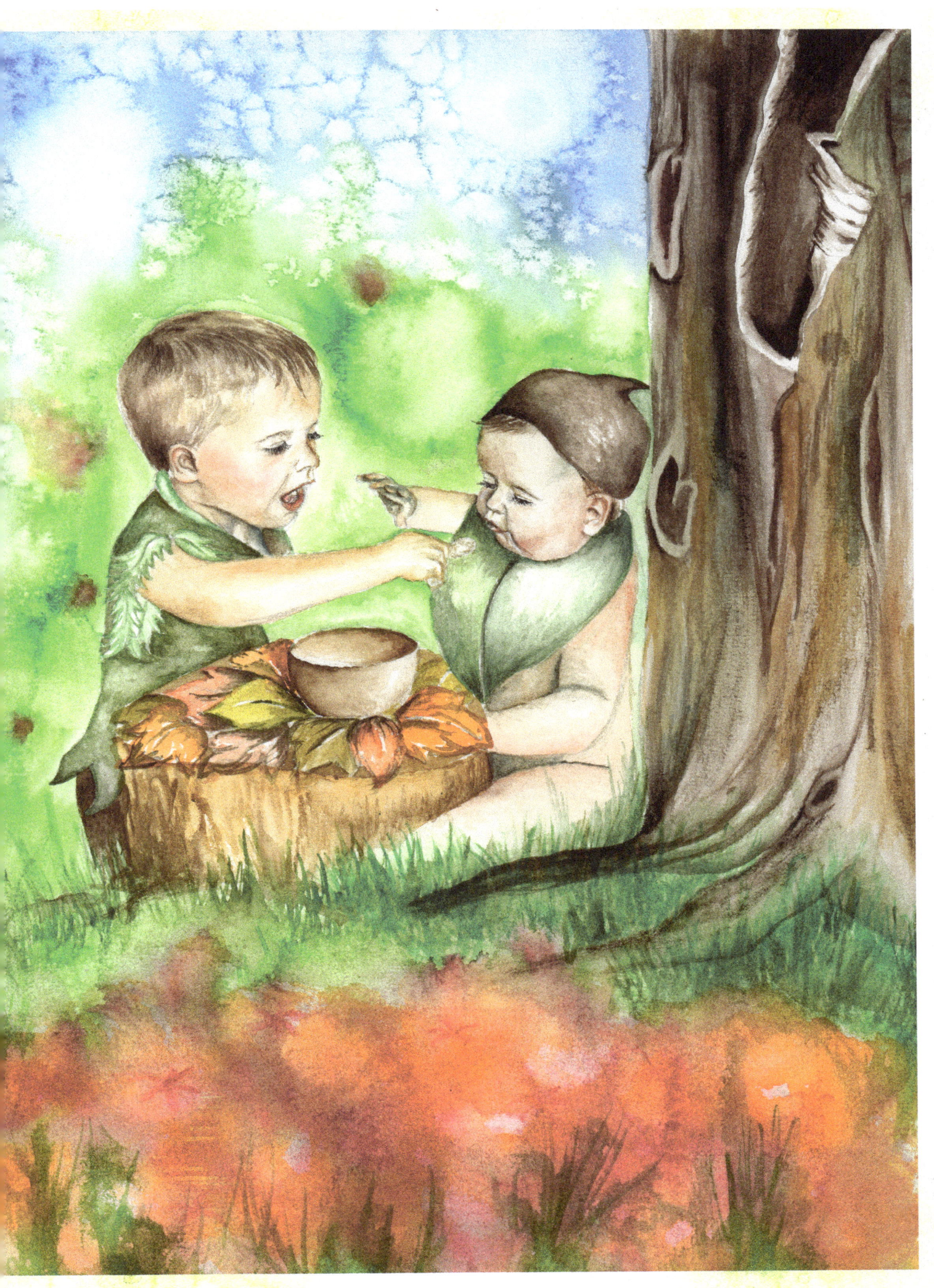

The Roots of Health

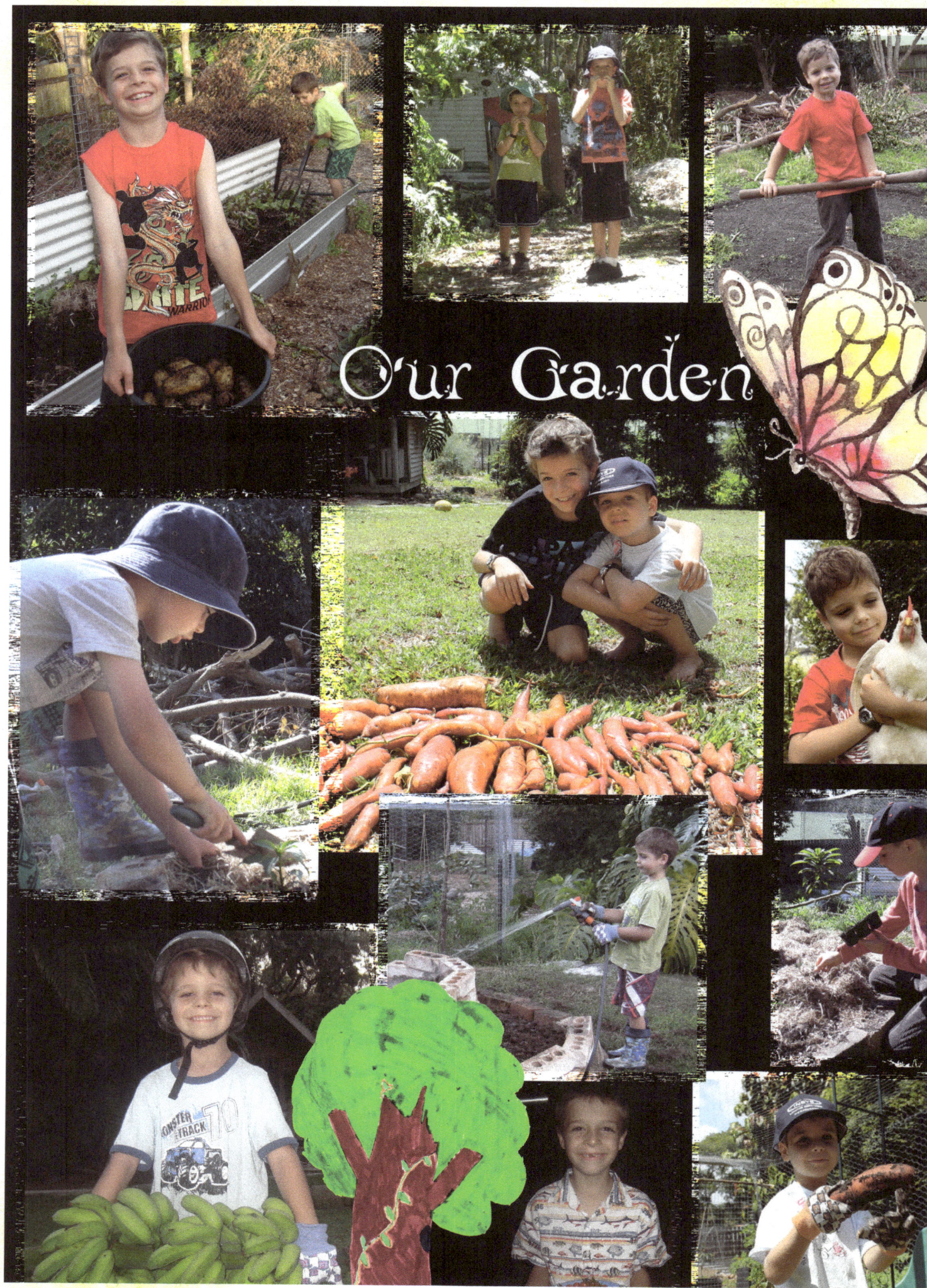

Where Does Food Come From?

We don't all have the inclination to become back yard gardeners, but as time moves on, it seems urban agriculture is the answer. With the majority of produce on the market being loaded with pesticides and deficient in nutrients, the importance of either finding an organic farmer's market or growing our own food, (even just a few vegetables) is significant. There is an abundant supply of resources on how to grow your own foods for those with only a patio and pots to those with sizeable yards. I will not cover that subject in this book, but we have found the benefits of our garden to be invaluable to our family.

I never really had an interest in gardening before I had children, however as I became more educated about healthy eating, I wanted our family to eat organic foods. As well as shopping at organic farmers markets, I saw that there would be benefit in growing a few of our own vegetables. The more I learned and tasted from our small garden, the more I loved the satisfaction of picking fresh foods and taking them straight to the kitchen. We soon created our own large garden, growing a variety of foods, and with my continuing education, I have involved my boys as much as I could in the gardening process.

Allowing children to get their hands into the earth and witness the growth cycle of seeds to shoots and then plants to vegetables is not only fascinating to them, but educational as well. They receive this learning directly from the garden and are more likely to eat foods that they, themselves, have had a hand in creating. Children, by nature are infinitely creative and this creativity does not have to be limited to pencil and paper. Allow them to be involved in designing your garden, choosing what to grow and nurturing the plants. There are few things more satisfying than looking out your window to see children eating cucumbers and tomatoes direct from the vine.

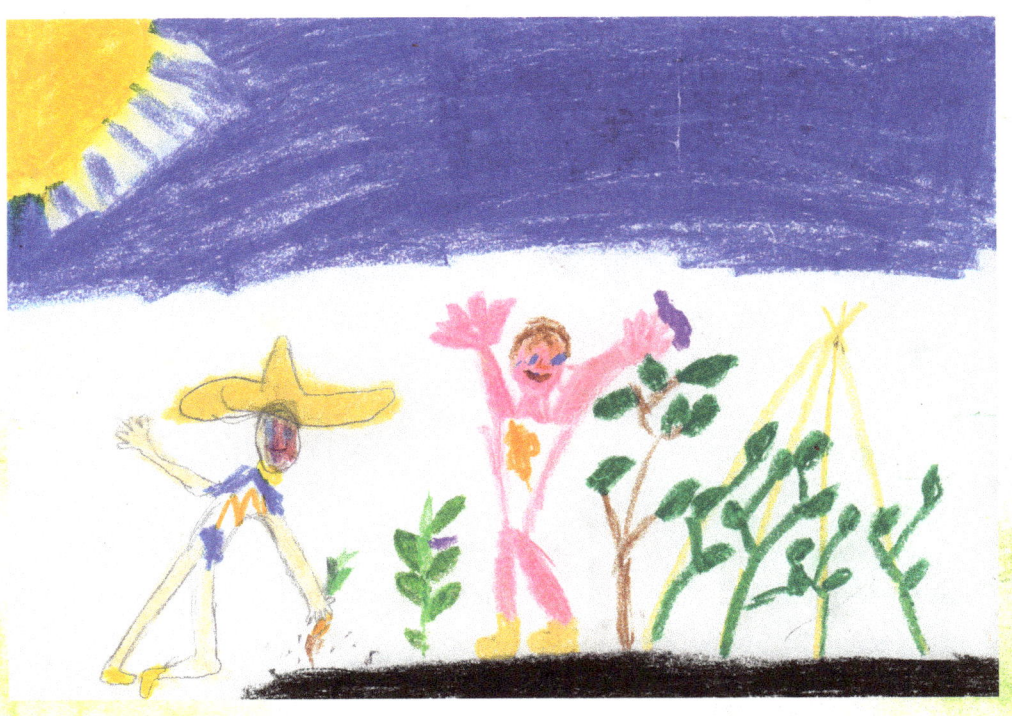

Healthy Children are Happy Children

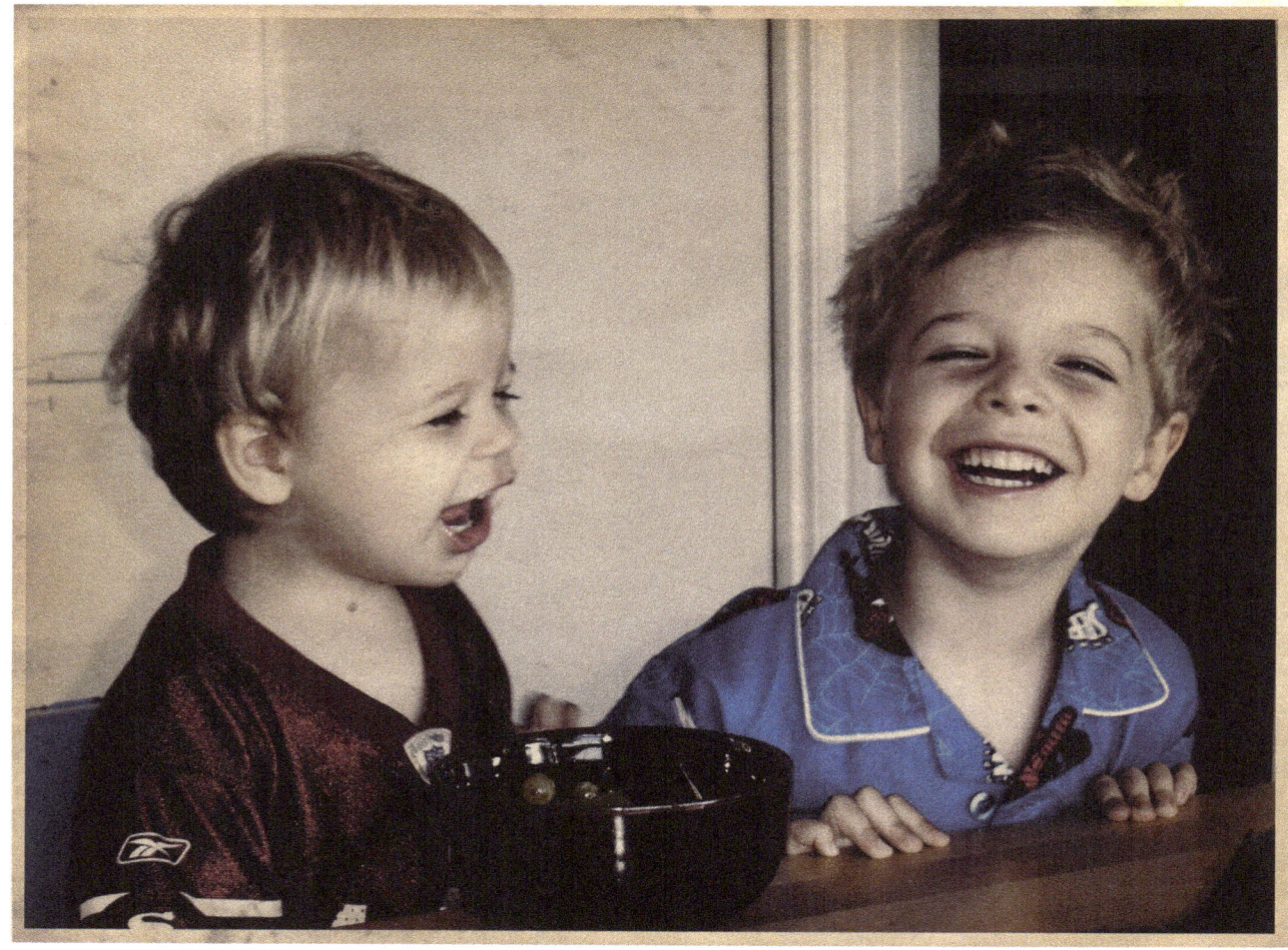

For many people, getting up in the morning is hard. Going to sleep at night can also be difficult. Even getting through the day without an ache or pain can be a challenge and getting through the winter without a flu or cold is not possible. It doesn't have to be this way.

Our bodies require an endless supply of nutrients in the form of vitamins, minerals, amino acids, antioxidants, complex carbohydrates, proteins and natural sugars. When your diet is depleted of these nutrients (and it is inevitable if you live on a diet made up of processed foods), the body will not function as it should. You will feel depleted. The immune system will be weak, energy levels low and moods up and down. Children's behaviour on a poor diet can manifest in a variety of ways, from lack of concentration to tantrums, mood swings and of course the endless snotty nose. So the question is, how can a person be truly happy in this state? I don't think they can.

It doesn't have to be about counting your nutrients either. For the majority of people, eating a well balanced diet of unprocessed foods, free from chemicals and including raw foods daily will meet your average requirements. You may choose to supplement during times of stress or winter to help the body's natural defences, but the majority of our nutrition is best taken in the form of food.

Dealing with Fussy Eaters

Of course every child is different and the reasons for a child's fussiness are not always the same. However, assuming your child is not sick, suffering from allergies or experiencing digestive problems, the main reason children seem to be fussy is for control purposes. Who has the strongest will? If you force feed a child when they are not hungry then it becomes a battle usually ending in an upset, which is not good for digestion. This then becomes a power play in future leading to a competition for power.

So my approach has always had two steps. First put the groundwork in by educating your child. (Use the first few points listed below). Next give a choice, but make that choice limited as in, "eat your dinner or go hungry" and don't back down. This may be considered a little old fashioned, but my children both enjoy their vegetables now, even greens and they are not a nightmare to take out because as long as there are vegetarian options, they are happy!

So here are the methods I have used. Some may take more willpower on your part than your child's (especially when you look at a beautiful little face, pleading for ice-cream in place of vegetables):

- Involve your child in growing and/or preparing the foods that you eat. Having a hand in the creation of a meal will often nudge a hesitant child towards at least trying foods they would otherwise refuse.
- Educate your child about nutrition. Why it is important that they eat healthy foods and what those foods are. Show them the results of eating junk foods (examples of this are everywhere in disease and obesity).
- Present foods that are pleasing to look at and give the meals enticing names. I have learned never to call a stew, "Stew". Much more imagination is needed.
- Help children to understand the work and love that goes into preparing the food so that they develop a respect and appreciation for what is given to them.
- Do not make special meals for fussy eaters. Adopt the rule that if they do not want to eat what is presented to them, they go without. (I do this unless a family member has a very strong dislike to one particular food that I know is genuine and not part of a control game).
- When it comes to new foods, adopt the rule, "you don't have to eat it all, but you are obliged to try it, every time...."
- When the fussiness gets extreme, as in my younger son Ryan refusing all vegetables at age 3, serve vegetables for every meal. Of course heat them and present them well as you usually would. At the heart of this situation it was easy to see the game of "who is in control". I did not make him eat the vegetables, I gave him a limited choice; eat or go hungry. The first time this happened he skipped dinner, but by breakfast was hungry enough to eat. The problem resurfaces every so often, but now all I need to do is remind him of the consequence and he changes his mind. Once the refusal is forgotten it is obvious that he actually enjoys vegetables, which is just another indicator that it is all a game!

Always Something Good to Eat

Short on time but don't want to resort to packets? Dread that morning rush when you need to get the kids out the door, but also want to put something nutritious into their lunch boxes? I now introduce you to "The Goodies Box", named by my son Ryan.

Whenever I get the chance (i.e. a couple of hours on the weekend or an hour here and there where I feel inspired to cook), I do some baking, cooking or raw food making. Whatever I make goes into a big plastic container and put straight into the freezer. This box can contain any number of different options for morning and/or afternoon tea, as most of the recipes in this book, (except salads) will freeze. Below is a list of foods that I put into the goodies box and other foods I freeze into portions for that quick grab in the morning. Many of these portions are good for lunch with a little salad or even on their own. The morning teas always consist of an item from the goodies box and a piece of fruit:

Goodies Box	Small Portions
Muffins	Dips
Muesli bars	Quiches
Bliss balls	Soups for the thermos
Raw brownies	Risotto patties
Biscuits	Lentil and other bean burgers (to go with a little salad)
Scones	Dahl and rice for the thermos

Never miss a chance to add to your stores, whether it is cooking dinner, an afternoon tea, or lunch on the weekend. You can always make double or even triple without it taking up much more time and it will save you resorting to processed foods. In this time-poor society it can be tricky to stay on top of family nutrition, but with a little organisation you will find that you feel better and your children will be happier!

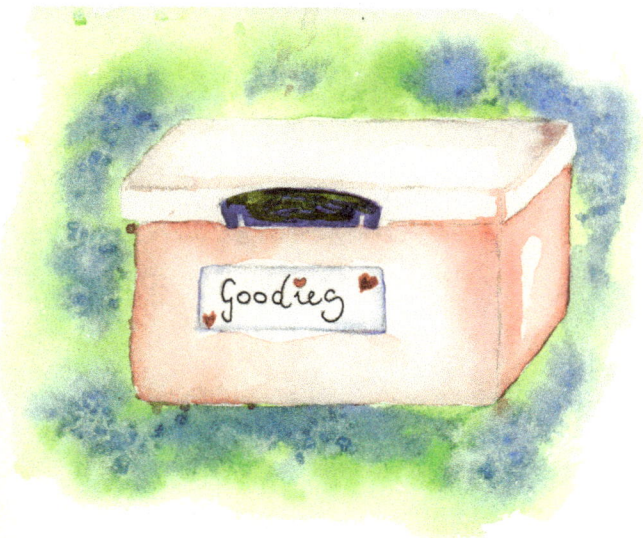

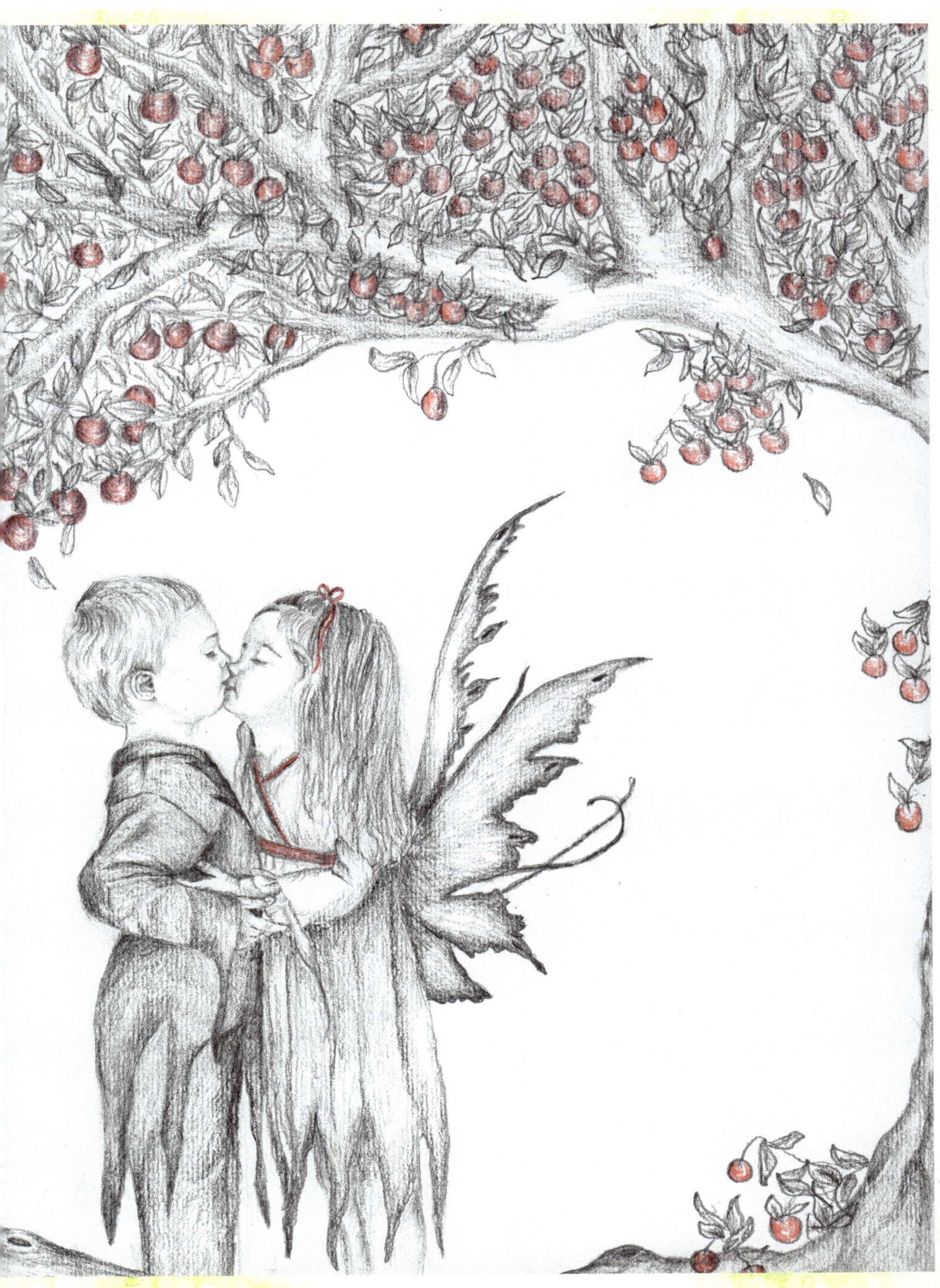

The Roots of Health

Kids in the Kitchen; Dinner Nights

It is important to me that by the time our boys leave home, they actually know their way around the kitchen, and are able to cook a variety of meals. They have always spent plenty of time in and around the kitchen but I wanted them to have a proper culinary education. Our solution has been to schedule dinner nights. They each choose a night during the week on which they are responsible for dinner. This responsibility includes:

- Choosing the meal and it has to be something different each time. (Usually a dessert is involved as well).
- Preparing the meal as much as possible on their own. (Their input increases with skill and age and I am always in the kitchen with them to make sure no fingers are severed).
- Setting the table and of course choosing where everyone sits (control, control and more control). We usually have about 10 candles lit and all the lights off so we eat in shadows.
- Dishing the meal out.

It is funny because sometimes they don't feel like following through with the commitment, but as soon as they start cooking they ALWAYS enjoy it. They are so proud of what they achieve thus it is a great way to build self-esteem and encourages them to try new things.

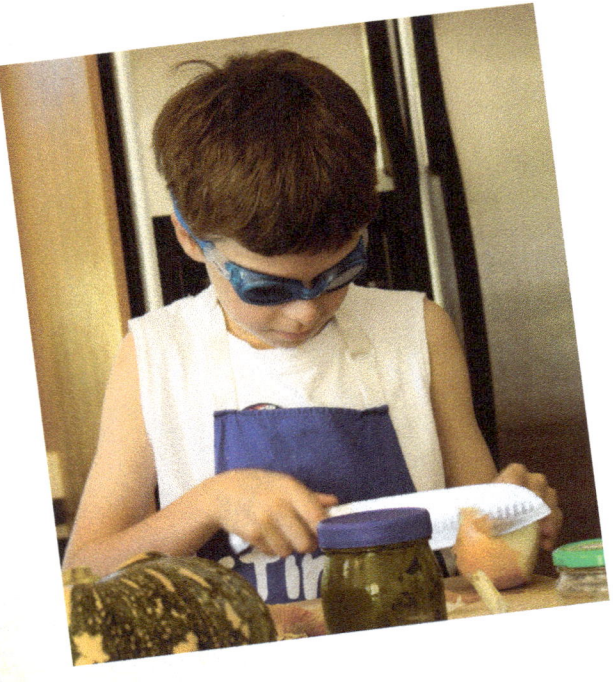

Trouble with cutting onions? Ethan uses goggles to deal with the problem.

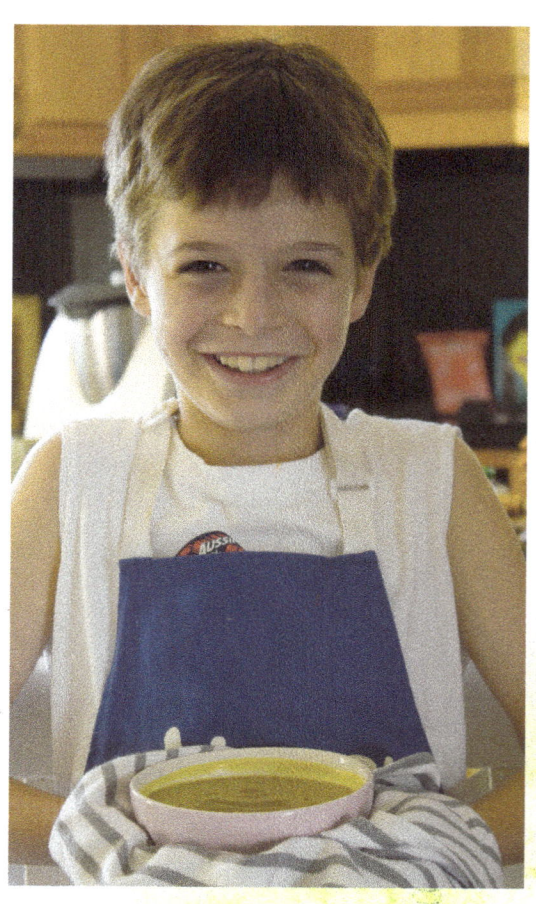

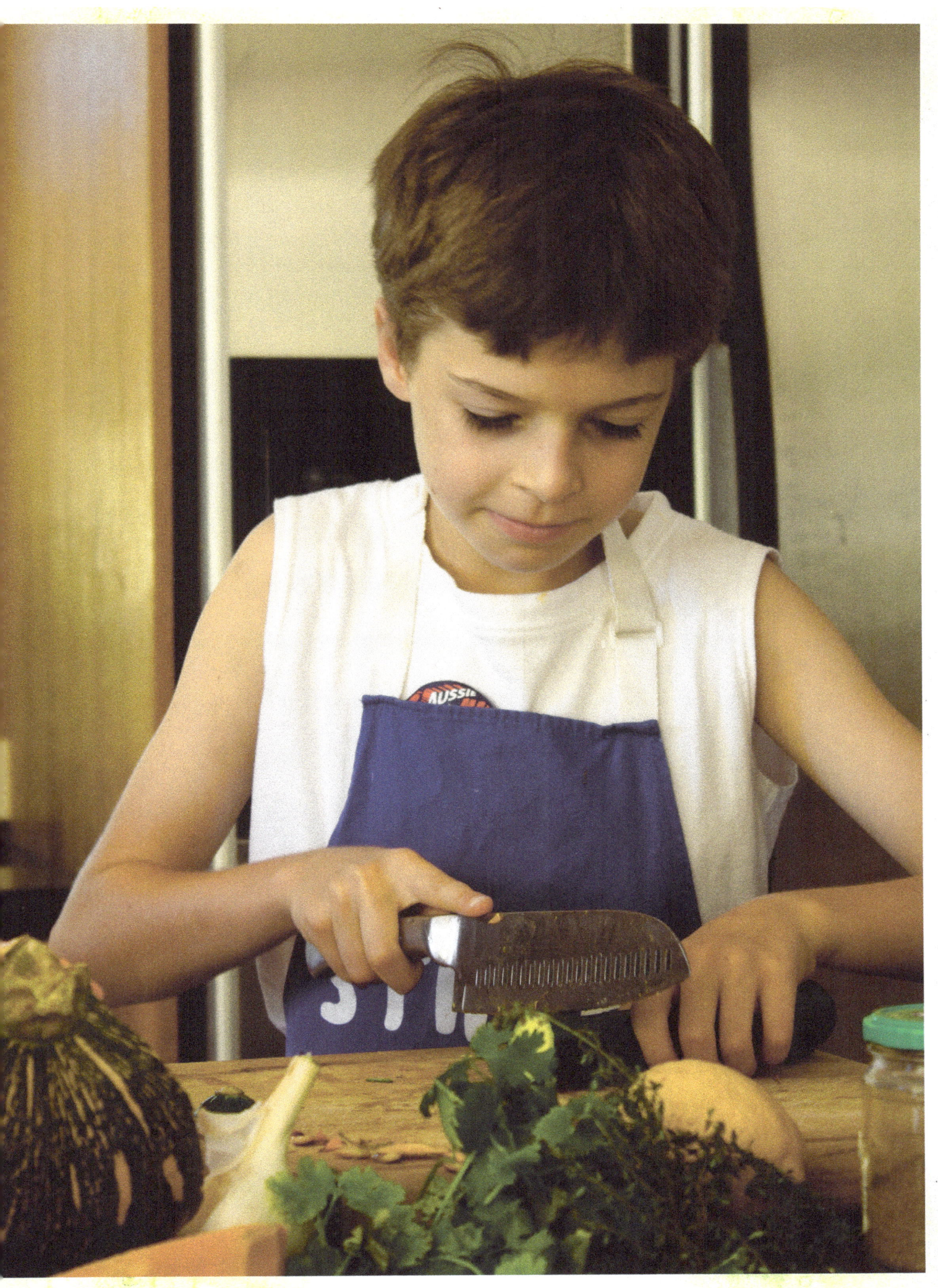

The Roots of Health

Glossary

Agave Syrup

A sweet syrup derived from the blue agave cactus that thrives in the volcanic soils of Southern Mexico. It was a food favoured by the Aztecs. It has the consistency of maple syrup and is one and a half times sweeter than sugar. Agave syrup is 80-90% fructose. Some say this makes it more healthy whilst others say it makes it less healthy. The jury is still out on this one. Like any sweetener, use in moderation.

Agave syrup is available from health food shops and some bulk food suppliers.

Arborio Rice

A short grain white rice used in risotto recipes. It undergoes less milling than other white rices and so has a higher content of starch. This starch is released as the rice is cooked, giving risotto its creamy consistency. Stirring the rice increases this release, thus the need to stir risotto constantly.

Arborio rice is available in supermarkets.

Arrowroot (Ground)

The ground powder made from the arrowroot plant. It is a starch thickener used in cooking. It will give sauces a glossy sheen and has advantages over corn flour. It will not lose its potency in an acidic liquid, it thickens at a lower temperature and has a more neutral taste. The downside is it does cost more.

Ground arrowroot is available from Asian supermarkets in larger quantities and regular supermarkets in small quantities.

Basmati Rice

Indian/Pakistani rice which is low GI and has a distinct flavour and scent. In fact, the Hindi translation of the word "basmati" is "queen of scents". It is not sticky at all and when cooked correctly, has separate, fluffy grains. It is considered the most gourmet of all the rices and is therefore, higher in price.

Basmati rice is available in supermarkets and Indian/Asian grocery stores.

Blackstrap Molasses

Molasses is an extremely mineral rich by-product of turning sugarcane into table sugar. There are three grades of molasses - sulphured, unsulphured and blackstrap. Sulphur is a chemical used to ripen sugarcane and is not good for us. Blackstrap molasses is produced from sun-ripened sugarcane and it has the highest nutrient content. It is very strong in flavour and does not cause an increase in blood sugar the way regular sugar does. It is used as a sweetener, but also has a very distinct flavour so needs to be used with some thought.

Blackstrap molasses is available in supermarkets and health food shops.

Cacao Powder
See Raw Cacao Powder.

Cacao Butter
See Raw Cacao Butter.

Coconut Oil
The benefits of this product are so numerous it is good to do some of your own research. Coconut oil is 90% raw unsaturated fat. This is different to animal derived saturated fat in that it is an important building block for every cell in the human body.
When purchasing coconut oil, make sure it is cold pressed extra virgin.
Cold pressed, extra virgin coconut oil is available from health food shops and some supermarkets.

Coconut Sugar
Made by collecting the sap from coconut blossoms and then boiling it until it reduces down to solids. It has been used in Asia for a long time, but is only just becoming popular in the west as it is a healthier alternative to table sugar and contains more minerals than most other sweeteners. It is also low GI and is reported to be the most sustainable sweetener in the world. The coconut palms this sugar is extracted from grow in diverse, wild-life supportive ecosystems, they are fast growing and require little water. They also produce a lot more sugar per hectare than sugarcane. More than one reason to make the switch!
Coconut sugar is available in health food shops, online and from some bulk food suppliers at the time of writing this book. It is only a matter of time before this product will be available in supermarkets.

Coconut Flour
A flour made from dried coconut meat. After it is dried, the fat is removed and the remaining coconut is ground into a fine meal, resembling wheat flour in appearance. Coconut flour is very absorbent, so it needs a much higher ratio of liquid to flour in recipes. Most cakes and biscuits made with coconut flour contain mainly eggs and liquid with a small amount of flour.
Coconut flour is available in health food shops, online and from some bulk food suppliers at the time of writing this book. It is only a matter of time before this product will be available in supermarkets.

Flaxseeds
See Linseeds.

Fruit spread
Fruit spreads are bottled and presented as jam, but have no table sugar added. They are made up of a puree of fruit, fruit pectin and usually a fruit sweetener such as grape juice.
Fruit spreads are available in the jam section of supermarkets or in health food shops.

Garam Masala

An Indian spice mix for which there is no set recipe, but which will usually include coriander, cumin, cardamom, cloves, black pepper, cinnamon and nutmeg. There are many different variations of Garam Masala as people adjust it to their own tastes.

Garam Masala is available in the spice section at the supermarket or Indian/Asian grocery stores. You could also try making your own if you have a coffee grinder or Thermomix.

Ghee

An ingredient used in Indian cooking, ghee is clarified butter. This is the butter oil without the lactose and other milk solids. Because the latter have been removed, ghee is not prone to spoilage and so does not need refrigeration. It has a unique flavour and is prized in Ayurvedic medicine.

Ghee is available in the international cooking section of supermarkets or Indian grocery stores.

Ground Arrowroot

See Arrowroot.

Linseeds

Also known as flaxseeds, linseeds are small brown seeds, very high in omega 3 and 6 fatty acids. They also contain significant amounts of calcium, magnesium, potassium and phosphorous. They may be eaten as they are, however the digestive system will not break the seed down and they will pass through as fibre. A more beneficial way to eat them is ground. They need to be either ground fresh or ground and then refrigerated so that the oils in them do not go rancid. Flaxseed oil is also prized as a valuable nutritional supplement due to the omega oil content. It also needs to be refrigerated.

Linseeds are available in supermarkets and health food shops.

Maple Syrup

A dark brown, viscous liquid made from the sap of maple trees. The sap, when first extracted is not very sweet, but after it has been boiled down to remove some of the water content, it becomes a thick sweet syrup. Maple syrup is high in manganese and is also a good source of zinc.

Maple syrup is available in supermarkets and health food shops.

Miso

Miso is an ingredient used in Japanese cooking. Soy beans and sometimes a grain are combined with salt and a beneficial mould culture. They are left to ferment, producing a paste that is used to season foods, particularly soups. Most misos available in supermarkets are pasteurised, meaning that the benefits of fermentation have been removed. It is possible to buy unpasteurised miso in some health food shops, or you can learn to make it yourself. Fermented foods are very good for the gut and therefore the immune system.

Pasteurised miso is available in supermarkets and unpasteurised miso is available in some health food stores.

Nigella Seeds

These are small black seeds from the Nigella plant, used in Indian and Middle Eastern cooking. They are often sprinkled on top of Turkish and naan breads. They are also known as black onion seeds or black cumin seeds and are thought to aid digestion.

Nigella seeds are available in Indian/Asian grocery stores and some supermarkets.

Pappadums

These are thin crackers (or flatbreads) made from gram flour, salt and water. Gram flour is made from ground lentils, which means pappadums are gluten free. They are cooked in hot oil to become a light, crispy chip and are served with accompaniments such as chutneys and mint sauce. We like to eat them with Dahl.

Pappadums are available in supermarkets and Indian grocery stores.

Quinoa

Quinoa is often mistaken for a grain. It is actually an ancient seed grown in the Andes, which was eaten by the Incas and has been known for it's superfood characteristics in that area for millennia. It is very high in protein, folate, magnesium, phosphorous, iron, copper, and manganese. Oh and it is gluten free! Each grain is small and round and when cooked, fluffs up like rice. It may be used as a substitute for rice or added to burgers, soups, stews, cakes, muffins and bread. It may be ground down to produce a gluten free flour as well. It is pretty hard to top!

Quinoa is available from supermarkets and health food shops.

Quorn Mince

"Quorn" is a trademark name for a vegetarian mycro-protein made from a fungus (Fusarium venenatum) with small amounts of egg white added. It comes in a variety of styles and flavours. For the purposes of this book, I have included it in only one recipe; "Not Sausage Rolls With a Twist" page 116. I did this because I prefer to use it over TVP which is often genetically modified. Quorn products are not genetically modified.

Quorn products are available in the frozen section at supermarkets.

Rapadura Sugar

An unrefined sugar that still contains the molasses and therefore mineral content from the sugarcane. Unlike white sugar, the making of rapadura involves squeezing the juice from the sugarcane, drying it and then grounding it finely. White sugar is produced by separating the sucrose from the molasses and mixing it with a host of chemicals (sulphur dioxide, lime, phosphoric acid, bleaching agents & viscosity reducers). White sugar looks better, pours better and stores for longer. Not so good for the insides though...Rapadura has a unique caramel flavour, fine grain and is a golden brown colour. Using rapadura sugar is a way of enjoying the benefits of blackstrap molasses without the overpowering taste that would come with using it in larger quantities.

Rapadura sugar is available from health food shops, online and some bulk food suppliers.

Raw Cacao Powder

Where do I start with this amazing superfood? Everyone knows what chocolate tastes like, but if you use the raw cacao powder in raw recipes you will reap the many rewards of the cacao bean. Of all the foods known to man, it is highest in antioxidants and vitamin C. It is also high in magnesium, chromium, iron, zinc, copper and manganese. According to David Wolfe, expert in superfoods, to eat raw cacao is to take a mineral supplement because the levels of the various minerals are so high in this one food. It also contains bliss chemicals; phenylethylamine (PEA – released when we fall in love), and anandamide. Remember most of this goodness is destroyed with high heat so consume raw or just warmed.

Raw cacao powder is available from health food shops and online.

Raw Cacao Butter

A pure vegetable fat extracted from the cocoa bean. It is high in antioxidants, including polyphenols, catechins and epicatechins that help to fight off free radicals. Flavonols in cacao butter also help the body produce Nitric Oxide, a compound essential for proper heart function. Cacao butter is solid at room temperature but will melt on a hot day. It can be used in raw chocolate recipes, homemade natural sweets, to set pie fillings and even as a skin moisturiser. Like the cacao powder it will lose its benefits if submitted to high temperatures.

Raw cacao butter is available from health food shops and online.

Rice Mirin

A Japanese condiment used in cooking. It is similar to a rice wine but with a much lower alcohol content.

Rice mirin is available in supermarkets and Asian grocery stores.

Rice Syrup

A sweetener made by culturing rice with enzymes to break down the starches. It is then cooked down to a syrup. It is not particularly high in nutrients, but is a lot better for you than white sugar. People who are gluten intolerant should check the label to make sure the product is gluten free. Sometimes the cultures for the syrup are grown using other grains.

Rice syrup is available from supermarkets and health food shops.

Sea Salt

Sea salt is not refined like table salt. It still contains high amounts of natural iodine, magnesium and trace minerals, essential for many functions in the body. Table salt is bleached and also contains additives such as aluminium compounds to keep it dry. In fact if you would like to know whether you have a salt that is good for you, leave a small amount out in the open overnight. If its texture is exactly the same the next day, the bin is the best place for it. Salt is not bad for you in moderation, in fact the body needs salt every day for many biological processes. It is "necessary for maintaining proper water balance and blood pH. It is also needed for stomach, nerve and muscle

function".[1] Make your salt count. Use a brand that is sourced naturally. I particularly recommend Celtic Sea Salt, a superior source of trace minerals.
Sea salt is available from supermarkets and health food shops.

Tahini
A paste made from ground sesame seeds. It comes in both hulled and unhulled versions. Hulled tahini has had the outside of the seed removed before grinding, making it lower in nutrition. However it is less bitter than unhulled tahini. Both pastes contain calcium, B vitamins, biotin, and choline. Tahini is also a source of vitamin A and is 20 percent complete protein.
Tahini is available from supermarkets and health food shops.

Tamari Sauce
Like Soy Sauce, Tamari sauce is made from fermented soy beans. The difference is in its richer, deeper flavour, lower salt content and the fact that it is gluten free.
Tamari Sauce is available from supermarkets and health food shops.

Textured Vegetable Protein (TVP)
A vegetarian protein made from soy flour. The soy bean oil is removed, the flour then pressure cooked and dried. On its own it is a good source of protein, however some of the TVP available has been enhanced with additives such as MSG, table salt, flavours and colours, so be careful what you buy. The other thing to look out for is genetically modified (GM) soy products. Most soy is now GM and so it is best to buy organic if you can find it. Organic products are not GM. TVP needs to be re-hydrated with boiling water before using.
TVP is available from supermarkets and health food shops.

Wild Rice
A different type of rice, as it is actually the seed of a grass plant. Its' grains are long, dark and chewy in texture and they have a nutty flavour. Wild rice is usually used sparingly with other rices, as it is very expensive and is mostly used only to complement other flavours.
Wild rice is available from supermarkets and health food shops.

---

1   Prescription for Nutritional Healing, Balch, Phillis A.

Bibliography

Books

Vitamins and Minerals; How to get the nutrients your body needs
Rose, Sara
Octopus Publishing Group, 2003

Guide to Nutritional Healing
Balch, Phyllis A.
Avery Books, 2000

Nourishing Traditions, revised second edition
Fallon, Sally
New Trends Publishing Inc. 2001

Sweet Poison; Why Sugar is Making You Fat
Gillespie, David
Penguin books, 2008

Principles of Anatomy and Physiology, 11th Edition
Tortora, Gerard J. & Derrickson, Bryan
John Wiley and Sons Inc.

The Okinawa Way; How to Improve Your Health and Longevity Dramatically
Wilcox, Bradley, Willcox, Craig D, Makoto Suzuki
Michael Joseph, 2001

Websites

www.truthinlabelling.org (information on food additives)
www.sbs.com.au (information for regional flavours)
www.foodmatters.tv
http://www.ricegourmet.com
http://www.pioneerthinking.com/beauty/skin/cellulite/lp-fatdetox.html
http://www.foodauthority.nsw.gov.au/consumers/other-food-topics/fats-and-trans-fats
http://www.bakeridi.edu.au/

Suggested Reading List

Sweet Poison: Why Sugar is Making You Fat
Gillespie, David
Penguin books, 2008

Excitotoxins: the taste that kills
Blaylock, Russell L.
Health Press, 1996

The pH miracle : balance your diet, reclaim your health
Young, Robert and Shelley
Piatkus, 2002

Superfoods: The Food and Medicine of the Future
Wolfe, David
North Atlantic Books, 2009

How Can I Use Herbs In My Daily Life, 5th Edition
Shipard, Isabell
Isabell Shipard, 2003

Skinny Bitch
Freedman, Rory and Barnouin, Kim
Griffin Press, 2007

Disease-Proof Your Child: Feeding Kids Right
Fuhrman, Joel, M.D
St Martin's Press, 2005

Diet For a New America
Robbins, John
H.J. Kramer Inc. 1987

Chook Book
French, Jackie
Manna Press 2005

Index

About the Author III
Agave Syrup, Glossary 284
Aladdin's Salad 148
All About Flour 46
Almonds
  Almondy Hummus 101
  Apricot and Almond Balls 223
  Almond and Cashew Balls 221
  Cranberry and Vanilla Cake Bars 239
Alternative Ingredients 46
Ambience in the Kitchen 38
Apple
  Blueberry and Apple Muffins 250
  Cranberry and Apple Balls 224
  Apple Crumble 268
  Honey and Apple Cake 240
Apricot and Almond Balls 223
Arborio Rice, Glossary 284
Arrowroot (Ground), Glossary 284
Asian Noodle Salad 160
Awesome Adzuki Curry 204

Baba Ganoush 94
Baby Bear Hummus 100
Baked Beans, Better 196
Baking
  A Great Tip 214
  Cake Tin Sizes 214
  Oven Settings 214
Banana
  Banana and Berry fluff 260
  Chocolate Banana Cream 260
  Green Smoothie 88
  Powerful Banana Smoothie 87
  Saucy Banana Pudding 262
Basmati Rice, Glossary 284
Beans
  Awesome Adzuki Curry 204
  Better Baked Beans 196
  Greek Beanies 120
Beans, Garlicky 130
Beautiful Bolognaise 192
Beautiful Brassicas 136
Beetroot
  Beetroot and Tomato Soup 176
  Heart's Desire Crackers 110
  Rainbow Spaghetti Salad 162
  Stain-Your-Clothes Dip 96
Berry Apple Porridge 78
Better Baked Beans 196
Better 'n' Bought Tomato Sauce 117
Bibliography 290
Biscuits
  Chocolate Chip Pecan 228
  Gingerbread 226
  Jam Drops 230
Blackstrap Molasses, Glossary 284
Bliss Balls
  Almond and Apricot Balls 223
  Almond and Cashew Balls 221
  Chocolate Goji Balls 220
  Chocolate, Honey Almond Balls 224

292   Endings

Chocolate Mint Balls **222**
Cranberry and Apple Balls **224**
The Original Bliss Ball **218**

Blood pH **24**

Blueberry
Blueberry and Apple Muffins **250**
Berry Apple Porridge **78**

Bolognaise, Beautiful **192**

Broccoli **16**

Brownies, Divine Raw **254**

Burgers
Garden **124**
Nutty Chick-a-pea **122**

C

Cacao Butter, Glossary **285**
Cacao Powder, Glossary **285**
Cacao, Raw **18**

Cakes
Carrot **242**
Chocolate Cupcakes **244**
Cranberry and Vanilla Cake Bars **239**
Honey and Apple **240**
Muffins **252**
Blueberry and Apple **250**
Lemon Syrup **248**
Once Upon a Time **246**
Saucy Banana Pudding **262**

Cake Tin Sizes **214**
Canned Food **54**
Carrots, Honeyed **134**

Cashews
Almond and Cashew Balls **221**
Chocolate Banana Cream **260**

Chocolate Chia Pudding **266**
Crispy Cashew Rice Treats **253**
Fruit Salad with Coconut Snow Cream **81**
Sunset Dip **92**

Cheesy Crackers **109**

Chia Seeds **18**
Chocolate Chia Pudding **266**

Chickens, Backyard **34**

Chickpeas
Baby Bear Hummus **100**
Cinderella Hummus **102**
Golden Chickpea Curry **198**
Herby Tomato Hummus **101**
Nutty Chick-a-pea Burgers **122**
Turkish Casserole **203**

Chocolate **256**
Chocolate Banana Cream **260**
Chocolate Chia Pudding **266**
Chocolate Chip Pecan Biscuits **228**
Cupcakes **244**
Divine Raw Brownies **254**
Goji Balls **220**
Honey Almond Balls **224**
Mint Balls **222**

Cinderella Custard **264**
Cinderella Hummus **102**

Coconut
Coconut Sugar, Glossary **285**
Crazy Coconut Rice **139**
Coconut Dahl **202**
Coconut Flour, Glossary **285**
Fruit Salad with Coconut Snow Cream **81**
Raw Coconut Rough **256**
Tropical Bliss Smoothie **88**

Cookies, *See* **Biscuits**
Cooking and Sprouting Techniques 64
Cooking Beans and Lentils 64
Cooking Equipment 38
Cooking Great Rice 68
Cooking Process, Starting 36
Cooking Terms 44
Cooking with Herbs 56
Corn Cakes, Golden 118
Couscous Medley 144
Crackers
    Cheesy 109
    Heart's Desire 110
    Making your own 104
    Popeye 108
    Potato and Rosemary 106

Cranberry and Apple Balls 224
Cranberry and Vanilla Cake Bars 239
Crazy Coconut Rice 139
Creating a Safe Kitchen 38
Crispy Cashew Rice Treats 253
Cucumber Salad, Posh 152
Custard, Cinderella 264

Definitions and Terms, cooking 44
Dips
    Almondy Hummus 101
    Baby Bear Hummus 100
    Cinderella Hummus 102
    Enchanted Forest 94
    Guacamole 98
    Herby Tomato Hummus 101
    Hummus 100
    Sassy Salsa 98
    Smoky Baba Ganoush 94
    Stain-Your-Clothes 96
    Sunset 92
    Tzatziki 120

Divine Raw Brownies 254
Dreamy Dahl 200

Eggs
    In Cooking 47
    Mini Quiches 126
    Omelettes 80
    Tomato Sunrise Slice 194
    Your Own Fresh Eggs 34

Enchanted Forest Dip 94
Equipment, cooking 38

Factory Farms 31
Farming
    Factory Farms 31
    Free-Range Animal Farms 30
    Non-Organic Farming 29
    Organic Farming 28
    Organic, Free-Range Farms 32
    Your Own Fresh Eggs 34

Fats
    Oil, Use in Cooking 53
    Omega Oils 20

Saturated Fats 20
  Trans Fats 22
Fire Engine Soup 170
Flaxseeds, Glossary 285
Flour
  All About 50
  Coconut, Glossary 285
  Wholemeal vs White 214
Free-Range Animal Farms 30
Frozen
  Banana and Berry Fluff 260
  Chocolate Banana Cream 260
  Fruit 258
  Home-Made Ice blocks 258
  Multicoloured Ice blocks 259
  Tropical Bliss 259
Fruit, Frozen 258
Fruit Salad with Coconut Snow Cream 81
Fruit spread, Glossary 285

G

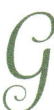

Gado Gado 208
Garam Masala, Glossary 286
Garden Burgers 124
Garden of Gratitude IV
Garlic 17
Garlicky Beans 130
Ghee, Glossary 286
Gingerbread Biscuits 226
Glossary 284
Gluten Free Toasted Muesli 77
Goji Berries 16
Golden Chickpea Curry 198

Golden Corn Cakes 118
Good Fats and Bad Fats 20
Great Baking Tip 214
Greek Beanies 120
Greens, kids eating 128
Greens, Lemony Peppered 138
Green Smoothie 88
Ground Arrowroot, Glossary 286
Guacamole 98

H

Happily Ever After Muffins 252
Heart's Desire Crackers 110
Hearty Lentil Soup 173
Herbs, Cooking With 56
Herby Tomato Hummus 101
Home-Made Ice Blocks 258
Honey
  and Apple Cake 240
  Chocolate, Honey Almond Balls 224
  Honeyed Carrots 134
How to Use This Book 8
Human Anatomy 14
Hummus 100

J

Ice blocks, Home-Made 258
Ice blocks, Multicoloured 259
Immune System 15

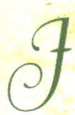

Jam Drops 230
Junk Food 23

Kids Eating Green! 128
Kitchen Safety 40

Lemon Syrup Muffins 248
Lemony Peppered Greens 138
Lentils
    Coconut Dahl 202
    Dreamy Dahl 200
    Fire Engine Soup 170
    Garden Burgers 124
    Hearty Lentil Soup 173
    Rainbow Salad 150
    Shepherd's Pie 190
    Turkish Red Lentil Soup 180
Lime, Pumpkin & Quinoa Salad 146
Linseeds, Glossary 286
LSA 86

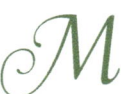

Making Your Own Crackers 104
Maple glazed Treasures 132
Maple Syrup, Glossary 286

Mexican
    Nachos 188
    Pie 206
    Seasoning
Milk
    Alternative Ingredients 47
    Which One to Use 53
Mini Quiches 126
Miso, Glossary 286
Muesli
    Bars 232
    Gluten Free Toasted 77
    Marvelous Toasted 74
    Swiss 76
Multicoloured Ice blocks 259
Mushroom Soup 174

Nachos 188
Name Variations, Ingredients 44
Nevery-lasting Nori Rolls 114
Nigella Seeds, Glossary 287
Non-Organic Farming 28
Noodle Salad, Asian 160
Nori Rolls 114
Not-Sausage Rolls with a Twist 116
Nutrition
    Immune System 15
    Processed Foods 12
    What Do Our Bodies Need 12
    Whole Foods 13
Nutty Chick-a-pea Burgers 122

O

Oil, Use in Cooking 53
Olives 18
Omega Oils 20
Omelettes 80
Once Upon a Time Muffins 246
Organic Farming 28
Organic, Free-Range Farms 32
Oven Settings 214

P

Pappadums, Glossary 287
Peach Pie 265
Perfect Pikelets 84
Personal Armies 15
Pies
   Mexican 206
   Peach 265
Pikelets 84
Pizzas 184
Platters and Other Savoury Snacks 111
Popeye Crackers 108
Porridge, Berry Apple 78
Posh Cucumber Salad 152
Potato and Rosemary Crackers 106
Potatoes, Rose-Married 135
Powerful Banana Smoothie 87
Processed Foods 12
Pudding
   Chocolate Chia 266
   Saucy Banana 262

Pumpkin

and Sweet Pea Risotto 210
Cinderella Hummus 102
Golden Corn Cakes 118
Lime, Pumpkin & Quinoa Salad 146
Scones 238
Soup 178
Sunset Dip 92

Q

Queen Bee Wedges 140
Quiches, Mini 126
Quick Ice Creams 259
Quinoa
   Glossary 287
   Lime, Pumpkin & Quinoa Salad 146
   Tabbouleh with a Spin 154
Quorn Mince, Glossary 287

R

Rainbow Salad 150
Rainbow Spaghetti Salad 162
Rapadura Sugar, Glossary 287
Raw Cacao 18
Raw Cacao Butter, Glossary 288
Raw Cacao Powder, Glossary 288
Raw Food 24
Raw-Some food 24
Raw Treats
   Almond and Apricot Balls 223
   Almond and Cashew Balls 221
   Banana and Berry fluff 260

Chocolate Banana Cream 260
Chocolate Goji Balls 220
Chocolate, Honey Almond Balls 224
Chocolate Mint Balls 222
Coconut Rough 256
Cranberry and Apple Balls 224
Crispy Cashew Rice Treats 253
Divine Raw Brownies 254
Home-Made Ice blocks 258
Multicoloured Ice blocks 259
Quick Ice Creams 259
The Original Bliss Ball 218
Tropical Bliss 259

Regional flavours 58

Rice
Arborio Rice, Glossary 284
Basmati Rice, Glossary 284
Cooking Great Rice 68
Crazy Coconut Rice 139
Crispy Cashew Rice Treats 253
Never-lasting Nori Rolls 114
Rice Mirin, Glossary 288
Rice Paper Spring Rolls 112
Rice Syrup 288
Sesame Rice Salad 156
Shanta's Sesame Rice 138
Varieties of 66
Wild Rice, Glossary 289
Wild Salad 158

Risotto, Pumpkin and Sweet Pea 210
Roasted Tomatoes 130
Rose-Married Potatoes 135

S

Safety in the Kitchen 40
Salsa 98
Sassy Salsa 98
Saturated Fats 20
Saucy Banana Pudding 262
Scones
Basic Scone 234
Lime and Coconut 236
Pumpkin 238
Sea Salt, Glossary 288
Sesame Rice Salad 156
Shanta's Sesame Rice 138
Shepherd's Pie 190
Slow Roasted Tomatoes 130
Smoky Baba Ganoush 94
Smoothies
Green 88
Powerful Banana 87
Tropical Bliss 88
Soup of Endless Possibilities 172
Spring Rolls, Rice Paper 112
Sprouting 64
Stain-Your-Clothes Dip 96
Stock Concentrate, Vegetable 166
Sugar
Blackstrap Molasses, Glossary 284
Coconut Sugar 285
Rapadura, Glossary 287
Sugar, definitions 48
Suggested Reading List 291
Sunset Dip 92
Superfoods
Blueberries 16

298 Endings

Broccoli 16
   Chia Seeds 18
   Garlic 17
   Goji Berries 16
   Kale 17
   Olives 18
   Raw Cacao 18
Sweeteners, Definitions 48
Swiss Muesli 76
Symbols
   Dietary Requirements 9
   Level of difficulty 8

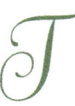

Tabbouleh with a Spin 154
Tahini, Glossary 289
Tamari Sauce, Glossary 289
Taste Bud Training 26
Textured Vegetable Protein (TVP), Glossary 289
The Forest King's Soup 168
Tomato
   and Beetroot Soup 176
   Better 'n' Bought Tomato Sauce 117
   Herby Tomato Hummus 101
   Salad 152
   Sassy Salsa 98
   Slow Roasted 130
   Sunrise Slice 194
Trans Fats 22
Tropical Bliss 259
Tropical Bliss Smoothie 88
Turkish Casserole 203
Turkish Red Lentil Soup 180

Tzatziki 120

Varieties of Rice 64, 66
Vegetable Stock Concentrate 166

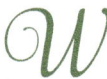

Waffles 82
Wedges, Queen Bee 140
Which Milk? 53
Which Oil? 53
Whole Foods 13
Wild Rice, Glossary 289
Wild Salad 158

Notes and Creative Ideas

Endings

www.ingramcontent.com/pod-product-compliance
Lightning Source LLC
Chambersburg PA
CBHW040233020526
44112CB00043B/2893